T0231166

Self-Assessment Color Review
Cattle and Sheep Medicine
Second Edition

Self-Assessment Color Review

Cattle and Sheep Medicine

Second Edition

Philip R. Scott

BVM&S, DVM&S, MPhil, DSHP, CertCHP, FHEA,
DiplECBHM, DiplECSRHM, FRCVS
Capital Veterinary Services
West Latchfields
Haddington
East Lothian, Scotland, UK
(formerly University of Edinburgh)

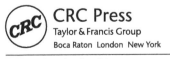

CRC Press
Taylor & Francis Group
Boca Raton London New York

CRC Press is an imprint of the
Taylor & Francis Group, an **Informa** business

CRC Press
Taylor & Francis Group
6000 Broken Sound Parkway NW, Suite 300
Boca Raton, FL 33487-2742

Printed on acid-free paper
Version Date: 20160223

International Standard Book Number-13: 978-1-4987-4737-0 (Paperback)

Visit the Taylor & Francis Web site at
http://www.taylorandfrancis.com

and the CRC Press Web site at
http://www.crcpress.com

Contents

Preface

This second edition of *Cattle and Sheep Medicine SACR* details the important clinical features of a range of common diseases of ruminants encountered in first-opinion practice in a problem-based format. The book contains many diseases not featured in the first edition. However, common diseases featured in the first edition are included, but the situations have been changed to mimic general practice; a disease does not always manifest the same clinical features every time. New images have been added for all the cases and multiple choice questions have been added for undergraduate revision purposes because this examination format is commonly adopted by many veterinary schools.

The clinical cases are not ordered in organ system, thereby mimicking the random presentation of cases during a busy round of calls in practice. The diagnosis and treatment regimens described herein are those used by the author over the past 30 years in commercial large animal practice in the UK; they acknowledge the time and financial restrictions in many situations but require no specialised facilities or equipment. The book is designed for veterinary undergraduates during their clinical rotations and for the recent graduate who encounters the occasional farm animal problem in mixed practice. All suggestions for further cases, comments and suggestions will be gratefully received and acknowledged by the author.

Philip R. Scott

Abbreviations

AGID	agar gel immunodiffusion	GGT	gamma glutamyltransferase
AP	alkaline phosphatase	GLDH	glutamate dehydrogenase
AST	aspartate aminotransferase	IBK	infectious bovine
BCS	body condition score		keratoconjunctivitis
BP	British Pharmacopoeia	IBR	infectious bovine
BRSV	bovine respiratory syncytial		rhinotracheitis
	virus	IKC	infectious keratoconjunctivitis
BUN	blood urea nitrogen	IM	intramusular/intramuscularly
BVD	bovine viral diarrhoea	IV	intravenous/intravenously
BVDV	bovine viral diarrhoea virus	IVRA	intravenous regional
CCN	cerebrocortical necrosis		anaesthesia
CFT	complement fixation test	JSRV	jaagsiekte sheep retrovirus
CLA	caseous lymphadenitis	L3	third-stage larva
CNS	central nervous system	LDA	left-displaced abomasum
CODD	contagious ovine digital	MCF	malignant catarrhal fever
	dermatitis	MD	mucosal disease
CPD	contagious pustular dermatitis	NEFA	non-esterified fatty acid
CSF	cerebrospinal fluid	NSAID	non-steroidal anti-
CVM	compressive cervical		inflammatory drug
	myelopathy	OPA	ovine pulmonary
DM	dry matter		adenocarcinoma
EAE	enzootic abortion of ewes	OPP	ovine progressive pneumonia
EBL	enzootic bovine leucosis	OPT	ovine pregnancy toxaemia
EBLV	enzootic bovine leucosis virus	PCV	packed cell volume
EDTA	ethylenediamine tetra-acetic	PEM	polioencephalomalacia
	acid	PGE	parasitic gastroenteritis
ELISA	enzyme-linked immunosorbent	RBC	red blood cell
	assay	SC	subcutaneous/subcutaneously
epg	eggs per gram	VMV	visna-maedi virus
EU	European Union	WBC	white blood cell
FAT	fluorescent antibody test	ZN	Ziehl–Neelsen (stain)
FECRT	faecal egg count reduction test		

Classification of cases: Cattle

Anaesthesia/analgesia
34, 67

Cardiovascular disease
7, 39, 50, 78, 80, 82, 91

Digestive system (mouth to anus)
3, 8, 12, 13, 19, 21, 26, 36, 40, 61, 63, 69, 72, 76, 77, 81, 83, 121

Eye disorders
57

Locomotor disease/disorders
1, 10, 11, 15, 18, 23, 29, 35, 43, 48, 53, 71, 75, 79, 85, 95, 100, 101, 102, 104, 105, 108, 109, 110, 111, 112, 114, 115, 117, 119

Husbandry/biosecurity
5, 6, 9, 27, 74, 98

Metabolic disease
38, 42, 56, 87, 106

Miscellaneous
31, 49, 65, 94, 113

Neoplastic disease
68, 97, 103, 116

Neurological disease
20, 24, 25, 28, 31, 46, 54, 55, 66, 93, 118, 123

Parasitic disease
45, 64, 73

Perinatal disease
14, 52, 88, 99

Reproductive system
4, 22, 33, 41, 44, 47, 60, 89, 92, 107, 122, 124, 125

Respiratory disease
2, 16, 17, 32, 37, 51, 58, 59, 86

Skin disease
62, 84, 96

Surgical procedure
120

Trace element disease
30, 126

Urinary tract
70, 90

Classification of cases: Sheep

Anaesthesia/analgesia
43, 99

Cardiovascular disease
29

Digestive system (mouth to anus)
1, 2, 5, 8, 19, 23, 40, 54, 60, 71, 80, 91, 112

Eye disorders
30, 59, 74

Locomotor disease/disorders
7, 15, 20, 27, 31, 32, 38, 44, 48, 77, 96, 98, 100, 101, 110, 113

Husbandry/biosecurity
35, 37, 41, 53, 57, 64, 66, 82, 87, 97, 121

Metabolic disease
62, 69

Miscellaneous
14, 21, 56

Neoplastic disease
4, 65, 88

Neurological disease
10, 11, 12, 58, 67, 68, 79, 90, 94, 109, 111, 118, 119

Parasitic disease
19, 24, 34, 49, 72, 83, 84, 86, 89, 108, 115

Perinatal disease
56, 93, 105, 120

Reproductive system
13, 16, 39, 45, 61, 78, 81, 103, 104, 107, 114, 116, 117

Respiratory disease
6, 9, 26, 33, 42, 47, 55, 70, 76, 85, 92

Skin disease
3, 17, 25, 35, 51, 52, 63, 73, 95, 102, 106, 123

Surgical procedure
99

Trace element disease
18, 22, 122

Urinary tract
28, 36, 46, 50, 75

CASE 1.1 A dairy cow presents with an extensive subcutaneous swelling in the stifle region of the left leg (**1.1a**). The swelling has gradually increased in size over the past 2 months. The swelling is fluid and the skin is under considerable pressure. No skin puncture wounds could be found. The cow is not lame and is otherwise healthy and eating well. Antibiotic therapy administered by the farmer has had no effect on the size of the mass. Ultrasound examination of the mass reveals a >25 cm diameter well-encapsulated anechoic area with multiple hyperechoic dots.

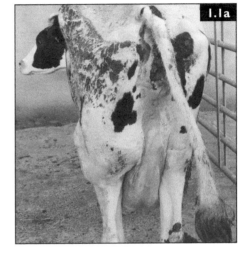

1 What is this lesion?
2 What is the likely cause?
3 What action would you take?

CASE 1.2 An aged beef cow treated previously for chronic suppurative pneumonia now presents with weight loss, ventral oedema and diarrhoea. Serum protein analysis reveals hypoproteinaemia caused by marked hypoalbuminaemia; proteinuria is also present. Rectal palpation reveals an enlarged left kidney; transabdominal ultrasonographic examination of the right kidney fails to reveal any other abnormality.

1 What conditions would you consider (most likely first)?
2 How could you confirm your diagnosis?
3 How can the condition be treated/prevented?

CASE 1.3 You are presented with a recumbent 10-day-old beef calf that has been scouring for the past 2 days (**1.3a**). The calf has not responded to oral rehydration solution administered twice daily and parenteral marbofloxacin administered by the farmer. Clinical examination fails to reveal any significant abnormalities other than abdominal distension detected by succussion and profound weakness. Analysis of blood samples reveals the following results:

Packed cell volume = 0.31 l/l (0.24–0.36) (31%, 24–36); total plasma protein = 68.0 g/l (60–75) (6.8 g/dl, 6–7.5); sodium = 128 mmol/l (128–145) (128 mEq/l, 128–145); potassium = 7.2 mmol/l (3.6–5.6) (7.2 mEq/l, 3.6–5.6); chloride = 105 mmol/l (94–111) (105 mEq/l, 94–111). Blood gas analysis: pH = 6.9 (7.35–7.45); pCO_2 = 46 mmHg; HCO_3 = 7 mmol/l (27–28) (7 mEq/l, 27–28); base deficit = 20 mmol/l (20 mEq/l).

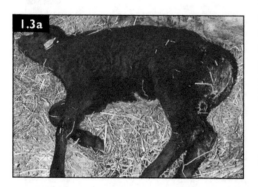

1 Comment on any clinically significant abnormalities.
2 What treatment(s) would you administer?

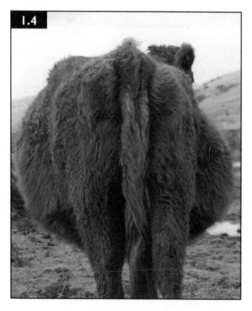

CASE 1.4 You are presented with an aged beef cow in poor body condition (BCS 1.5/5) with a 'papple-shaped' abdomen when viewed from behind (**1.4**). The abdominal distension has not increased much over the past few weeks. The cows in the herd are due to start calving within 3 weeks and are grazing poor pasture and fed barley straw and 1 kg of concentrates. This cow appears otherwise well and came to the feed trough this morning as usual.

1 What conditions would you consider?
2 What action would you take?

CASE 1.5 A farmer feeds a total mixed ration to his dairy cows; the straights are stored on the floor of a large multi-purpose shed (**1.5a**).

1 List the disease risks, and potential vectors, associated with this method of feed storage.
2 How could these disease risks be reduced?

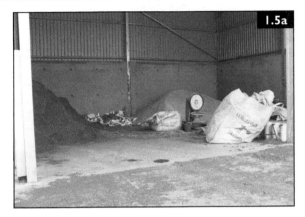

CASE 1.6 You are called to assist a cow calving on a beef farm. Approaching the calving pens you notice an old wheelbarrow used to store the 'essentials' (**1.6**).

1 Comment on the suitability of antibiotic storage and syringe and needle use/disposal. What are the risks associated with this practice?
2 Comment on the bottle and teat used to ensure passive antibody transfer. Are there any risks you can foresee?
3 Any other comments?

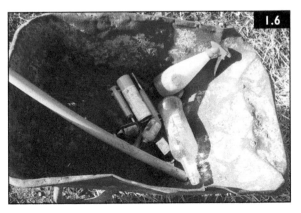

3

CASE 1.7 You are presented with a non-pregnant beef cow in poor body condition (BCS 1.5/5) with submandibular oedema and what appears to be a distended abdomen. This cow is bright and alert and is eating well. Ballottement of the abdomen is difficult to interpret. Transabdominal ultrasound examination of the cranial lower quadrant on the right-hand side yields the sonogram shown (1.7a).

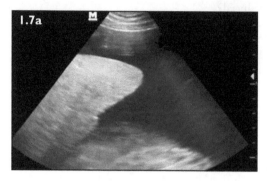

1 Describe the important findings.
2 What conditions would you consider?
3 What action would you take?

CASE 1.8 A beef farmer reports that several of his fattening cattle are dull, inappetent and scouring (1.8). The cattle were housed 4 weeks ago and the

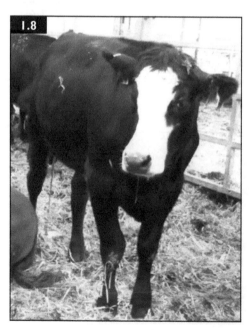

barley component of the ration steadily increased to *ad-libitum* feeding 2 days ago. When walking, several affected cattle appear weak and often stumble. They have distended abdomens due to an enlarged static rumen; bruxism is frequently heard. Auscultation reveals no rumen motility; succussion reveals tinkling sounds due to the sequestration of fluid and gas. There is profuse very fluid, foetid diarrhoea, which has a sweet-sour odour and contains whole grains.

1 What conditions would you consider (most likely first), and what is the pathogenesis?
2 What action would you take?

CASE 1.9 On a hot summer day you drive past a field with beef cattle standing in surface water draining from a midden (**1.9**). The cattle co-graze with sheep.

1 List the potential disease risks.
2 What immediate action would you recommend?

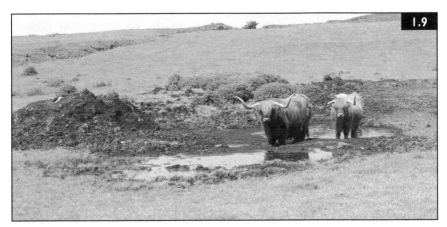

CASE 1.10 A 15-month-old Holstein heifer at pasture with 45 others presents with severe (10/10) lameness of the left hind leg with considerable swelling of the left gluteal region (**1.10a**). The heifer is so painful that she is unable to walk more than a few paces. Examination in the field reveals a raised rectal temperature of 41.5°C (106.7°F), congested mucous membranes and a crepitant feel over the swollen gluteal region.

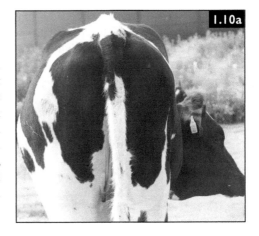

1 What conditions would you consider (most likely first)?
2 What treatment would you recommend?
3 What control measures would you recommend?

CASE 1.11 You are presented with a beef bull that is 9/10 lame on the right hind leg. The bull is at pasture with 30 cows and presented acutely lame

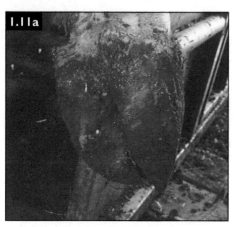

2 days ago and now spends most of his time lying down. When forced to walk the bull abducts the affected leg, placing most of his weight on the medial claw. The bull just squeezes into cattle stocks designed for cows. There are no palpable joint swellings. Raising the affected foot reveals a grossly overgrown lateral wall almost completely covering the sole (**1.11a**).

1 Describe what you will do.

CASE 1.12 A 5-year-old beef bull presents with a 3-month history of increasing abdominal distension and loss of condition (**1.12a**). The bull's appetite is poor and there are scant hard faecal balls coated in mucus in the rectum. The bull has a roached-back appearance and an anxious expression. The abdomen is markedly distended and 'papple-shaped' (10 to 4 distension; **1.12a**). Rectal temperature is normal. Heart rate is 72 beats per minute. The force and rate of rumen contractions

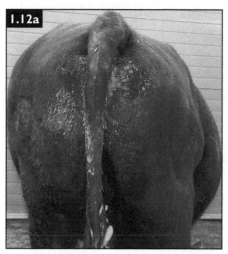

is increased to approximately 3–4 cycles per minute (normal rate is one cycle every 40 seconds or so). The withers pinch test (Williams' test) is negative. Passage of a stomach tube releases only a small amount of gas.

1 What conditions would you consider (most likely first)?
2 How would you confirm your diagnosis?
3 What actions/treatments would you recommend?

CASE 1.13 A 5-month-old beef calf in a group of 20 presents with free gas bloat (**1.13a**). The cattle are housed and fed silage plus 2 kg (4.4 lb) of concentrates per day. There is no history of bloat in this group.

1 What are the possible causes?
2 What action would you take?
3 How can you tell when the problem has resolved?

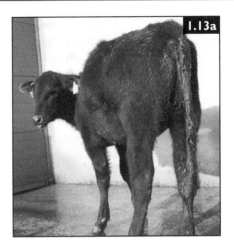

CASE 1.14 A 10-day-old beef calf presents with sudden-onset lethargy with bleeding from both nostrils and prolonged bleeding from a jugular IV injection site (**1.14a**). The herd comprises 130 spring calving cows and 82 calves have been born in the past 3 weeks. There have been two similarly affected calves in the last week; both calves were 10–14 days old and died within 2 days of initial clinical signs despite antibiotic and NSAID therapy. The farmer had noted that there was prolonged bleeding after inserting ear tags in these calves. The present calf had been normal since birth but has stopped sucking and is lying around most of the time. Rectal temperature is 40°C (104°F). There are petechial haemorrhages on the sclerae, hard palate and beneath the tongue. The heart rate and respiratory rate are increased but there are no adventitious sounds. The umbilicus is normal and there are no joint swellings.

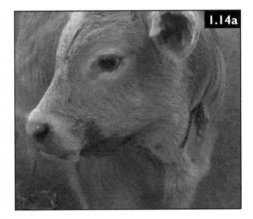

1 What conditions would you consider (most likely first)?
2 What treatments would you consider?
3 How would you confirm your diagnosis?
4 What preventive measures could be adopted?

CASE 1.15 You are presented with an aged beef cow with a large 10 cm diameter mass (**1.15a**) firmly attached to the medial aspect of the third metatarsal bone of the left hind leg. The mass has been slowly increasing in size for the past 2–3 months. The cow is not lame, but there is palpable enlargement of the popliteal lymph node.

1 What conditions would you consider (most likely first)?
2 What further examination could you undertake?
3 What action would you take?

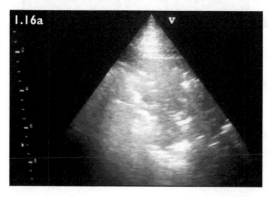

CASE 1.16 A 2-year-old Holstein heifer presents with history of poor appetite and low milk yield having calved 6 weeks ago. Rectal temperature is 38.9°C (102°F). Heart rate is 72 beats per minute; respiratory rate is 36 breaths per minute with an abdominal component. Auscultation of the chest reveals no adventitious sounds but the heifer has an occasional soft cough and mucopurulent nasal discharge. Ultrasonography approximately half way up the right chest wall over the sixth intercostal space produces the image shown (**1.16a**).

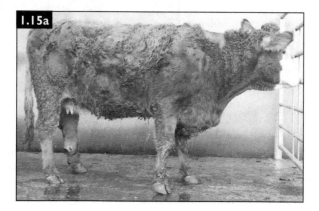

1 Describe the important sonographic findings and your interpretation.
2 What pathology does the sonogram represent?
3 What treatment would you give?

CASE 1.17 You are requested to undertake a necropsy of a 5-month-old home-bred Limousin-cross beef calf, housed 2 weeks ago, that died after a short period of marked respiratory distress manifest as an increased respiratory rate with abdominal breathing efforts and open mouth breathing. The calf was one of six that had been treated yesterday by the farmer with tulathromycin. Postmortem examination of the lungs reveals marked anteroventral consolidation but also extensive caudodorsal emphysema/bullae formation (**1.17**).

1 What condition would you consider the most likely cause?
2 What action should the farmer have taken?
3 What control measures could be adopted for future years?

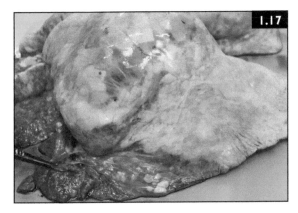

CASE 1.18 A beef farmer with a spring calving herd reports that approximately 20% of his calves show severe shortening of long bones (**1.18a**), tendon laxity and occasionally brachygnathia. This is the first time this problem has been recognised on this farm. No new bulls have been added to the herd recently and the calves are the progeny of cows of all breeds and ages.

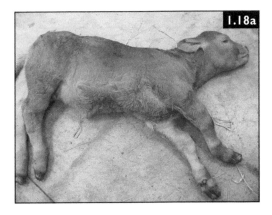

1 What is this condition?
2 How can the problem be investigated?
3 What control measures can be introduced?

CASE 1.19 You are presented with a 9-month-old beef heifer that is much smaller than other heifers in the group (170 kg [375 lb] versus 320 kg [700 lb]; [**1.19**, animal on left]). The calf and her dam were purchased when the calf was approximately 2 weeks old. This is the only animal in the group affected. Clinical examination fails to reveal any significant abnormalities; there is no history of illness for this calf.

1 What conditions would you consider (most likely first)?
2 What tests would you undertake?
3 What other clinical problems could be expected?
4 How could this scenario have been prevented?

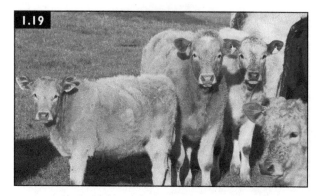

CASE 1.20 A 4-month-old Charolais beef calf has had difficulty bearing weight on the fore legs for approximately 1 week. The calf appeared normal for the first 3 months of life and is in excellent body condition. The calf spends a lot of time in sternal recumbency and has difficulty raising itself. The calf is bright and alert and propels itself along on its knees using its hind legs (**1.20a**). There are reduced reflexes and flaccid paralysis of the fore legs and increased reflexes and spastic paralysis of the hind legs.

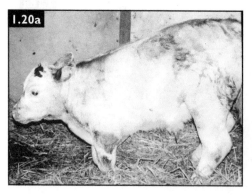

1 Where is the lesion?
2 What lesion would you suspect (most likely first)?
3 What ancillary tests could you undertake?
4 What is the prognosis?

CASE 1.21 A beef farmer reports that two of 15 young beef calves have a wet lower jaw with drooling of saliva. There is a large firm swelling in one cheek of each of the affected calves (**1.21**). Digital palpation of the cheek via the mouth reveals loss of mucosa and a necrotic plug of muscle in the centre of the diphtheritic mucosal lesion. There is halitosis and swelling of the drainage submandibular lymph node. Rectal temperature is marginally elevated at 39.2°C (102.6°F).

1 What is the cause (most likely first)?
2 What treatment would you recommend?
3 Are there any control measures?

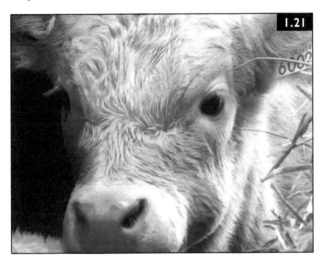

CASE 1.22 You are called to examine a scouring calf on a beef farm. Walking to the calving pens you observe the calving jack used by the farmer to assist delivery of oversized calves (**1.22a**). When asked, the farmer states that he assists more than 50% of cows to calve, although many of those cows 'assisted' occur late in the evening so that he can go to bed.

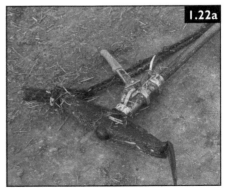

1 What are your observations/ comments?

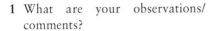

11

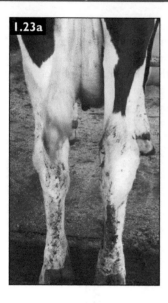

CASE 1.23 During a routine visit to a dairy farm you notice that a large number of cows have large swellings over the lateral aspect of the hock joints (1.23a). The affected cows are not lame.

1 What are these lesions?
2 What is the likely cause?
3 What action should be taken?

CASE 1.24 Following bulling activity yesterday, a farmer comments that one of his dairy cows has developed a ventral depression of the tail head with the hind legs drawn well forward under the body (1.24a). The cow appears to be in considerable discomfort. Clinical examination reveals complete lack of tail tone, a rectum distended with firm faeces and a full urinary bladder extending well forward over the brim of the pelvis.

1 What is the cause of this problem (most likely first)?
2 What treatment would you administer?
3 What action would you take?

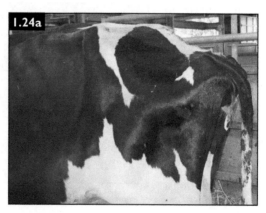

CASE 1.25 You are presented with a valuable 4-month-old bull calf, which the farmer reports has become increasingly unsteady on its legs over the past month (**1.25a**). The calf has a good appetite and is growing well. He has a lowered head carriage and a wide-based stance and is ataxic with hypermetria of the fore legs, with these changes more pronounced when he trots. There is normal strength in all four legs. The hind leg ataxia results in the calf occasionally falling over, especially when turning quickly. The calf has a normal menace and pupillary light reflexes in both eyes. No cranial nerve deficits are detected. No other animals in the group show similar clinical signs.

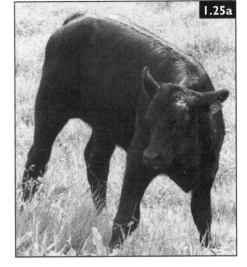

1 What area of the brain could be involved?
2 What conditions would you consider?
3 What tests could be undertaken?
4 What action would you take?

CASE 1.26 A group of housed dairy calves, weaned 3 weeks previously and then mixed together, present with chronic weight loss, poor appetite with chronic faecal staining of the tail and perineum (**1.26a**). Rectal temperatures are normal.

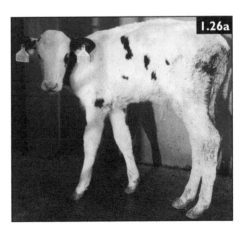

1 What conditions would you consider (most likely first)?
2 How would you confirm the diagnosis?
3 What treatment would you recommend?

13

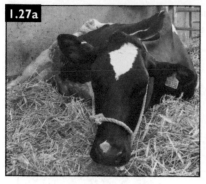

CASE 1.27 A 6-year-old Holstein cow that calved 12 hours earlier is presented in sternal recumbency, profoundly depressed, dehydrated, afebrile (37.8°C [100.1°F]), with toxic mucous membranes, an elevated heart rate of 96 beats per minute and an increased respiratory rate (34 breaths per minute) (**1.27a**). The cow is too weak to stand. The udder is soft but a pale, serum-like secretion can be drawn from one quarter. There is profuse diarrhoea but no blood is present in the faeces.

1 What diseases would you consider (most likely first)?
2 Which disease(s) is most likely?
3 What treatments would you administer?
4 What control measures could be adopted?

CASE 1.28 You are presented with a 2-week-old Holstein bull calf, which the farmer reports has been unsteady on its legs since birth, which was unassisted. The calf has a good appetite and is growing well. He has a lowered head carriage and a wide-based stance (**1.28a**). The calf is ataxic with hypermetria of the fore legs, with these changes more pronounced when the calf trots. The ataxia occasionally results in the calf falling over, especially when turning quickly in the pen. Fine muscle

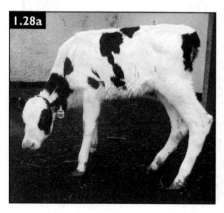

fasciculations are sometimes present in the neck and head, which become more pronounced during handling and resemble coarse muscle tremors causing vigorous jerking movements of the head. The calf has normal menace and pupillary light responses in both eyes. No cranial nerve deficits are detected.

1 What area of the brain could be involved?
2 What conditions would you consider?
3 What action would you take?

CASE 1.29 While attending to a lame bull, a beef client comments that he has a month-old suckled heifer calf that collapses onto the ground when stressed. This behaviour was first observed soon after birth and has not worsened. When the herd is moved to another field, the affected calf lags behind the others and after 50 metres (55 yards) or so suddenly develops hind leg rigidity, propelling itself forwards with the nose almost touching the ground, and then falls into lateral recumbency (**1.29a**). There is no seizure activity and the calf stands within 10–20 seconds and walks away, albeit with a stilted gait and low head carriage (**1.29b**). The affected calf is bright, alert and responsive but appears to have exaggerated double muscling compared with herd mates of similar breeding. The tail is not lifted normally when defaecating/urinating, resulting in faecal and urine contamination of the base and tip of the tail, respectively.

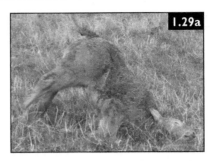

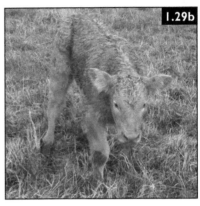

1 What conditions would you consider?
2 What tests could be undertaken?
3 What action would you take?

CASE 1.30 A beef farmer complains that several of his 30 5-month-old winter-born calves have disappointing growth rates after turnout to permanent pasture 2 months previously (**1.30**). He believes that there is depigmentation around the ear margins and eyes, giving a 'spectacle-eye' appearance in these calves, and there is a sparse hair coat. There is some evidence of diarrhoea but no widening of the epiphyses of the distal leg bones.

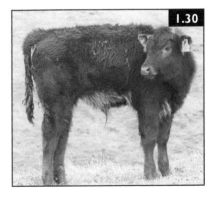

1 What conditions would you consider (most likely first)?
2 What samples could you collect?
3 What advice would you offer?

15

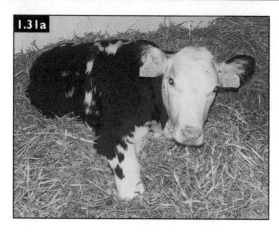

CASE 1.31 You are presented with a stirk with a suspected compressive spinal lesion between T2 and L3 (upper motor neuron signs in both hind legs) and need to collect a CSF sample to aid diagnosis (**1.31a**).

1 How would you collect a lumbar CSF sample?

CASE 1.32 A 2 year-old Holstein heifer presents with a 10-day history of poor appetite and weight loss (**1.32a**). The heifer produced a live calf unaided 3 weeks previously but is yielding only 16 litres per day (heifer average = 32 litres 3 weeks after calving). The heifer is dull and depressed. Rectal temperature is 38.9°C (102°F). Ocular and oral mucous membranes appear slightly congested. Heart rate is 72 beats per minute; respiratory rate is 36 breaths per minute with an abdominal component. Auscultation of the chest reveals increased wheezes anteroventrally on both sides. The heifer has an occasional soft cough and mucopurulent nasal discharge. The ruminal contractions are normal, occurring once per minute. The heifer has been treated with marbofloxacin for 5 days prior to examination without apparent improvement.

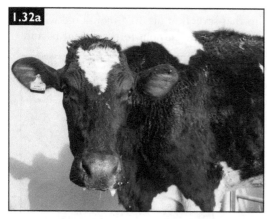

1 What conditions would you consider (most likely first)?
2 How could you confirm your provisional diagnosis?
3 What treatment would you recommend?
4 What is the prognosis for this heifer?

CASE 1.33 During a routine fertility visit to a dairy herd you are presented with a cow that calved 78 days ago showing recurrent and irregular oestrous activity (nymphomania). The cow has a particularly prominent tail head (**1.33a**). The farmer describes the cow as 'cystic'.

1 What condition is the farmer talking about?
2 What causes the abnormal oestrous behaviour?
3 What treatment would you administer?
4 What advice would you offer?

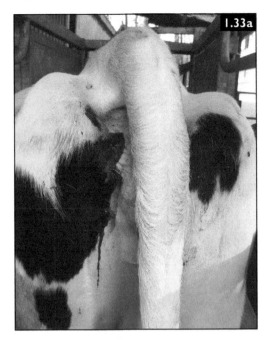

CASE 1.34 You are told by the principal of the practice to dehorn a group of beef heifers intended for breeding (**1.34a**). Your client has just purchased these cattle because they were cheap. The cattle weigh approximately 350 kg (770 lb).

1 While this barbaric practice is not now as common as 20–30 years ago, what analgesic protocol would you adopt?

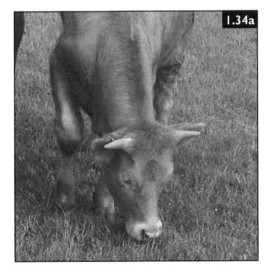

17

CASE 1.35 During late summer a beef cow at pasture presents with severe (10/10) lameness of the right hind leg with marked muscle atrophy over the right hip. The

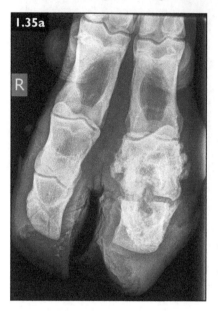

right hind foot is swollen above the coronary band with marked widening of the interdigital space. The farmer reports that the cow has been lame for 4 weeks and failed to improve after a single injection of long-acting oxytetracycline administered using a pole lance 3 weeks ago. A dorsoplantar view of the right hind foot is shown (**1.35a**).

1 Comment on the significant radiographic abnormalities.
2 What is the likely cause(s) of this condition?
3 What is the likely duration of this condition?
4 Has this cow received appropriate treatment and care?
5 How can this problem be resolved?

CASE 1.36 You are presented with a 2-year-old pedigree beef bull with a 2-day history of drooling saliva and quidding. The bull had been purchased 6 months earlier and is insured for loss of use and mortality/euthanasia for welfare reasons. The farmer noted a large firm swelling of the left mandible and treated the bull with a single injection of long-acting oxytetracycline. The bull is otherwise

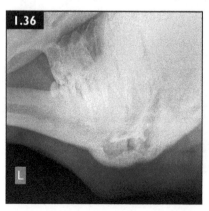

bright and alert. On clinical examination there is marked enlargement of the horizontal ramus of the left mandible, with surrounding painful soft tissue swelling. There is enlargement of the left submandibular lymph node. A lateral radiograph of the left mandible is shown (**1.36**).

1 Describe the important features shown.
2 What conditions would you consider (most likely first)?
3 What treatment would you recommend?

CASE 1.37 A 320 kg (700 lb) bulling heifer presents with a 10-day history of poor appetite and weight loss. The heifer is dull and depressed with a rectal temperature of 39.1°C (102.4°F). Ocular and oral mucous membranes appear slightly congested. Heart rate is 72 beats per minute; respiratory rate is 32 breaths per minute with an abdominal component. The heifer has an occasional soft cough and

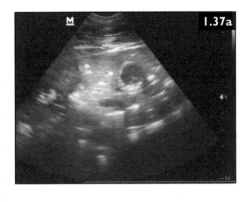

mucopurulent nasal discharge. Auscultation of the chest reveals increased wheezes anteroventrally on both sides. Ruminal contractions are normal, occurring once per minute. The heifer was treated as a calf for suspected respiratory disease with marbofloxacin (for 3 consecutive days on two separate occasions). Ultrasound examination of the chest using a 5 MHz sector scanner positioned on the chest wall 10 cm above the point of the elbow reveals the image shown (**1.37a**).

1 Describe the sonogram.
2 What conditions would you consider?
3 What treatment would you recommend?
4 What is the prognosis for this heifer?

CASE 1.38 During summer you are presented with a recumbent 6-year-old dairy cow. The cow presented with suspected hypocalcaemia early in the morning having calved unaided during the night. The cow could have been recumbent for up to 8 hours in a sparsely bedded calving pen. The cow was treated with 40% calcium borogluconate (IV and SC) by the farmer for suspected hypocalcaemia, but has not regained its feet (**1.38**). The cow has cleansed (passed the placenta) and there is no mastitis. The farmer describes the cow as a 'downer' and has moved her outdoors using a tractor to a grass paddock.

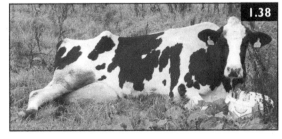

1 What is the definition of a downer cow?
2 What is the likely cause?
3 What treatment would you administer?
4 What is the prognosis for this cow?

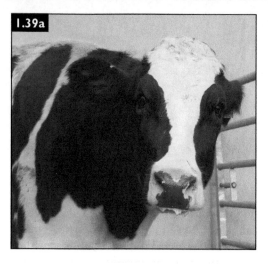

CASE 1.39 A 7-year-old Holstein cow presents with a 2-week history of poor milk yield, reduced appetite, marked weight loss and a painful expression (**1.39a**). The cow is dull and stands with a roached back and abducts the elbows. There is marked jugular distension. Rectal temperature is 39.1°C (102.4°F). Heart rate is 96 beats per minute and irregular but there are no audible murmurs. Respiratory rate is 36 breaths per minute.

1 What conditions would you consider (most likely first)?
2 What treatment would you recommend?
3 What is the prognosis?

CASE 1.40 A beef cow presents dull, anorexic with continuous salivation and staining of the lower jaw. An extended neck and 'anxious' expression are present (**1.40a**). Closer examination of the mouth reveals halitosis and pain on palpation

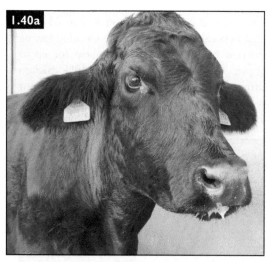

of the pharyngeal region. There has been a rapid loss of body condition and the cow has a gaunt appearance.

1 What conditions would you consider (most likely first)?
2 How would you confirm your diagnosis?
3 What treatment(s) would you administer?

CASE 1.41 You are presented with a 600 kg (1,320 lb) fattening bull that is not eating. The farmer has noted that the bull is slightly stiff when walking and has a swollen scrotum (**1.41a**). Clinical examination reveals an elevated rectal temperature of 40.1°C (104.2°F) and a hot and painful scrotum, but detailed palpation of the contents is not possible because of the oedematous scrotal skin.

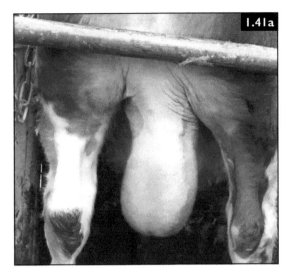

1.41a

1 What conditions would you consider (most likely first)?
2 What further investigations would you undertake?
3 What is the likely cause?
4 What treatment would you administer?

CASE 1.42 At a weekly routine fertility visit to a 600 cow dairy you are presented with a recently-calved 6-year-old Holstein cow that has stopped eating and is yielding only 12 litres per day. The cow had a BCS of 4/5 at calving, suffered from hypocalcaemia and has lost considerable body condition in the past 2 weeks. The cow is dull and appears unsteady on her legs. She has been observed licking at walls, cubicle partitions and her own flanks for long periods of time. Rectal temperature is normal. The cow has a gaunt appearance with sunken sublumbar fossae consistent with a much reduced appetite. The cow is constipated while other cows in the high yielding group have soft faeces. There are high-pitched tinkling sounds in the left flank extending under the rib cage.

1 What conditions would you consider (most likely first)?
2 How could you confirm your diagnosis?
3 What treatment would you administer?
4 How could this condition be prevented?

21

CASE 1.43 You are presented with a 2-hour-old pedigree bull calf that will not bear weight on the left hind leg. The cow was restrained standing in cattle stocks during delivery of the calf. The calf was in posterior presentation and delivered with considerable difficulty by the farmer using a calving jack. There is considerable swelling proximal to the stifle region.

1 What conditions would you consider?
2 How could you confirm your diagnosis?
3 What is the prognosis?
4 How could this situation have been prevented?

CASE 1.44 Interpret these data compiled from commercial beef herds in the UK.

1 Age at first calving. According to the English Beef and Lamb Executive (EBLEX), the age at calving in beef heifers is approximately 34 months.
2 Calving period. In England, surveys show calving periods in the range of 20–22 weeks for 2010/11. Calving periods for beef suckler herds in Scotland were 14–16 weeks for 2010. The average calving intervals for suckler cows calving in England and Wales in 2010 were broadly similar, ranging from 440 to 446 days.
3 Barren rate. Data from enterprise costing surveys show barren cow rates in the range of 6.3 to 8.1 barren cows per 100 cows exposed to the bull in 2010.
4 Bull infertility. Up to 40% of bulls are subfertile.

CASE 1.45 During late winter a farmer complains that some of his autumn calving beef cows are in poorer body condition than expected and have diarrhoea (1.45a). He has also noted that not as many cows as usual are bulling. The herd is managed outdoors and co-grazes pastures with sheep. The cows are fed *ab-libitum* good quality big bale silage and 2 kg of barley per head per day. The average rainfall during the previous summer and autumn was much higher than normal.

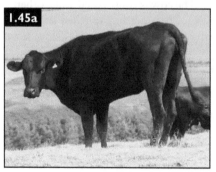

1.45a

1 What conditions would you consider (most likely first)?
2 How would you confirm your diagnosis?
3 What treatment would you administer?
4 What advice would you give to the farmer?

CASE 1.46 You are presented with a recumbent 3-day-old beef calf that has been unable to stand following assisted delivery in anterior presentation when the calf 'stuck at the hips' (**1.46**). Clinical examination reveals that the calf is unable to extend the left stifle joint, bear weight and extend the leg; the right leg is less severely affected.

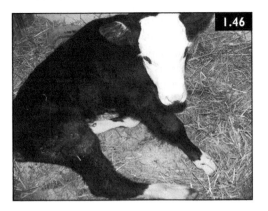

1 What conditions would you consider (most likely first)?
2 What treatment would you administer?
3 How could this problem have been prevented?

CASE 1.47 A 15-month-old pedigree heifer in a group of 15 other heifers at pasture presents with increasing udder development and enlargement of all four teats despite not having been mated (**1.47a**); transrectal ultrasound examination reveals that the heifer is not pregnant.

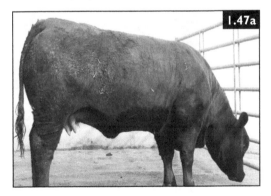

1 What is the likely cause?
2 How would confirm your diagnosis?
3 What action could be taken?

CASE 1.48 A 10-month-old heifer presents with severe (8/10) lameness of the right hind leg. The heifer was examined by a colleague 10 days ago after sudden-onset lameness; no cause was found, including detailed examination of the foot, and the animal was treated with meloxicam and amoxicillin/clavulanic acid combination for 4 days without improvement. Clinical examination of the heifer reveals considerable soft tissue swelling immediately proximal to the tibiotarsal joint, but the joint itself is not distended. Radiographs of this region are shown (1.48a, b).

1 Describe the abnormal radiographic findings.
2 What is the likely cause?
3 What action should have been taken at the first veterinary examination?

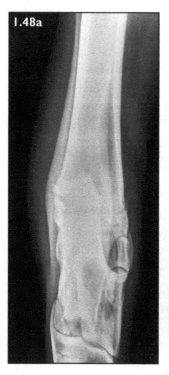
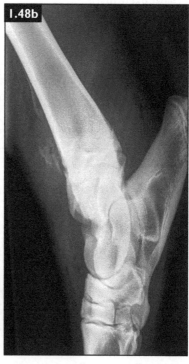

CASE 1.49 A 15-month-old fattening heifer presents with an extensive swelling over much of the left flank estimated to represent about one-third of the animal's bodyweight. The swelling appeared suddenly 2 months ago and has increased slightly in size since. The swelling is very firm and the skin is under considerable pressure. The heifer has difficulty rising to her feet and spends most of the time standing. The heifer is otherwise

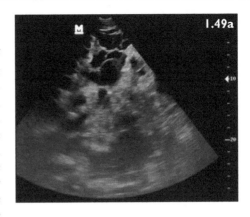

healthy and eating well. Antibiotic therapy administered by the farmer has had no effect on the size of the mass. An ultrasonogram of the mass is shown (**1.49a**).

1 What is this lesion?
2 What is the likely cause?
3 What action should be taken?

CASE 1.50 A 6-year-old beef cow presents with extensive brisket oedema and distended jugular veins. This condition has developed slowly over several months but has become pronounced in the last 2 weeks. Rectal temperature is normal. Heart rate is 100 beats per minute but the heart sounds are muffled on both sides of the chest. Respiratory rate is elevated to 40 breaths per minute with a slight abdominal component. Lung sounds are heard only in the dorsal lung fields.

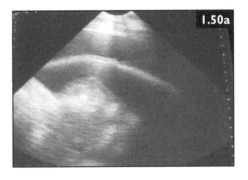

1 Describe the important features of the sonogram obtained using a 5 MHz sector scanner in the sixth intercostal space approximately half way up the chest wall (**1.50a**).
2 What conditions would you consider (most likely first)?
3 What treatment would you administer?

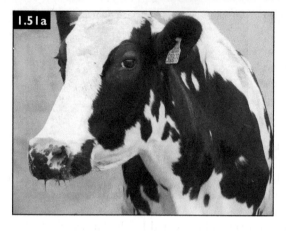

CASE 1.51 A 3-year-old cow presents with a poor milk yield and reduced appetite. The cow was treated for suspected respiratory disease by the farmer with oxytetracycline, with a short-term response. Today, the farmer is concerned because the cow has a bright red discharge from both nostrils (1.51a). On clinical examination the heifer is bright and alert with a rectal temperature of 39.2°C (102.6°F). Heart rate is 88 beats per minutes with no audible murmur. There are no increased respiratory sounds. Rumen motility is normal.

1 What conditions would you consider (most likely first)?
2 What tests could be undertaken to confirm your provisional diagnosis?
3 What treatment would you administer?
4 What control measures would you recommend?

CASE 1.52 You are called to replace the small intestines herniated through the umbilicus of a beef calf born 1 hour earlier (1.52).

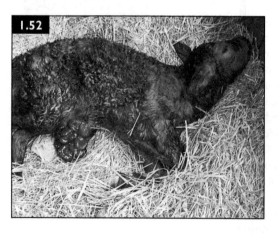

1 What is the prognosis for this calf?
2 What action would you take, including details of your anaesthetic approach?
3 How can this problem be prevented?

CASE 1.53 During late summer you are presented with a recently weaned 9-month-old beef calf that has had an usual gait for the past 3 months. The calf is poorly grown compared with its peers and has a stilted gait on both hind legs. The calf spends a lot of time in sternal recumbency and has great difficulty raising itself. There is no history of a previous disease episode affecting this calf. There are no effusions in any of the palpable joints (stifle joints distally). You suspect a lesion affecting both hips and decide to radiograph the hip joints/pelvis (**1.53a**).

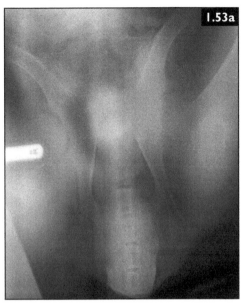

1 Describe the radiographic findings.
2 What conditions would you consider?
3 What action would you take?

CASE 1.54 During a routine fertility visit to a dairy herd you are presented with a heifer 72 days in milk that has not yet been served. The heifer has hobbles on her hind legs (**1.54a**).

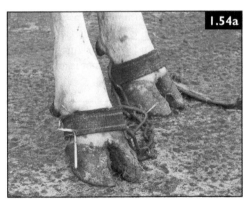

1 Why would the farmer apply hobbles?
2 Are the hobbles fitted correctly?
3 How long should hobbles remain in place?
4 How could the risk of this problem be reduced?

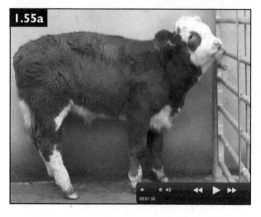

CASE 1.55 During winter you are presented with a 7-month-old spring-born beef heifer still sucking its dam (**1.55a**). Since housing the cattle 2 months ago, the farmer has noted that the calf is dull and wanders aimlessly around the pen, often walking into corners, and not reversing out like normal cattle. The calf often holds its head up when wandering around such that the farmer thinks it is blind. Clinical examination reveals absence of menace response in both eyes but normal papillary light reflexes. There are no other cranial nerve defects. The calf had been treated by a practice colleague with vitamin B1 2 weeks earlier but without improvement.

1 What conditions would you consider (most likely first)?
2 What tests would you undertake?
3 What treatment would you administer?

CASE 1.56 During summer you are called to attend a recumbent 10-year-old beef suckler cow. The cow is at pasture with a 3-month-old calf at foot. The cow is in lateral recumbency and shows seizure activity (**1.56a**), which makes further clinical examination difficult. The farmer is anxious that you treat the cow immediately to prevent imminent death.

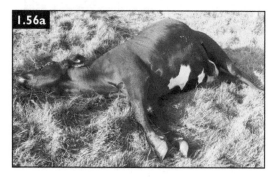

1 What conditions would you consider (most likely first)?
2 What treatment would you administer immediately?
3 What samples would you collect to confirm your diagnosis?
4 What control measures could be adopted for the rest of the herd?

CASE 1.57 During summer a farmer complains that several cattle at pasture show epiphora with tear-staining of the face, initially serous but becoming increasingly purulent and matting the lashes and hair of the face. On closer examination there is marked conjunctivitis with injected tortuous scleral vessels and hyperaemic conjunctivae. Affected cattle show marked photophobia with blepharospasm (1.57).

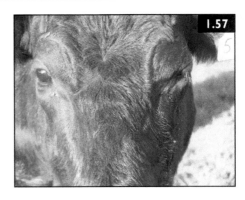

1 What conditions would you consider (most likely first)?
2 What treatment would you administer?
3 What action would you take?

CASE 1.58 During late October you are asked to examine a young Charolais bull purchased from a pedigree sale 2 months ago. The bull was introduced into a group of four cull cows 3 weeks ago to make sure he was able to serve normally before being transferred to the main herd. Clinical examination reveals pyrexia (40.4°C [104.7°F]) and purulent bilateral nasal discharges (1.58). The respiratory rate is increased and auscultation of the chest reveals crackles, but these sounds are probably transferred from the upper respiratory tract because transthoracic ultrasonography fails to reveal any abnormality of the visceral pleurae. Visual inspection of the cows in the group reveals no abnormalities.

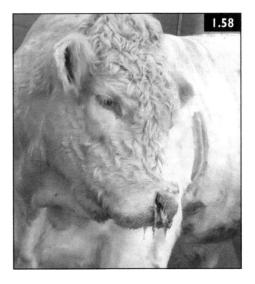

1 What conditions would you consider (most likely first)?
2 How would you confirm your diagnosis?
3 What treatment(s) would you recommend?
4 What control measures could be adopted for future years?

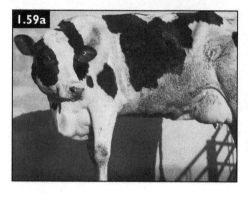

CASE 1.59 You are presented with a dairy cow with a 2-week history of lethargy, poor appetite and reduced milk yield. The cow now stands with a roached back stance with the neck extended and the head held lowered (**1.59a**). Rectal temperature is elevated (39.4°C [102.9°F]). Ocular and oral mucous membranes are congested. Heart rate is 92 beats per minute. Respiratory rate is elevated to 44 breaths per minute with an obvious abdominal component. Auscultation of the left chest reveals widespread high-pitched tinkling/splashing sounds two-thirds the way up the chest wall, with normal breath sounds on the right-hand side of the chest. Pinching over the withers elicits a painful expression. Ruminal contractions are reduced in strength and frequency. The farmer is unaware that the dairyman had treated the cow for hypocalcaemia immediately after calving when she was found cast on her back and extremely bloated. The cow responded well to IV calcium borogluconate.

1 What conditions would you consider (most likely first)?
2 What tests would you undertake?
3 What treatment would you recommend?
4 How could this condition have been prevented?

CASE 1.60 A 6-year-old beef cow presents with 2-month history of weight loss and diarrhoea despite anthelmintic treatment by the farmer. The cow calved 1 week ago and her calf is much smaller (27 kg [60 lb]) than the other calves in the group (**1.60a**).

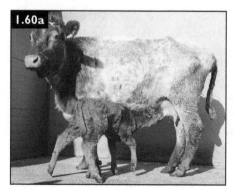

The cow's rectal temperature is normal. No significant clinical signs are found except for diarrhoea without blood or mucosal casts.

1 What conditions would cause weight loss and diarrhoea (most likely first)?
2 What further tests could be undertaken?
3 Why is the calf much smaller than other calves in the group?
4 What is the prognosis for the calf?

CASE 1.61 You are presented with a 10-year-old Friesian cow that is in very poor condition (BCS 1/5). The cow is yielding only 18 litres per day when normally 40–45 litres per day would be expected 2 weeks after calving. Clinical examination reveals a normal rectal temperature. The cow is slightly constipated. A sweet ketotic smell is obvious on the cow's breath. The sublumar fossae are markedly sunken (**1.61a**), indicative of a small rumen and poor appetite over the previous 2–3 days. Normal rumen movements can be heard caudally in the left sublumbar fossa. On percussion, high-pitched metallic sounds ('ping, ping, ping') can be heard high up on the left-hand side of the abdomen under the caudal ribcage. Rectal examination fails to reveal any abnormality. There is no evidence of mastitis or metritis.

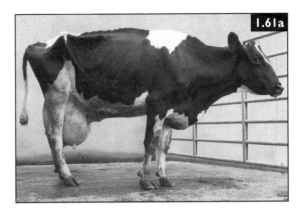

1 What is your diagnosis?
2 What other conditions could cause tympany in this area?
3 What action would you take?
4 What treatment(s) would you administer?

CASE 1.62 During winter a beef farmer complains that his bulls are constantly rubbing against gateposts and fences causing extensive hair loss, especially over the shoulder, neck and ears (**1.62**). The bulls are in excellent body condition. The cows and calves in the same groups are much less affected.

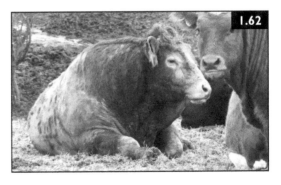

1 What conditions would you consider?
2 What further tests could be undertaken?
3 What actions/treatments would you recommend?
4 Are there any consequences of this problem?

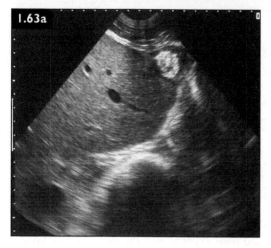

CASE 1.63 A Holstein cow presents with history of poor appetite, poor milk yield and weight loss over several weeks. Antibiotic therapy (5 consecutive days' penicillin injections) has effected some improvement. Blood samples collected by a colleague reveal a marked neutrophilia with left shift and hypoalbuminaemia (17 g/l [1.7 g/dl]) and hyperglobulinaemia (67 g/l [6.7 g/dl]). Your colleague suspects a focal infection and requests help scanning the cow's liver (1.63a).

1 Describe the sonogram.
2 What conditions would you consider (most likely first)?
3 What treatment would you recommend?

CASE 1.64 During mid summer a beef farmer complains about sudden onset of frequent coughing in a group of cows (1.64) grazing permanent pasture. This pasture has been rented for the first time this year and has been previously grazed by yearling beef cattle. Some cows show an increased respiratory rate at rest with an abdominal component. Clinical examination reveals that the cattle are afebrile.

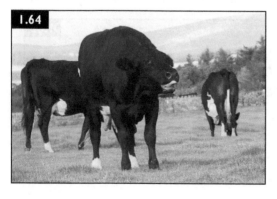

1 What conditions would you consider (most likely first)?
2 What laboratory tests could be undertaken to confirm your provisional diagnosis?
3 What treatment would you administer?
4 What control measures would you recommend?

CASE 1.65 During summer grazing an adult beef cow presents with sudden-onset profound depression, anorexia and pyrexia (41.5°C [106.0°F]). There is intense scleral congestion, bilateral keratitis and corneal opacity. There is marked photophobia and blepharospasm. There is copious purulent nasal discharge (**1.65**). Examination of the mouth reveals halitosis from an erosive stomatitis. There is crusting of the muzzle and sloughing of the mucosa. There is a generalised peripheral lymphadenopathy. The cow is hyperaesthetic to touch, especially around the poll.

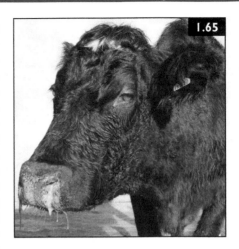

1 What conditions would you consider (most likely first)?
2 How could you confirm your suspicions?
3 What treatment would you administer?
4 List any preventive/control measures.

CASE 1.66 A 4-day-old Charolais-cross beef calf presents in opisthotonus (**1.66a**) and handling produces paddling movements. The calf was born indoors and transferred to pasture when 36 hours old. Rectal temperature is 39.2°C (102.6°F). The menace response is absent and there is marked episcleral congestion and dorsomedial strabismus. Respiratory rate is increased at 60 breaths per minute. The umbilicus had been treated with strong iodine solution and appears normal. There is no evidence of diarrhoea. The lymph nodes are not enlarged.

1 What conditions would you consider?
2 How could you confirm your diagnosis?
3 What is the likely cause?
4 What treatment(s) would you administer?
5 What recommendations would you offer?

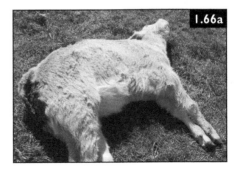

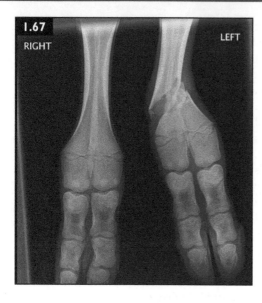

CASE 1.67 A day-old beef calf has been found 10/10 lame on the left hind leg. Radiography confirms a fracture through the distal third metatarsal bone (**1.67**).

1 How could effective analgesia be achieved?
2 What action would you take?
3 What is the likely prognosis?

CASE 1.68 A 10-year-old beef cow in good condition presents with a 2-week history of a protruding left eye and mucopurulent ocular discharge. The farmer has also noticed a blood-tinged serous discharge from the right nostril. Clinical examination reveals a normal respiratory rate (24 breaths per minute) but little or no air movement via the left nostril (**1.68a**). There is swelling of

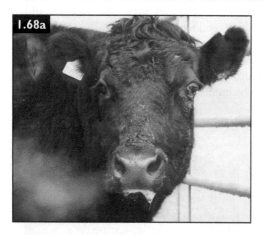

the left maxillary region. The submandibular lymph nodes are normal size. Auscultation of the chest fails to reveal any abnormality. Rectal temperature is normal.

1 What conditions would you consider (most likely first)?
2 What further tests could be undertaken?
3 What action would you take?

CASE 1.69 During summer a 3-month-old beef calf at pasture presents with scant mucohaemorrhagic faeces. The calf shows tenesmus causing temporary rectal prolapse. Mucous membranes are slightly pale and the calf is approximately 7% dehydrated. Rectal temperature is 40.0°C (104°F). There is crusting of the nasal mucosa (**1.69a**) with oral ulcers, most prominent on the hard palate, which are overlain by necrotic debris. All other calves in the group healthy are growing well.

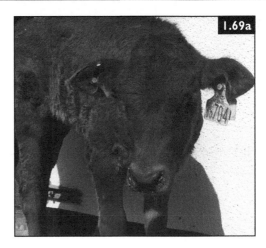

1 What conditions would you consider (most likely first)?
2 How could you confirm your suspicions?
3 What necropsy findings would confirm your suspicions?
4 List any preventive/control measures.

CASE 1.70 A 6-month-old beef calf presents with a history of poor growth; the calf weighs only 150 kg (330 lb) whereas contemporary animals in the group weigh >280 kg (615 lb). The calf is dull and depressed with a poor appetite. Transthoracic ultrasonography reveals normal lungs. Transabdominal ultrasonography in the right sublumbar fossa fails to immediately identify the right kidney, instead this image (**1.70a**) is found.

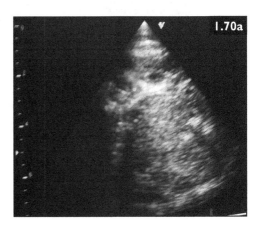

1 Describe the sonogram.
2 What could this structure represent?
3 What action would you take?

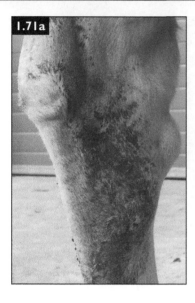

CASE 1.71 A rapidly growing yearling beef bull presents with marked effusion of the tibiotarsal and tarsometatarsal joints of both hind legs (left hock joint shown in **1.71a**) 1 month before a major bull breeding sale. The owner reports insidious onset of mild lameness. He considers this normal for all young bulls reared intensively for breeding sales, but had one bull rejected for a similar presentation last year.

1 What conditions would you consider?
2 Is this bull fit for sale as a breeding bull?
3 How could this problem be reduced/prevented?

CASE 1.72 You are presented with a 2-week-old pedigree beef bull with an umbilical swelling. The swelling is firm, painful and cannot be reduced. The calf has not been sucking well for the past 2 days. Ultrasound examination of the swelling produces this image (**1.72a**).

1 What are the important sonographic features seen in the sonogram?
2 What action would you take?

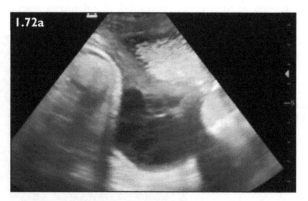

CASE 1.73 During late summer several 8-month-old dairy-cross heifers present with rapid condition loss and diarrhoea (**1.73**). The heifers are set-stocked at three animals per hectare on permanent pasture. Clinical examination reveals normal rectal temperatures, absence of either ocular or nasal discharges and no adventitious sounds on auscultation of the chest. The calves were vaccinated against lungworm 6 and 2 weeks before turnout to pasture in the spring.

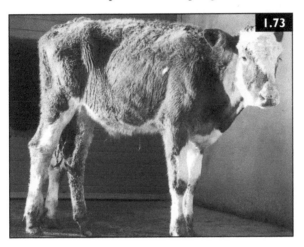

1 What conditions would you consider (most likely first)?
2 What further tests could be undertaken?
3 What treatment(s) should be administered?
4 Could this problem(s) be prevented next year?

CASE 1.74 A beef farmer is experiencing problems with cryptosporidiosis towards the end of a 9-week indoor calving period during the spring. He notices that his neighbour is calving outdoors without such a problem and asks you for advice about whether he should turn all remaining pregnant cows out to pasture.

1 What are the potential benefits and risks?

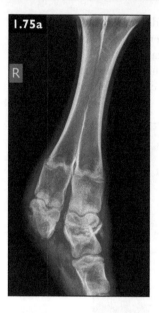

CASE 1.75 A month-old beef calf presents with severe (10/10) lameness of the right fore leg. The calf had previously been diagnosed with septic pedal arthritis of the lateral claw, which had been amputated through distal P1 10 days previously. Clinical examination reveals swelling and pain associated with P1 of the medial claw. A dorsopalmar radiograph of this region is shown (**1.75a**).

1 Describe the abnormal radiographic findings.
2 What action should be taken?

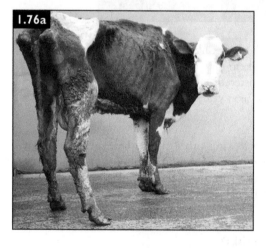

CASE 1.76 During summer you are presented with a 6-year-old beef cow with a 3-month history of weight loss and diarrhoea (**1.76a**) despite flukicide treatment by the farmer. The cow calved 4 months ago and her calf is much smaller than the other calves in the group because of poor milk supply. The cow's rectal temperature is normal. No significant clinical signs are found except for diarrhoea without blood or mucosal casts.

1 What conditions would cause such weight loss and diarrhoea (most likely first)?
2 What further tests could be undertaken?
3 What control measures could be adopted?

CASE 1.77 During the summer you are presented with a valuable pedigree beef bull at pasture that is slow to move and stands with an arched back. The farmer comments that the bull has shown tenesmus over the past 2 days but passes only mucus (**1.77**). For the past 3 days the bull has refused the 2 kg (4.4 lb) of concentrates offered daily. The farmer suspected 'an impaction' and has stomach-tubed the bull with 50 litres of electrolytes once daily for the past 2 days but without improvement. Rectal temperature is normal. Mucous membranes appear congested. The abdomen is markedly distended but rumen motility is absent. The bull does not dip his back when the withers are pinched. Auscultation of

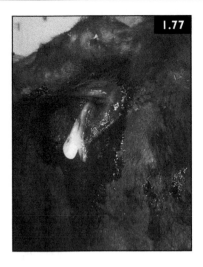

the heart and lungs reveals no abnormality except for an elevated heart rate of 98 beats per minute. No abnormality is felt on rectal palpation. The farmer has treated the bull with penicillin for the previous 2 days without improvement.

1 What conditions would you consider (most likely first)?
2 What further tests would you undertake?
3 What action would you take?

CASE 1.78 During winter a dairy cow presents with chronic weight loss, poor appetite and reduced milk production. No other cows in the group are affected. This morning, the farmer has noted bright red arterial blood at the cow's nostrils (**1.78a**). On clinical examination the cow is dull with a rectal temperature of 39.2°C (102.6°F). Mucous membranes appear normal. Heart rate is 88 beats per minutes with no audible murmur. There are no adventitious lung sounds. Rumen motility is reduced.

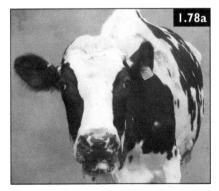

1 What conditions would you consider (most likely first)?
2 How can you confirm your provisional diagnosis?
3 What treatment would you administer?
4 What action would you recommend?

39

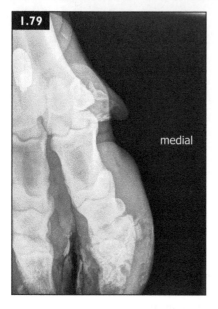

CASE 1.79 You are presented with a valuable beef bull that has been 9/10 lame on the right fore leg for the past 2 months. A professional foot trimmer has attended the bull on two previous occasions but without improvement. The lameness was sudden in onset. On clinical examination the bull adducts the right fore leg and adopts a 'crossed leg' stance with weight borne on the sound lateral claw. Examination of the bull in a turning foot crate reveals a very thin sole of both claws of the right fore foot. A dorsopalmar radiograph is shown (**1.79**).

1 What conditions would you consider (most likely first)?
2 What action would you take?

CASE 1.80 A 6-year-old Holstein cow presents with a 2-week history of poor appetite, weight loss and poor milk yield. The cow has a painful facial expression, and walks slowly. There is obvious brisket oedema and distended jugular veins. Rectal temperature is elevated (39.2°C [102.6°F]). Heart rate is 80 beats per minute but the heart sounds are muffled on both sides of the chest. Respiratory rate is elevated to 40 breaths per minute with a slight abdominal component.

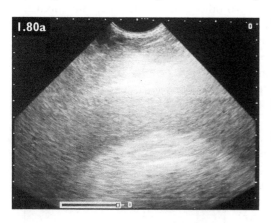

1 Describe the important features of the sonogram obtained at the sixth intercostal space using a 5 MHz sector scanner (**1.80a**).
2 What treatment would you administer?
3 Could this situation have been prevented?

CASE 1.81 A colleague requests an opinion regarding a beef cow that has been off colour for the past 4 days. The cow has not eaten for 3 days and presents with an arched back. There are no rumen contractions, but auscultation of the right sublumbar fossa reveals a large area of high-pitched resonant sounds in the site consistent with a very distended caecum. No abnormality could be

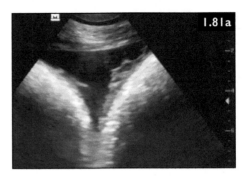

palpated on rectal examination. Rectal temperature is 39.1°C (102.4°F). Heart rate is 90 beats per minute. Your colleague would like to perform an exploratory laparotomy on the basis that "there is nothing to lose". You recommend further examination and this sonogram (1.81a) was obtained with a 5.0 MHz sector transducer connected to a real-time, B-mode ultrasound machine placed in the lower right sublumbar fossa; the examination took 3 minutes.

1 Describe the important sonographic findings.
2 What further tests might you undertake?
3 What action would you take?
4 Comment on the value of an exploratory laparotomy in this case.

CASE 1.82 A 3-year-old Holstein cow presents with a 4-week history of brisket and submandibular oedema (1.82a). The cow is in the far dry group (cows 8 to 3 weeks pre-partum) at pasture. They are examined every day by the tractor driver, who simply counts the number of cows in the field. On clinical examination the cow is dull and depressed and stands with a roached back with the head lowered. There is marked jugular distension and a jugular pulse. Rectal temperature is 39.1°C (102.4°F). The heart is barely audible, being replaced by high-pitched splashing sounds present on both sides of the chest loudest about half way up the chest wall. Respiratory rate is 40 breaths per minute with normal breath sounds limited to the dorsal lung field.

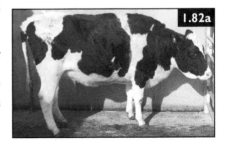

1 What conditions would you consider (most likely first)?
2 What treatment would you recommend?
3 What recommendations would you make?

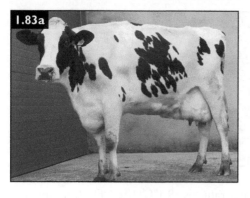

CASE 1.83 You are presented with a dairy cow that is slow to move and stands with an arched back (**1.83a**). The farmer complains that the cow has reduced her milk yield from 35 litres per day to less than 10 litres per day. The rectal temperature is marginally elevated (39.2°C [102.6°F]). Mucous membranes appear congested. Rumen motility is reduced. The cow does not dip her back when the withers are pinched.

Auscultation of the heart and lungs reveals no abnormality. The farmer has treated the cow with ceftiofur for the previous 3 days without improvement.

1 What conditions would you consider (most likely first)?
2 What furthers tests would you undertake?
3 What treatment would you administer?
4 What action would you take?

CASE 1.84 A 5-year-old cow presents with skin lesions confined to the non-pigmented white areas (**1.84**). The affected skin is dry and raised at the periphery from normal healthy pigmented skin. The skin of the teats appears dry and 'papery'. The farmer also reports that this cow often has a red nose during the summer.

1 What conditions would you consider (most likely first)?
2 What are the possible causes?
3 What advice would you offer?

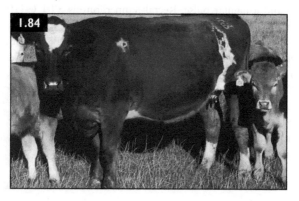

CASE 1.85 While out walking on a summer's afternoon you observe a herd of dairy cows coming in for afternoon milking. Approximately 40% of the herd is either score 2/3 or 3/3 lame (DairyCo lameness scale). One cow lags well behind the remainder of the herd (**1.85**).

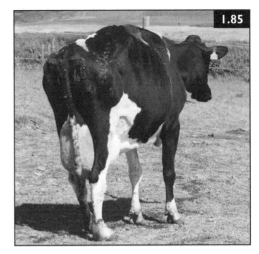

1 List four important observations.
2 What conditions would you consider (most likely first)?
3 What other tests could you employ?
4 What treatment would you administer?
5 What action would you take?

CASE 1.86 A Holstein heifer presents with a history of poor appetite and weight loss. The heifer produced a live calf unaided 3 weeks previously but is yielding only 18 litres per day when the herd average is 32 litres. The heifer is dull and the rectal temperature is 39.2°C (102.6°F). Heart rate is 86 beats per minute. Respiratory rate is 38 breaths per minute. Auscultation of the chest reveals no breath sounds over the right chest and reduced sounds on percussion. The heifer has a soft productive cough. Ruminal contractions are normal, occurring once per minute. The heifer has been treated with marbofloxacin for 3 days prior to examination without apparent improvement. A transthoracic ultrasonogram of the right chest is shown (**1.86a**).

1 Describe the sonogram and the likely cause.
2 What treatment(s) would you administer?
3 What changes would you expect with successful treatment?

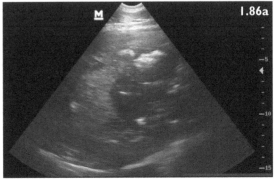

43

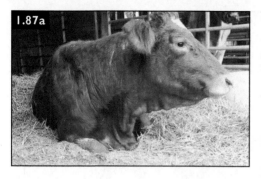

CASE 1.87 A beef cow presents in sternal recumbency after assisted delivery of dead full-term twins by the farmer. The cow (**1.87a**) is in much poorer body condition (BCS 1.5/5) than the remainder of the group (appropriate BCS of 2.5–3.0/5). The cow is very dull with little ruminal activity and the faeces are hard, dry and coated in mucus. Mucous membranes are pale yellow. There is submandibular and brisket oedema. There are retained fetal membranes and a foetid vaginal discharge. The udder is flaccid and contains little colostrum.

1 What conditions would you consider (most likely first)?
2 What tests would you undertake?
3 What treatments would you administer?
4 What control measures would you recommend?

CASE 1.88 A dairy farm with an intensive block calving pattern is experiencing pre-weaning calf mortality in excess of 12%, with most losses occurring within the first 5 days after birth (**1.88**). The cows calve in a large communal area with the calves removed after about 4–6 hours. Calves born between 10 pm and 8 am are removed from their dams after morning milking and transferred to individual pens. All calves are then fed a proprietary milk replacer, with *ad-libitum* concentrates, until weaning at 6 weeks old.

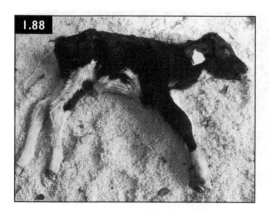

1 What is the likely cause of such mortality?
2 How would you investigate this problem?
3 What simple practical recommendations would you make?

CASE 1.89 You are presented with a dull dairy cow that calved twins 3 days ago. The cow is yielding only 18 litres per day, has a fever (39.9°C [103.8°F]) and retained fetal membranes (**1.89**). Mucous membranes are congested and there is reduced ruminal motility. Rectal examination reveals an enlarged uterus. There is profuse diarrhoea without blood or mucosal casts. There is also a foetid watery red-brown vaginal discharge.

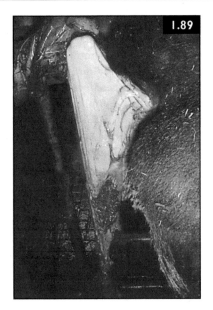

1 What conditions would you consider (most likely first)?
2 What treatments would you administer?
3 What follow-up treatment would you recommend?

CASE 1.90 A 6-year-old Limousin beef cow presents with 6-week history of weight loss. The cow calved 6 months ago and is 4 months pregnant. Rectal temperature is marginally elevated (39.2°C [102.6°F]). The ocular and oral mucous membranes are pale. Heart rate is 70 beats per minute. Respiratory rate is 24 breaths per minute with no abnormal sounds detected on auscultation of the chest. The cow has a poor appetite and the rumen is shrunken, giving the abdomen a drawn-up appearance (**1.90a**); ruminal contractions are reduced in strength and frequency. The cow is passing normal faeces. The cow makes frequent attempts to urinate but only a small amount of urine is voided. The cow resents rectal palpation, which reveals a thickened bladder wall and enlarged ureters.

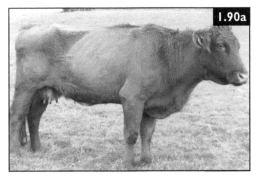

1 What conditions would you consider (most likely first)?
2 How could you confirm your provisional diagnosis?
3 What is the prognosis?
4 What treatment would you recommend?

CASE 1.91 You are presented with a 2-year-old Holstein heifer that has developed obvious brisket, submandibular and fore leg oedema over the past 2 months. Rectal temperature is normal. The heifer has an increased respiratory rate (44 breaths per minute) with frequent non-productive coughing. Auscultation of the chest reveals reduced audibility of lung sounds and reduced resonance on percussion of the ventral third on both sides of the chest. Heart rate is 90 beats per minute and slightly irregular; the sounds are also reduced in volume. The jugular veins are distended. Transthoracic ultrasonography half way up both sides of the chest reveals the same image (**1.91a**).

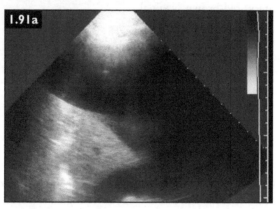

1 Describe the important sonographic findings.
2 What are the possible causes?
3 What action would you take?

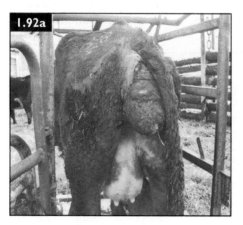

CASE 1.92 You are presented with an aged beef cow with a cervicovaginal prolapse (**1.92a**). The cow calved unaided 10 days previously and passed the placenta within 2 hours.

1 How would you correct this problem?
2 What is your advice regarding the management of this cow?

CASE 1.93 A beef cow with a month-old calf at foot has been unable to fully extend and bear weight on the right fore leg since colliding with a fence during handling through the cattle stocks 2 weeks ago. The cow is otherwise well and eating normally. There is obvious loss of muscle over the scapula with a more prominent spine than on the left side. There is a dropped elbow, flexion of the distal leg joints and scuffing of the hooves as the right leg is moved forward (**1.93**). The foot is knuckled over at rest. The right prescapular lymph node is not swollen. Muscle tone is reduced but withdrawal reflexes appear normal.

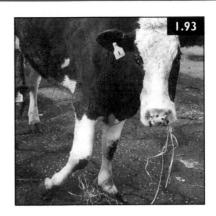

1 What conditions would you consider (most likely first)?
2 What treatment(s) would you administer?
3 What is the prognosis for this cow?

CASE 1.94 You are attending a lame bull on a beef farm and drive past cattle grazing poor quality pasture (**1.94**).

1 Identify the potentially toxic plant present in the field?
2 What clinical signs might be expected?
3 How is the diagnosis confirmed?
4 What treatment and control measures could be adopted?

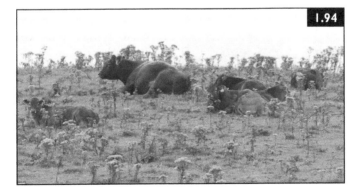

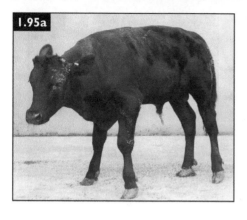

CASE 1.95 A farmer reports that two approximately 6-month-old intensively-reared beef bulls have been found with a mid-shaft femoral fracture without apparent cause, necessitating immediate slaughter for welfare reasons. Several other young bulls in this group of 30 are lame with swelling of the carpal and hock joints (**1.95a**). The cattle are fed *ad-libitum* cereals with access to barley straw. Clinical examination of two bulls reveals severe lameness with widening of the metaphyses, particularly of the third metacarpal and third metatarsal bones.

1 What conditions would you consider (most likely first)?
2 What further examinations could you undertake to confirm your diagnosis?
3 What treatment would you administer?

CASE 1.96 During winter, several animals in a group of 40 housed 4–6-month-old beef calves present with skin lesions distributed over the whole body, but

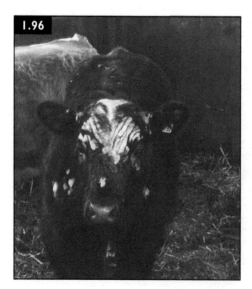

especially the head and neck (**1.96**). The lesions are superficial, dry, white, scaly and non-pruritic. The affected skin is not thickened.

1 What conditions would you consider (most likely first)?
2 What further tests could be undertaken?
3 What actions/treatments would you recommend?
4 Are there any special concerns?

CASE 1.97 A 6-year-old dairy cow presents with chronic weight loss and poor production since calving 2 months ago. The cow has an increased respiratory rate of 34 breaths per minute with an increased abdominal component. There are reduced lung sounds in the ventral third of the chest on both sides. Heart rate is slightly muffled and elevated at 88 beats per minute. There is an obvious jugular pulse extending half way up the cow's neck. No other abnormalities are detected on clinical examination. Rectal temperature is normal. Further examination of the chest using a 5 MHz sector scanner on the lower right side reveals this image (**1.97a**, dorsal to the left).

1 Describe the abnormal findings in the sonogram.
2 What is this lesion?
3 What is the likely cause?
4 What action should be taken?

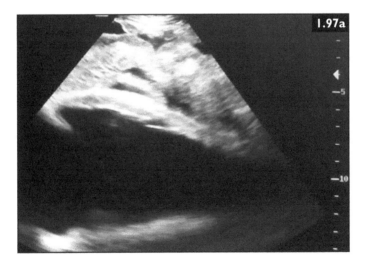

CASE 1.98 List five biosecurity measures and five biocontainment measures that will reduce the risk of *Salmonella dublin* infection in a dairy herd.

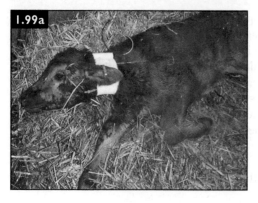

CASE 1.99 You are presented with a 3-day-old beef calf showing seizure activity (**1.99a**). The calf was normal for the first 36 hours of life but then appeared dull for about 12 hours and was not sucking. On clinical examination there is marked episcleral injection, toxic mucous membranes and mild/moderate dehydration. There is slight distension of the hock and fetlock joints and the calf's extremities feel cold. Rectal temperature is 37°C (98.6°F). The navel feels normal. Palpation and succussion of the abdomen reveals no fluid distension of the abomasum and no distended small intestines.

1 What conditions would you consider (most likely first)?
2 What is the cause of this problem?
3 What treatment would you administer, and what is the prognosis?
4 What control measures would you implement?

CASE 1.100 A pedigree beef bull calf presents with non-weight-bearing lameness (10/10) of the left hind leg of several months' duration (**1.100a**). The bull has been attended by a colleague who believes the bull has a septic pedal arthritis, but cannot decide which digit is affected and asks for your opinion. The bull has been treated with amoxicillin plus clavulanic acid for 7 consecutive days, and tilmicosin on two separate occasions; both treatments have failed to effect any improvement. There is marked muscle atrophy over the gluteal region. The popliteal lymph node cannot be palpated. There is marked oedema extending from the coronary

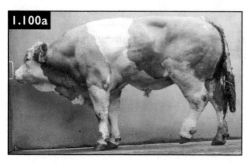

band to the mid-third metatarsal region (**1.100a**). This swelling is very painful and the bull kicks aggressively, preventing detailed palpation of the fetlock joint. There is no evidence of a puncture wound.

1 What action would you take?

CASE 1.101 A beef calf aged 6 months presents with severe lameness (8/10) of the left fore leg of several weeks' duration. The calf was normal for the first 3 months or so, but has failed to grow as well as other calves in the group and is in poor body condition. The calf has been treated by the farmer with amoxicillin plus clavulanic acid administered for 5 days without improvement, and subsequently by a veterinary colleague with marbofloxacin. There is obvious muscle atrophy over the shoulder and the prescapular lymph node is 10 times its normal size. There is firm swelling surrounding the carpus, which is painful on palpation. There is no evidence of a puncture wound. A dorsoventral radiograph of the left carpus is shown (**1.101a**).

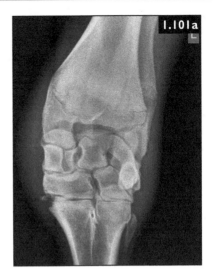

1 Describe the abnormalities present.
2 What action would you take?
3 Are there any specific control measures?

CASE 1.102 You are presented with a 9-month-old beef calf that has become increasingly 'lame' (**1.102a**) over the past 4 months such that the right hind foot does not contact the ground. Clinical examination reveals contraction of the gastrocnemius muscle causing gross overextension of the hock such that the affected leg is held caudally 15–20 cm off the ground. There is pronounced circumduction of the leg as the calf struggles to walk.

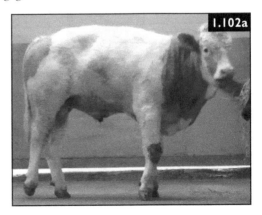

1 What conditions would you consider (most likely first)?
2 What options would you consider?
3 What control measures could be implemented?

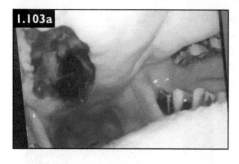

CASE 1.103 An 8-year-old beef cow in poor condition presents with a 2-week history of weight loss. The farmer had noticed excessive salivation 3 days previously and had instigated daily treatment with penicillin without improvement. Clinical examination reveals tachypnoea (40 breaths per minute) and stertor. Nasal airflow is reduced and the animal breathes through the mouth when stressed. There is marked halitosis. After placing a Drinkwater gag, a 6 × 3 cm area of ulceration with impacted food material in the centre is visible in the caudal hard palate (**1.103a**). The submandibular lymph nodes are approximately twice normal size.

1 What conditions would you consider (most likely first)?
2 What further tests could be undertaken?
3 What action would you take?

CASE 1.104 You are presented with an aged beef cow that has been 6/10 lame on the left hind leg for the past few months. There is extensive muscle wastage

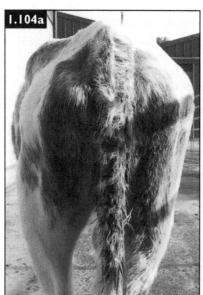

over the gluteal region (**1.104a**). Clinical examination reveals marked thickening of the stifle joint capsule and obvious joint effusion. No other joint lesions can be palpated, although assessment of the hip joint proves difficult.

1 What conditions would you consider (most likely first)?
2 What other tests could you employ?
3 What treatment would you administer?
4 What action would you take?

CASE 1.105 A beef bull calf aged 3 months presents with non-weight-bearing lameness (10/10) of the right hind leg of 10 days' duration. The calf has been treated by the farmer with amoxicillin plus clavulanic acid administered for 5 days without improvement. There is marked muscle atrophy over the gluteal region. The popliteal lymph node cannot be palpated. There is swelling (oedema) surrounding the fetlock joint, which is painful on palpation. The surrounding oedema prevents accurate palpation of the fetlock joint and no joint effusion can be appreciated. There is no evidence of a puncture wound. A dorsoplantar radiograph of the right fetlock region is shown (**1.105a**).

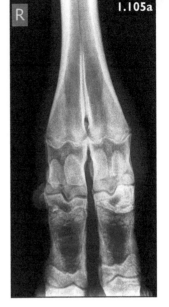

1 Describe the abnormalities present.
2 What action would you take?
3 Are there any specific control measures?

CASE 1.106 At a post-calving check at 21 days you notice a large (30 cm diameter) swelling over the left chest wall of a Holstein cow (**1.106**, arrow). The swelling is firm, fluid-filled, hot and slightly painful. It does not appear to be attached to the chest wall. No obvious skin puncture wound could be found. The cow is otherwise healthy and milking well.

1 What is the likely cause?
2 What action would you take?
3 How can this problem be prevented?

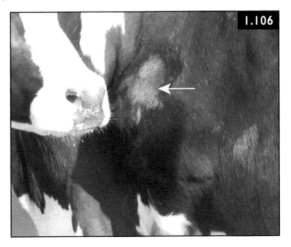

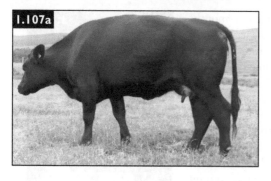

CASE 1.107 During summer a beef farmer complains that a cow is isolated from the group and is dull and depressed. The cow has a gaunt appearance and is reluctant to walk. There is obvious distension of all four fetlock joints and both hock joints. Rectal temperature is 40.0°C (104°F). Mucous membranes are congested. Rumen contractions are reduced. Respiratory rate is raised to 40 breaths per minute. The cow did not conceive last year and therefore did not calve this spring. Despite not lactating, the right forequarter is enlarged and the teat is very swollen, with flies clustered at the teat orifice (1.107a).

1 What conditions would you consider (most likely first)?
2 What is the cause?
3 What treatments would you administer?
4 What control measures would you recommend?

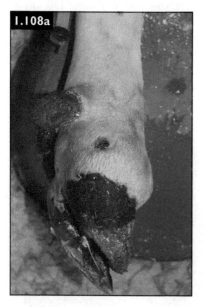

CASE 1.108 You are presented with a 9-month-old Holstein bull, intensively reared on *ad-libitum* cereals, that shows moderate (6/10) lameness of the left hind leg. The bull was purchased 1 month previously when the lameness was attributed to digital dermatitis, which was prevalent in the group at that time. The bull failed to improve after a single injection of long-acting oxytetracycline. Clinical examination reveals a discharging sinus over the lateral aspect of the distal leg midway between the coronary band and the fetlock joint. There is also marked swelling immediately above the coronary band (1.108a).

1 What conditions would you consider (most likely first)?
2 What action would you take?

CASE 1.109 You are presented with a severely lame (10/10) beef cow that became suddenly lame 2 weeks ago. The cow was treated with procaine penicillin for 3 consecutive days without improvement. The cow was examined 1 week ago by a colleague and treated with tilmicosin but without improvement. There is now marked swelling and widening of the interdigital space, with extensive tissue necrosis and discharging sinuses above the coronary band of both digits (**1.109a, b**).

1 What is your diagnosis?
2 How could you confirm your diagnosis?
3 What action would you take?
4 List any management, prevention and control measures.

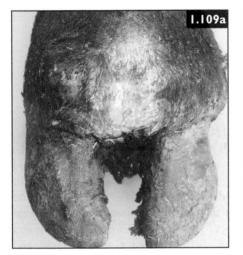 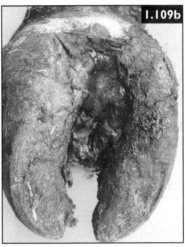

CASE 1.110 A beef bull calf aged 3 days presents with sudden-onset lameness (8/10) of the right hind leg. The calf was treated by the farmer yesterday with amoxicillin plus clavulanic acid without improvement. There is mild distension of the right stifle joint; no other joint lesions can be palpated. Rectal temperature is normal. There is no umbilical swelling.

1 What action would you take?
2 Are there any specific control measures?

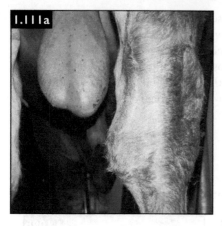

CASE 1.111 You are presented with a 6-year-old beef bull with 3/10 lameness of the right hind leg. The bull has shown intermittently low-grade lameness for about 6 months. There is slight effusion of the tibiotarsal and tarsometatarsal joints of both hind legs but marked bony swelling on the lateral aspect in the region of the tarsometatarsal joint (**1.111a**). This bony swelling appears smooth and is not painful to the touch. The owner asks your opinion on the future breeding prospects of this bull.

1 What conditions would you consider?
2 What assessment could you undertake?
3 Is this bull fit for future breeding?
4 How could this problem be reduced/prevented?

CASE 1.112 During early summer a beef cow at pasture presents with moderate (6/10) lameness of the right hind leg with muscle atrophy over the right hip. The farmer intends to cull the cow as soon as possible as she is not pregnant and

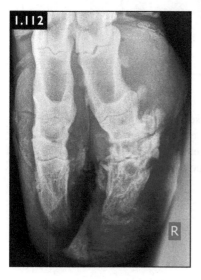

her calf has just been weaned. The right hindfoot is swollen above the coronary band but there is no widening of the interdigital space. The farmer reports that the cow has been slightly lame for several weeks and failed to improve after a single injection of long-acting oxytetracycline. A dorsoplantar view of the right hind foot is shown (**1.112**).

1 Comment on the significant radiographic abnormalities.
2 What treatment would you administer?
3 How should this problem have been treated when the cow first presented lame?

CASE 1.113 A 2-month-old beef calf presents in opisthotonus (**1.113a**). The calf was found 2 days ago in lateral recumbency and was treated with penicillin by the farmer without improvement. The calf shows severe muscle rigidity such that the joints cannot be flexed. The calf is afebrile.

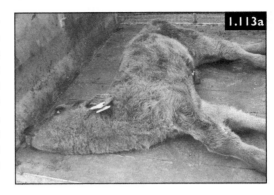

1 What conditions would you consider (most likely first)?
2 What laboratory tests could be undertaken to confirm your provisional diagnosis?
3 What treatment would you administer?
4 What control measures would you recommend?

CASE 1.114 A dairy cow presents with a horizontal hoof defect affecting all eight digits (**1.114a, b**); the cow is not lame.

1 What is this defect?
2 What is the likely cause?
3 What action would you take?
4 Are there any specific control measures?

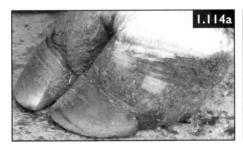
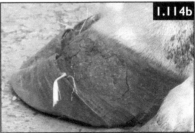

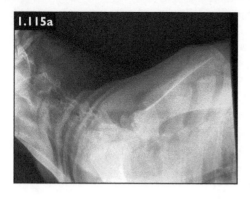

CASE 1.115 A pedigree beef bull calf aged 3 months presents with severe (9/10) lameness of the right fore leg of 4 weeks' duration. The calf has been treated with at least three courses of antibiotics, including amoxicillin plus clavulanic acid and tilmicosin, without improvement. There is marked muscle atrophy and the spine of the scapula is prominent. The prescapular lymph node is markedly enlarged (four times normal size). There is thickening of the joint capsule of the shoulder joint; no other joints are abnormal on palpation. An oblique radiograph of the right shoulder is shown (**1.115a**).

1 Describe the abnormalities present.
2 What is the likely cause?
3 What action would you take?
4 Are there any specific control measures?

CASE 1.116 A bright, alert 11-month-old beef stirk presents with a 2-month history of mild bloat and brisket oedema (**1.116a**). Rectal temperature is normal. The stirk has an increased respiratory rate (30 breaths per minute) and is noted to eructate frequently. Auscultation of the chest fails to reveal any abnormal lung sounds, but there is reduced resonance on percussion of the ventral third of the chest on both sides. The heart is clearly audible with a rate of 72 beats per minute. Rumen motility is normal and the stirk has passed normal faeces. The peripheral lymph nodes are normal.

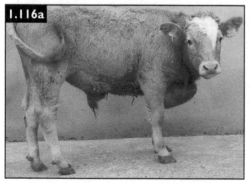

1 What conditions would you consider (most likely first)?
2 How could you confirm your diagnosis?
3 What action should you take?

CASE 1.117 You are presented with a 2-hour-old pedigree bull calf unable to bear weight on the left hind leg after forced extraction by the farmer using a calving jack. The cow was restrained in cattle stocks during delivery of the calf. The calf was in posterior presentation. The cow fell down when considerable traction was applied using a calving jack with the calf 'half way out'. There is considerable swelling distal to the calf's left stifle region.

1 Interpret the radiographic findings (**1.117a, b**).
2 What is the prognosis?
3 How could this situation have been prevented?

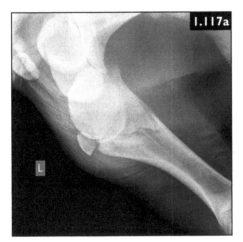
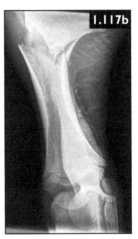

CASE 1.118 Following a difficult calving a beef cow presents with weakness of both hind legs and, most noticeably, increased flexion and knuckling of both hind fetlock joints (**1.118**).

1 What are the possible causes (most likely first)?
2 What treatment would you administer?
3 How could this problem have been avoided?

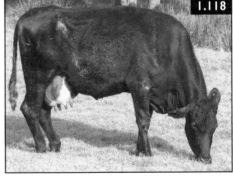

CASE 1.119 A dairy cow presents with lameness of the right hind foot (scale 3/3; DairyCo scale 0–3, where 3 is severe lameness). The foot has been examined by the farmer on two previous occasions over the past 6 weeks but without improvement. Farm records show that the cow has a toe lesion, possibly a deep white line

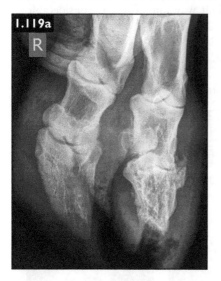

abscess. The cow has lost considerable body condition and is yielding less than 50% of predicted yield. The foot is raised and, after removing debris from the large cavity previously created by the farmer's foot paring, it is possible to probe bone beneath a small layer of granulation tissue. A dorsoplantar radiograph of the foot is shown (**1.119a**).

1 Describe the important radiographic findings.
2 What is this defect, and what is the likely cause?
3 What action would you take?
4 Are there any specific control measures?

CASE 1.120 You are presented with a Holstein heifer 5 days after toggling (Grymer/Sterner method) for a LDA. The cow has a poor appetite, a disappointing milk yield (less than 5 litres per day) and has lost considerable weight since the toggling, leading to a very gaunt appearance. The cow stands with an arched back with the head held lowered. Rectal temperature is 39.2°C (102.6°F). Mucous membranes are congested and there is severe dehydration. Respiratory and heart rates are elevated. There are no rumen contractions. Scant mucus-coated faeces are present in the rectum.

1 What conditions would you consider (most likely first)?
2 What laboratory tests could be undertaken to confirm your provisional diagnosis?
3 What treatment would you administer?
4 What is the prognosis?
5 What alternative surgical approach could have been undertaken?

CASE 1.121 You suspect traumatic reticulitis in a beef cow that is dull and inappetent with a static rumen. The cow has been ill for 5 days and unresponsive to an injection of long-acting oxytetracycline administered by the farmer on the second day of illness. Transabdominal ultrasonography using a 5 MHz sector scanner immediately caudal to the xiphisternum yields this sonogram (**1.121a**). No reticular contractions are noted during the 2 minutes' ultrasound examination.

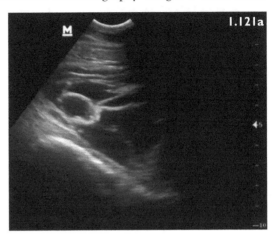

1 Describe the sonogram.
2 What is the prognosis for surgery?
3 What action would you take?
4 What control measures could be employed?

CASE 1.122 You are presented with a 16-month-old pedigree beef bull with a large swelling around the prepuce (**1.122a**). The swelling has gradually increased in size over the past 3 months. The swelling is very firm and the skin is under considerable pressure. No skin puncture wounds can be found. The bull is otherwise healthy and eating well; urination is not affected (**1.122a**). Antibiotic therapy administered by the farmer about 2 months ago initially caused reduction of the mass, but it is now larger than ever.

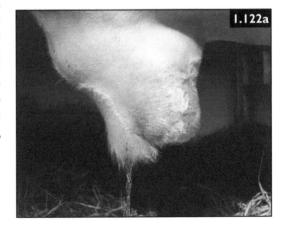

1 What is the likely cause?
2 What action would you take?

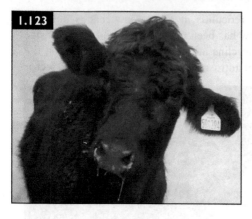

CASE 1.123 An 8-month-old steer presents with a head tilt towards the left side and drooping of the left ear and left upper eyelid (ptosis) (**1.123**). There is normal cheek muscle tone. The steer is bright and alert but appears unsteady when trotting out of the cattle stocks. Rectal temperature is normal.

1 What conditions would you consider (most likely first)?
2 What is the likely cause?
3 What treatment would you administer?
4 What is the prognosis for this case?

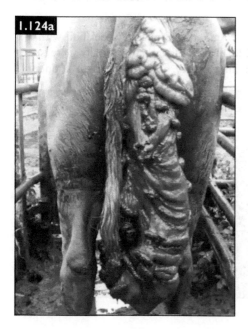

CASE 1.124 You are presented with a young beef cow that calved some hours ago and has just been found with a uterine prolapse (**1.124a**). The fetal membranes are not attached.

1 How would you correct this problem?
2 What treatments will you administer?

CASE 1.125 When loading cattle for transport to the slaughter plant a beef farmer notices a swollen scrotum in one of the steers. The steer was purchased 6 months ago and now weighs 800 kg (1,760 lb) and has been growing at a similar rate to its peers. The farmer has not noted any illness but is concerned

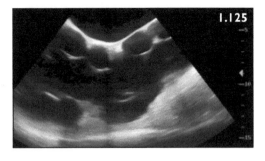

because the animal has been consigned as a steer and will be downgraded as a bull, incurring considerable financial penalty. Rectal temperature is 38.6°C (101.5°F). The scrotum is approximately 25 cm in diameter and is soft on palpation and feels fluid-filled rather than containing fat. No testicles can be palpated. The scrotum is neither hot nor painful. Ultrasound examination of both sides of the scrotum yields the same sonographic findings (**1.125**).

1 Describe the important sonographic findings.
2 What conditions would you consider (most likely first)?
3 What further investigations would you undertake?

CASE 1.126 When loading four 13-month-old intensively-reared beef bulls for transport to the slaughter plant, a farmer notes that one of the bulls (**1.126**, arrow) appears blind and walks into gates and other obstacles. The cattle are in excellent body condition and have grown at more than 1.4 kg/day. The cattle are fed *ad-libitum* cereals with access

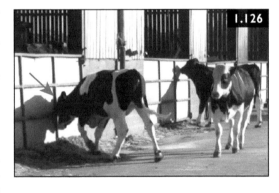

to barley straw. Clinical examination of two bulls reveals bilateral lack of menace response and papillary light reflexes. Inspection of other groups fails to reveal any abnormal behaviour or lameness.

1 What conditions would you consider (most likely first)?
2 What further examinations could you undertake to confirm your diagnosis?
3 What treatment would you administer?
4 What other problems might be expected?

CASE 1.1

1 What is this lesion? A large subcutaneous abscess.
2 What is the likely cause? There are no obvious skin puncture wounds. A contaminated IM injection into the gluteal region, which has tracked distally, is likely.

3 What action would you take? Lance the abscess (**1.1b**) near its ventral margin to ensure complete drainage. The abscess cavity should be irrigated with very dilute povidone–iodine daily for the next few days. Parenteral antibiotic therapy is not necessary. Check whether the cow was injected IM 2–3 months ago and review injection technique where necessary.

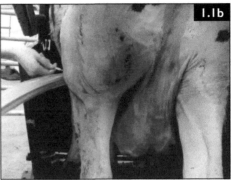

CASE 1.2

1 What conditions would you consider (most likely first)? Amyloidosis (secondary to chronic pneumonia); right-sided heart failure; chronic liver pathology such as chronic severe fasciolosis; pyelonephritis; paratuberculosis; endocarditis.

Extracellular deposition of amyloid (abnormal deposits of glycoprotein) occurs mainly in the kidney, but also in the gut, liver, adrenal gland, spleen, and other tissues. Both primary and secondary forms of amyloidosis exist. Primary amyloidosis is likely an immune-mediated or metabolic storage disease, whereas secondary amyloidosis has been associated with chronic infections in various organ systems (in this case chronic suppurative pneumonia).

2 How could you confirm your diagnosis? Renal biopsy is rarely indicated. The poor condition of cows at presentation means that most are culled and the diagnosis confirmed at necropsy (**1.2**).

3 How can the condition be treated/prevented? There is no effective treatment as the condition is irreversible. Early treatment of chronic infection may reduce the risk of secondary amyloidosis, but the condition is uncommon and secondary in clinical significance to the primary lesion.

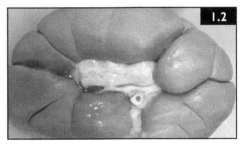

CASE 1.3

1 Comment on any clinically significant abnormalities. The calf does not appear dehydrated. The total plasma protein concentration is consistent with adequate passive antibody transfer (colostrum ingestion). The sodium and chloride concentrations are normal. The very low bicarbonate concentration and pH value indicate metabolic acidosis probably as a consequence of diarrhoea and loss of bicarbonate/production of organic acids from secondary milk fermentation in large intestine. The calf is hyperkalaemic following compensatory exchange of hydrogen ions for intracellular potassium ions, although there may be whole body depletion of potassium.

2 What treatment(s) would you administer? Treatment must correct the acidosis. Total base deficit (or negative base excess) is calculated as:

$$\text{base deficit} \times \text{bicarbonate space (ECF)} \times \text{dehydrated calf weight}$$
$$= 20 \times (0.5) \times 40 = 400 \text{ mmol bicarbonate}$$

ECF = extracellular fluid volume

32–48 g of sodium bicarbonate yielding 400–600 mmol can be added to 3 litres of isotonic saline and administered over 3 hours, with the first litre given over 20 minutes or so. There is a marked improvement within this time period (**1.3b**). The higher bicarbonate content takes into account potential underestimation of the base deficit and ongoing losses.

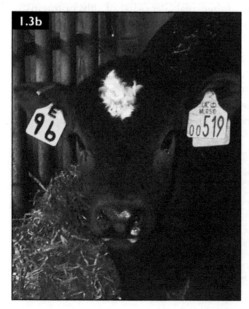

1.3b

There is debate whether follow-up fluids should comprise a high alkalinising oral rehydration solution (ORS) because the severe acidosis has already been corrected by IV bicarbonate administration. One litre of milk should be alternated with ORS to prevent starvation, because the ORS has a low energy content. There is no justification for antibiotic administration unless there is evidence of focal bacterial infection such as omphalophlebitis or polyarthritis.

Scouring was the most common disease reported in young calves and the greatest single cause of death in the UK. Between 2003 and 2012 around 10,000 faecal samples from neonatal calves with diarrhoea were tested. A diagnosis was reached in approximately 75% of submissions with isolation rates of rotavirus (42%), cryptosporidiosis (40%), bovine coronavirus (9%) and colibacillosis (8%).

CASE 1.4

1 What conditions would you consider? Advanced (possible twin pregnancy) in an old cow; distended rumen due to poor fibrous diet and advanced pregnancy; hydrallantois; vagus indigestion; ascites (right-sided heart failure); hydramnion.

This is probably a twin pregnancy in an old cow coupled with a high fibre diet with inadequate supplementary feeding. Hydrallantois is caused by abnormal placental function with severe abdominal distension caused by the massive accumulation of allantoic fluid (up to 250 litres) that occurs over a short period during the last trimester.

2 What action would you take? Recommend replacing barley straw with grass silage or increasing concentrate feeding to prevent further loss of the cow's body condition and to ensure sufficient colostrum accumulation at calving. Energy requirements for dam maintenance and advanced pregnancy are approximately 80–90 MJ/day, typically afforded by *ad-libitum* good quality silage and 2–3 kg (4.4–6.6 lb) of barley per day. If straw is fed, this should be supplemented with urea or other protein source to improve intake. Failure to feed adequate energy levels may lead to starvation ketosis (pregnancy toxaemia) in cattle carrying twins.

Live twin calves were born 14 days later.

CASE 1.5

1 List the disease risks, and potential vectors, associated with this method of feed storage. A range of *Salmonella* species transmitted by wild birds; tuberculosis transmitted by badgers; paratuberculosis transmitted to feed from vehicle wheels, boots, etc; *Neospora caninum* transmitted by dogs and foxes; botulism following the death of wild birds; mycotoxicosis from mouldy grain and wet storage conditions.

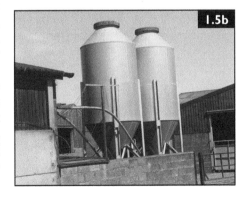

2 How could these disease risks be reduced? The building should be vermin proof. Doors must be kept closed whenever access is not required, otherwise there is no advantage of having doors. Storage bins (**1.5b**) should be used wherever possible.

CASE 1.6

1 Comment on the suitability of antibiotic storage and syringe and needle use/disposal. What are the risks associated with this practice? Needles and syringes are designed for single use, although farmers often use them on multiple occasions (there are no new syringes/needles on view). Several antibiotics, including the penicillin preparation in this situation, require storage between 2 and 8°C (35.6 and 46.4°F) (in a refrigerator for most months of the year). Exposure to high environmental temperatures could adversely affect drug efficacy. There is increased risk of contaminated injection sites, with dirty needles/syringes leading to abscesses/cellulitis. There is no sharps disposable receptacle. A 16 gauge needle is not suitable for injecting a cow; an 18 gauge needle would be more appropriate.

2 Comment on the bottle and teat used to ensure passive antibody transfer. Are there any risks you can foresee? It is good practice to encourage the calf to suck colostrum rather than use an oesophageal feeder, but the bottle and teat are filthy. As well as colostrum, the calf is likely to ingest bacteria contaminating the teat and bottle. Calf diphtheria could result from repeated use of a contaminated teat.

3 Any other comments? There is an antibiotic aerosol can in the wheelbarrow presumably to spray the umbilicus of newborn calves; however, there is also a spray bottle, but the contents do not look like strong veterinary iodine. A teat dip bottle may be easier to disinfect the umbilical remnant.

CASE 1.7

1 Describe the important findings. There is a large amount of free fluid within the abdominal cavity, with dorsal displacement of viscera including the liver (**1.7b**). There is no fibrin present, therefore the fluid is likely to be a transudate. The liver has very rounded margins consistent with chronic venous congestion (nutmeg liver).

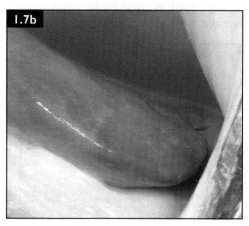

Amyloidosis could also explain the hepatomegaly and ascites, but is uncommon in cattle.

2 What conditions would you consider? Ascites as a consequence of right-sided heart failure or hypoproteinaemia (hypoalbuminaemia). Causes of right-sided heart failure could include: chronic respiratory disease such as chronic suppurative pneumonia and diffuse fibrosing alveolitis; mediastinal mass such as thymic lymphosarcoma or abscess; endocarditis; pericarditis; dilated cardiomyopathy (DCM). Causes of hypoalbuminaemia could include: chronic fasciolosis; amyloidosis; pyelonephritis; paratuberculosis; gut tumour (uncommon in cattle compared with sheep).

3 What action would you take? Careful auscultation of the chest would detect septic pericarditis, but there may be no audible murmur in cattle with endocarditis and DCM. Transthoracic ultrasonography to check for pleural effusion and superficial lung pathology. Ultrasonographic examination of heart valves. Serum protein analysis. Sedimentation test for fluke eggs in faeces. Transabdominal examination of the right kidney.

Any action would be based on the findings of these examinations. Vegetative endocarditis of the tricuspid valve was confirmed in this cow.

CASE 1.8

1 What conditions would you consider (most likely first), and what is the pathogenesis? Barley poisoning/ruminal acidosis; salmonellosis. The sudden and unaccustomed ingestion and fermentation of large quantities of carbohydrate-rich feeds results in increased lactic acid production accompanied by a fall in rumen pH, which kills many cellulolytic bacteria and protozoa. Acid-tolerant bacteria such as *Streptococcus bovis* survive, producing more lactic acid. There is a marked increase in rumen liquor osmolarity, with fluid drawn in from the extracellular space causing dehydration. Low rumen pH reduces motility, causing stasis and mild bloat. Lactate is absorbed into the circulation, leading to the development of a metabolic acidosis. This metabolic crisis is further compounded by toxin absorption through the compromised rumen mucosa.

2 What action would you take? In most situations therapy is restricted to oral fluids, IV multivitamin preparations and antibiotic therapy. Proprietary antacid products contain 220 g sodium bicarbonate, 110 g magnesium oxide and 40 g yeast cell extract diluted in 20 litres for a cow. Antacid drenches, including 500 g of magnesium hydroxide/450 kg, are also recommended to counter the acidosis. Penicillin injections are given daily for up to 10 days in severely affected cattle to counter potential bacteraemia via the hepatic portal vein.

Intravenous fluids should contain bicarbonate, and in an emergency situation it would be safe to administer 10 mmol/l of bicarbonate over 2–3 hours and monitor progress. In practical situations: 16 g of sodium bicarbonate = 200 mmol of bicarbonate, therefore a 320 kg heifer estimated to be 7% dehydrated would require:

$$\text{Estimated base deficit} \times \text{dehydrated body weight} \times \text{extracellular fluid volume}$$
$$(\text{i.e. } 10 \times 300 \times 0.3)$$
$$= 900 \text{ mmol of bicarbonate}$$

Thus 72 g of sodium bicarbonate in 5 litres of saline would approximate a 10 mmol/l base deficit in a 320 kg animal.

Siphoning off ruminal contents (rumen lavage) is described. Large volumes of warm tap water are repeatedly forced down a very wide bore stomach tube, and are then siphoned off. A rumenotomy to remove the rumen contents using a siphon can be attempted, but considerable care is needed to prevent leakage into the abdominal cavity during surgery because affected cattle are recumbent, and it is usually not possible to exteriorise much of the rumen wall due to the large fluid contents.

Management/prevention/control measures: grain/concentrate feeding must be gradually increased over a minimum of 6 weeks before *ad-libitum* feeding. Allow more than 10% of the diet as good quality roughage.

CASE 1.9

1 List the potential disease risks. Coccidiosis in calves (*Eimeria alabamensis*); leptospirosis; *S. typhimurium* and *S. dublin*; exotic serotypes from wildlife/vermin; cryptosporidiosis (calves); paratuberculosis (calves infected from midden); abortion caused by *Neospora caninum* if the midden is used as a latrine by dogs/foxes; nitrate poisoning where surface water drains grassland area recently fertilised; *Mycobacterium* tuberculosis (infected cattle/badgers using midden as a latrine).

2 What immediate action would you recommend? The surface water must be fenced off immediately and mains water supply established. Livestock should not have access to a midden.

CASE 1.10

1 What conditions would you consider (most likely first)? Include: blackleg (clostridial myositis); femoral fracture; cellulitis/penetration wound; tetanus.

2 What treatment would you recommend? There is no effective treatment for blackleg when the condition is so far advanced and the heifer should be euthanased for welfare reasons. Treatment could be attempted with penicillin and supportive therapy such as oral fluids and an IV NSAID injection, but subsequent necropsy examination in this case revealed that this would not have worked and only have prolonged the animal's suffering, whereby the musculature is dry and dark purple with numerous gas pockets (**1.10b**). The lungs are congested and oedematous. Recent earth works with piles of excavated soil in the field could have been the source of the clostridia, with trauma to the musculature during bulling behaviour providing an anaerobic site for bacterial multiplication.

3 What control measures would you recommend? The farmer was advised to vaccinate the remaining cattle against *Clostridium chauvoei* (blackleg) immediately. In addition, all cattle were injected with procaine penicillin at the time of vaccination to prevent the handling procedure from precipitating further cases. The second blackleg vaccine was given 2 weeks later. No further losses resulted in this group. Blackleg vaccine is cheap and a valuable insurance policy if losses from blackleg have previously occurred on the farm.

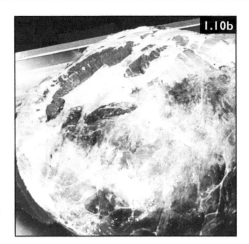

CASE 1.11

1 Describe what you will do? The bull's gait indicates a lesion affecting the lateral claw. The most likely lesion is a white line abscess, which occurs most commonly in the abaxial white line towards the sole. An abscess of the sole is also possible. Sole ulcers and digital dermatitis are uncommon in beef cattle and would be obvious on close inspection of the soles and bulbs of the heel, respectively.

The overgrown wall horn covering the sole is quickly removed using a hoof knife and the white line searched for the presence of any penetrating small sharp stones/black marks. Where present, the white line abscess ascends towards the coronary band, therefore the wall rather than the sole should be removed. There should be no damage to the corium and therefore no bleeding when paring the foot. A considerable amount of the wall horn has been removed to release the abscess (**1.11b**), which was under considerable pressure. There is no need to bandage the foot in this case because the corium has not been damaged. There is no requirement to administer antibiotics.

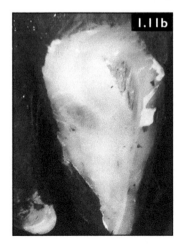

The bull was sound within 24 hours and the lameness did not recur. Haemorrhage is evident in the sole of this claw at the site of a sole ulcer and the farmer was advised regarding routine foot trimming in a tilting crush specifically designed for bulls.

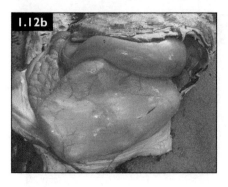

CASE 1.12

1 What conditions would you consider (most likely first)? Include: vagus indigestion; localised peritonitis; LDA; traumatic reticulitis.

2 How would you confirm your diagnosis? A diagnosis of vagus indigestion is based on the clinical findings (rumen hypermotility and abdominal shape) and exclusion of other conditions. Localised peritonitis, often arising from traumatic reticulitis, is considered to be the most common cause of vagus indigestion where the heart rate is normal. Ultrasonographic examination of the anterior abdomen using a 5 MHz sector scanner failed to detect any abnormality. Ultrasound-guided abdominocentesis yielded a small quantity of straw-coloured peritoneal fluid with a low protein concentration and low cell count comprised mainly of lymphocytes (normal values).

3 What actions/treatments would you recommend? The prognosis for this bull was considered to be very poor due to the chronicity and severity of the abdominal distension and he was sent for slaughter, therefore no necropsy findings were available. Postmortem examination often fails to reveal any significant gross lesion other than massive distension of the forestomachs (**1.12b**, gas has been released from the rumen).

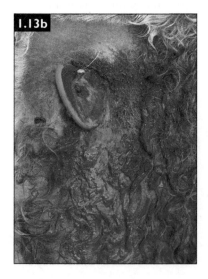

CASE 1.13

1 What are the possible causes? Physical obstruction/choke; pressure on the oesophagus by enlarged mediastinal and bronchial lymph nodes related to previous bout of bronchopneumonia; thoracic mass (thymic lymphosarcoma); poor diet. It is often not possible to diagnose a specific cause.

2 What action would you take? Pass an orogastric tube to relieve accumulated gas. Insert a trochar/cannula (**1.13b**) or create a rumen fistula if the problem recurs more than once per day over the following 3–4 days. Check for presence of chronic pneumonia; may ultrasound scan chest and treat accordingly (e.g. prolonged penicillin therapy for chronic suppurative pneumonia). If a trochar is inserted in the summer months, check regularly for cutaneous myiasis of the wound edges. Review diet, especially protein content, if no cause of the bloat is found. However, a single case in a group of growing cattle suggests that diet would be an unlikely cause.

3 How can you tell when the problem has resolved? Plug the trochar after 2–3 weeks to check whether the bloat returns or if the primary problem has been successfully treated. If the bloat does not return after several days, remove the trochar and the flank wound will quickly seal the rumen, which is now firmly adherent to the abdominal wall. A rumen fistula will close by granulation tissue from the wound edges after approximately 2–3 months.

CASE 1.14

1 What conditions would you consider (most likely first)? Bovine neonatal pancytopenia (BNP); coagulopathy associated with septicaemia.

BNP is a recently emerged disease of calves that has been described across Europe since 2007. It presents as a bleeding disorder of calves less than 1 month old resulting in a high level of mortality due to bone marrow trilineage hypoplasia accompanied by depletion of peripheral thrombocytes and leucocytes. The disease is mediated by ingestion of alloantibodies in colostrum from particular cows and the subsequent binding of these alloantibodies to calf haematopoietic cells. BNP is strongly associated with the use of a particular BVDV vaccine (Pregsure® BVD; Pfizer Animal Health) in the dams of affected calves.

2 What treatments would you consider? There is no treatment and affected calves should be euthanased for welfare reasons. Where doubt exists over the diagnosis, symptomatic treatment with antibiotics and NSAIDs could be considered.

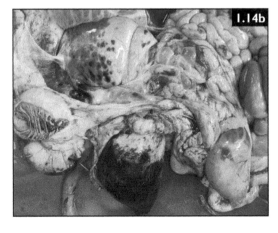

3 How would you confirm your diagnosis? Haematology reveals a massive leucopenia and thrombocytopenia. The disease is characterised by a hypoplastic or aplastic bone marrow at necropsy with multifocal petechial, ecchymotic and suffusive haemorrhages (**1.14b**).

4 What preventive measures could be adopted? In this beef herd BNP cases stopped when colostrum ingestion was prevented by muzzling the calf for the first 36 hours of life, and feeding colostrum obtained from a dairy herd not vaccinated with Pregsure® BVD. The beef cows were milked for 36 hours after calving and the colostrum and milk discarded.

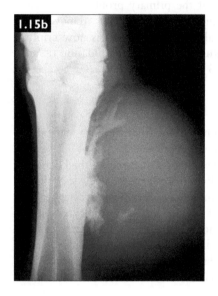

1.15b

CASE 1.15

1 What conditions would you consider (most likely first)? Tumour arising from the periosteum; granulation tissue associated with penetrating foreign body; sequestrum.

Sequestrum formation in the mid-third metatarsal/metacarpal region is occasionally encountered in 1–2-year-old cattle, with bulls more commonly presented than heifers/steers.

2 What further examination could you undertake? Radiography reveals thickening of the cortex underlying the well-circumscribed soft mass and marked periosteal reaction (**1.15b**). There is mineralisation of the mass where it is adherent to the periosteum.

3 What action would you take? The cow is not lame and removal of the mass would be neither simple nor inexpensive. Regrowth would be a possibility. Analgesia could be achieved under deep xylazine sedation and large volume (3 mg/kg lidocaine) low extradural block. IVRA would be difficult to achieve with the lesion so high up the third metatarsal bone. Perhaps the pragmatic approach to cull the cow and use the sale value to part finance the purchase of a replacement heifer would be the best option. A biopsy might give a more informed prognosis but the farmer decided to cull the cow without incurring further expense.

CASE 1.16

1 Describe the important sonographic findings and your interpretation. The bright linear echo formed by normal visceral pleura is present in the dorsal lung field but is replaced ventrally by hypoechoic areas extending up to 4–8 cm into the lung parenchyma, consistent with extensive lung consolidation.

2 What pathology does the sonogram represent? There is extensive lung consolidation consistent with chronic bronchopneumonia and subsequent bronchiectasis. Bronchiectasis has been defined as a dilation of a segment of a bronchus and is the result of a chronic bacterial or mycotic infection with destructive inflammation of the wall of the bronchus in chronic, undrained, purulent bronchitis with or without bronchopneumonia. Grossly dilated bronchi are filled with a viscous, purulent, yellow–green exudate comprising of large collections of inflammatory cells with collapse of the surrounding parenchyma (**1.16b**). These permanently dilated small bronchi and bronchioles, located in ventral parts of the lungs, contain a range of microorganisms including *Mannheimia hemolytica* and *Pasteurella multocida*, but especially *Trueperella pyogenes*.

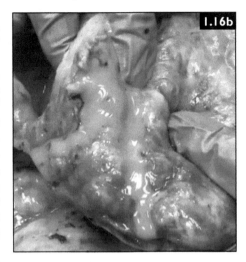

T. pyogenes is a gram-positive coccobacillus that becomes established only following compromise of the host's physical, cellular or secretory defence mechanisms, often after viral, mycoplasmal and bacterial infections. Infection with *T. pyogenes* is commonly associated with persistent BVDV infection in growing cattle. Concurrent infection with *Fusobacterium* and other anaerobic bacteria is not uncommon, causing halitosis.

3 What treatment would you give? The most effective (and inexpensive) treatment is 22,000 IU/kg procaine penicillin administered IM daily for up to 6 weeks, with a good treatment response within 2–3 days. However, this heifer failed to respond to antibiotic therapy due to extensive lung pathology and was euthanased for welfare reasons; bronchiectasis was demonstrated at necropsy by squeezing the consolidated lung areas with pus expressed from the lower airways (**1.16b**).

CASE 1.17

1 What condition would you consider the most likely cause? Peracute bovine respiratory syncytial virus (BRSV) infection (with secondary bacterial infection).
2 What action should the farmer have taken? The first few clinical cases in a respiratory disease outbreak are typically the most severely affected, therefore veterinary attendance is essential at the start of any respiratory disease problem. Veterinary examination is essential to identify the likely cause, exclude other

potential causes of this outbreak, such as IBR, collect appropriate samples and decide on the best antibiotic therapy.

In this calf that died, a single injection of a soluble corticosteroid, such as dexamethasone, was indicated to reduce the immune-mediated/allergic type reaction associated with inhalation of viral antigen into the caudodorsal lung that occurs in severe cases of BRSV-induced respiratory disease. Such treatment may have been life-saving. The benefits of NSAIDs such as ketoprofen and flunixin meglumine remain equivocal in such cases of severe respiratory disease caused by BRSV.

Few farmers request veterinary attendance at the beginning of a respiratory disease outbreak; instead they rely on whole group antibiotic injection without any monitoring, which is not only more costly but often results in chronic cases. From the farmer's perspective, whole group antibiotic injection requires much less labour/time. Whole group antibiotic therapy is contrary to the policy of veterinary organisations in many countries worldwide, including the British Veterinary Association, on antibiotic usage and the One Health concept on antibiotic resistance. There can be little justification for the use of fluoroquinolone antibiotics in bovine respiratory disease, especially when used in a metaphylaxis approach.

3 What control measures could be adopted for future years? Vaccination against BRSV, preferably by the intranasal route, should be completed at least 2 weeks prior to housing. The enterprise should be evaluated for risk factors such as high stocking density, high humidity and poor ventilation of farm buildings, mixed age housing and weaning/dietary stress factors after housing. Purchased cattle must not be mixed with homebred cattle.

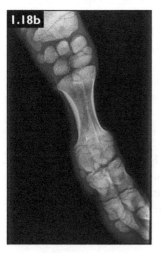

CASE 1.18

1 What is this condition? Congenital joint laxity and dwarfism (CJLD). CJLD is a congenital (non-inherited) skeletal anomaly reported in beef herds worldwide, with clusters of calves born with severe shortening of long bones, tendon laxity and occasionally brachygnathia.

2 How can the problem be investigated? Calves are born with disproportionate dwarfism, shortening of the diaphyses, misshapen epiphyses and variable joint laxity (**1.18b**).

3 What control measures can be introduced? The aetiology is unknown, although some authors have suggested manganese deficiency as a possible cause.

The problem is associated almost exclusively with spring calving beef herds where cows are fed a silage-based diet without straw or cereal supplementation during the winter months. Damage to the developing fetus probably occurs between 3 and 6 months of gestation. An unknown dietary teratogenic factor may be involved, but none has been identified.

There is no treatment and although joints stabilise and calves may walk normally, they remain chronically stunted and have no value for beef production. In herds where the disease has occurred, problems in subsequent years can normally be prevented by supplementing the silage-based diet during mid trimester with some hay/straw and cereals.

CASE 1.19

1 What conditions would you consider (most likely first)? Include: persistent infection with BVDV; chronic suppurative pneumonia or other septic focus; poor dam milk yield/mastitis; congenital abnormality.

2 What tests would you undertake? A blood sample result was BVDV antibody negative/antigen positive, (probably) indicating a persistently infected BVDV animal. While retesting would be necessary in 1 month's time to differentiate from a transiently viraemic animal, this would be unlikely when the calf shows typical clinical signs of persistent BVDV infection. The faecal worm egg count was low at 100 strongyle epg (probably *Ostertagia* spp.).

3 What other clinical problems could be expected? Potential problems include a poor pregnancy rate in the breeding cattle in the group due to embryonic/early fetal death if infected by BVDV. *In-utero* infection of the developing fetus in seronegative females between 45 and 135 days results in the birth of a persistently infected calf with cerebellar hypoplasia/hydranencephaly, a common manifestation of fetal infection later in this period. Transient infertility of the bull could result after virus infection if he was seronegative. Abortions can be expected at 4–7 months of gestation in susceptible animals.

4 How could this scenario have been prevented? National eradication programmes have proved very successful in several countries in the EU and are progressing well in other member states. In other countries, prevention of disease could involve establishment and maintenance of a BVDV-free herd by serological screening of all purchased cattle and strict biosecurity including double fencing of all perimeters. A concurrent vaccination programme of all breeding cattle would appear to be the safest option where doubts exist over herd biosecurity. However, a recent study revealed that 21% of farmers vaccinated cattle using the incorrect dose of vaccine or by the wrong route, and nearly 50% had the wrong interval between doses.

CASE 1.20

1 Where is the lesion? The lesion lies between in the spinal cord between C6 and T2.

2 What lesion would you suspect (most likely first)? The most likely lesion is vertebral empyema originating in one of the articular facets extending to involve the vertebral body and into the vertebral canal causing cord compression (**1.20b**). Despite the chronic nature of the empyema (several weeks to months), the calf may present with sudden onset of neurological signs. Certain *Salmonella* serotypes, especially *S. dublin*, can cause such bone infections.

Other lesions include: vertebral body fracture - sudden onset of neurological signs and pain associated with movement of the head (more commonly affects C4/C5); vitamin E/selenium deficiency - recumbency caused by white muscle disease presents as a bright, alert calf weak on all four legs.

3 What ancillary tests could you undertake? Further tests to identify a vertebral body lesion (bone lysis) are difficult even with excellent quality radiographs. Myelography can be performed but is expensive and not without risk. Lumbar CSF

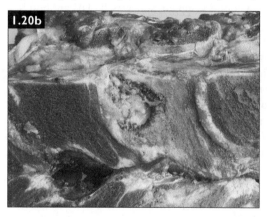

analysis is a useful indicator of an inflammatory lesion causing spinal cord compression with an increase in protein from 0.3 g/l to >1.2 g/l (30 mg/dl to >120 mg/dl).

4 What is the prognosis? Compressive spinal cord lesions (see **1.20b**), whether traumatic or inflammatory in origin, offer a grave prognosis and this calf was euthanased for welfare reasons.

CASE 1.21

1 What is the cause (most likely first)? Necrotic stomatitis (calf diphtheria); actinobacillosis.

Fusobacterium necrophorum causes a necrotic stomatitis typically seen in young dairy calves kept under unhygienic conditions with dirty feeding equipment. Lesions may also follow trauma to the buccal cavity caused by oesophageal feeders used to administer either colostrum or oral electrolyte solutions, and dosing gun injuries. Infection may extend to involve the larynx, causing anorexia, pyrexia, frequent harsh coughing, inspiratory stridor (roaring, honking) audible from a considerable distance and dyspnoea. The laryngeal region is swollen and palpation is resented. Death due to asphyxiation with necrotic debris occluding the lumen may occur if animals remain untreated for several days.

2 What treatment would you recommend? Calf diphtheria is treated with procaine penicillin (IM injection for 5–7 consecutive days). Parenteral potentiated sulphonamides and oxytetracycline are also effective.

3 Are there any control measures? The disease is prevented by high standards of hygiene when rearing dairy calves. In this situation the farmer was administering colostrum to calves slow to suck by an oesophageal feeder, which was never cleaned or disinfected.

CASE 1.22

1 What are your observations/comments? The calving ropes and calving aid are filthy, which could introduce infection into the posterior reproductive tract/uterus when placing them around the calf's legs and/or head. Any unnecessary manual interference at calving greatly increases the risk of puerperal metritis, although the farmer says that few cows are sick after calving. You recommend that you review the calving records to compare those cows that calve unaided with those requiring 'assistance', but only the minimum data of the birth dates of the calves are recorded.

Puerperal metritis commonly affects cows after unhygienic manual interference to correct fetal malpresentation/malposture, after delivery of twins or a dead calf and following infectious causes of abortion. In most of these situations, there is retention of some, or all, of the fetal membranes. Cows suffering hypocalcaemia during second stage labour have an increased incidence of retained fetal membranes (RFM) and metritis. Bacterial entry and multiplication within the uterus produces toxins, which are absorbed across the damaged endometrium. Vaginal examination often stimulates discomfort and vigorous straining, and reveals copious amounts of red–brown foetid fluid.

RFM should only be removed if they come away with gentle traction, but this is rarely undertaken in beef cattle and the placenta(e) are passed after 5–7 days without apparent adverse effects (**1.22b**). This situation differs significantly from dairy cattle, where retained placentae often give rise to clinical illness. The future reproductive performance of beef cows in relation to calving ease is rarely investigated in beef herds apart from comments on caesarean operations if the cow fails to become pregnant. Surprisingly, cystitis progressing to pyelonephritis appears to be unrelated to dystocia.

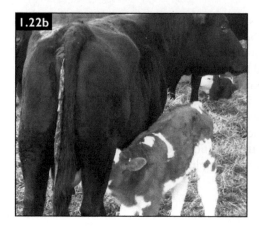

Assisting more than 50% of the herd to calve is far too high a percentage; ideally this figure should be zero, but twins and those calves in posterior presentation often need assistance. Selecting a bull based on calving ease would be a significant step forward, not least for animal welfare reasons.

CASE 1.23

1 What are these lesions? Capped hocks, cellulitis and effusion of the hock joint. Capped hocks are common in dairy cows caused by repeated trauma from unyielding (concrete) lying surfaces.

2 What is the likely cause? Poor cubicle design coupled with insufficient or inappropriate bedding material leads to repeated trauma and skin damage; skin penetration and development of cellulitis may result.

3 What action should be taken? Hock swellings are an indication of poor housing and can be readily prevented by good cubicle design, maintenance and amount and type of bedding material. The prevalence of hock swellings in dairy cattle has been used as an outcome measure of cow welfare. An example of very poor maintenance of sand bedded cubicles is shown (**1.23b**). Prevalence of hock and carpal lesions should be interpreted alongside whole herd lameness scoring. No treatment is necessary; prevention is important.

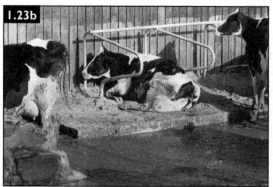

Infected (cellulitis) lesions are best treated with procaine penicillin or cephalosporin, the latter having no milk-withhold restriction in many countries. Lancing any large lesion should be carefully considered because this often results in considerable haemorrhage from blood vessels in the thick fibrous capsular wall. Furthermore, the incision site quickly seals over. Prior ultrasound scanning of the lesion would identify the nature of the swelling and the extent of any subcutaneous abscess.

CASE 1.24

1 What is the cause of this problem (most likely first)? Fracture of sacral vertebra(e) (crushed tail head syndrome, a vague term that refers to an injury to the sacral or coccygeal vertebrae of dairy cows following mounting activity, causing variable spinal nerve injury leading to tail paresis/paralysis and, in some cases, bladder dysfunction and sciatic nerve deficits). A lesion at S2–S4 would explain the clinical signs shown by this cow.

2 What treatment would you administer? In acute cases, treatment with NSAIDs or corticosteroids may reduce the local inflammation and improve neurological function temporarily, but the prognosis for full recovery is guarded. Careful palpation of the ventral surface of vertebral column per rectum may reveal the sacral fracture (**1.24b**).

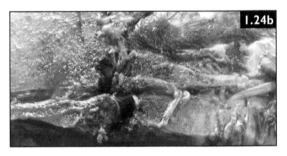

3 What action would you take? This cow was euthanased and the sacral fracture confirmed at necropsy. Emergency on-farm slaughter could be considered but the carcass value of a dairy cow is often too low to be financially viable; transport to a slaughter plant cannot be justified for welfare reasons.

CASE 1.25

1 What area of the brain could be involved? The clinical signs are suggestive of a cerebellar lesion. The calf has shown clinical signs for the past month only, therefore a developmental lesion rather than a congenital lesion would be suspected.

2 What conditions would you consider? Cerebellar abscess; cerebellar abiotrophy.

3 What tests could be undertaken? A cerebellar abscess was considered to be the more likely diagnosis. A lumbar CSF sample collected under local anaesthesia revealed a clear and colourless sample, but laboratory examination showed increased protein and white cell concentration comprised almost exclusively of

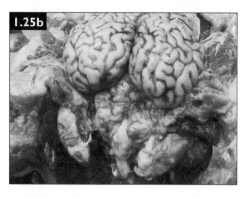

neutrophils. There was no history of BVDV infection on this closed unit.

4 What action would you take? Antibiotic therapy is ineffective in treating large abscess(es) in the brain regardless of location and the calf was euthanased because of the hopeless prognosis. An abscess in the cerebellum was identified at necropsy (**1.25b**).

CASE 1.26

1 What conditions would you consider (most likely first)? Coccidiosis; poor nutrition; salmonellosis. Coccidiosis is caused by infection by the protozoan *Eimeria* spp., which parasitize the epithelium lining of the alimentary tract. *E. zuernii, E. bovis* and *E. alabamensis* are the most common and pathogenic. Infection causes loss of epithelial cells and villous atrophy, with consequent diarrhoea and possibly dysentery. Outbreaks of disease are commonly seen 3–4 weeks after mixing groups of dairy calves.

2 How would you confirm the diagnosis? Diagnosis is based on epidemiological and clinical findings affecting most calves in a group. Demonstration of large numbers of oocysts in faecal samples is helpful, but speciation is rarely undertaken in field outbreaks because of laboratory costs. Remember that small numbers of oocysts are

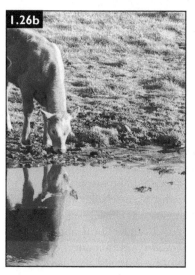

present in the faeces of many normal calves and the stage of infestation greatly influences the number of oocysts present in faeces. There is a good response to specific anticoccidial therapy. Histopathology findings in a dead calf confirm the clinical diagnosis.

3 What treatment would you recommend? Move calves from the infected building immediately. A sulpha drug given orally for 3–5 days is a common treatment. Toltrazuril and diclazuril can be used for both treatment and prophylaxis. Oral fluid therapy may be indicated in certain cases. Decoquinate can be used in-feed for prevention of coccidiosis in diary calves. Monensin sodium is used as a coccidiostat in many countries, but is not licensed within the EU.

Strict attention to disinfection of buildings between batches of calves and clean feeding areas mean that coccidiosis is uncommon in modern dairy units. Disease caused by *E. alabamensis* may result from contaminated water courses in pastured calves during summer months (**1.26b**). As survival of oocysts is possible from one year to another, calving on the same pasture each year may increase the disease risk.

CASE 1.27

1 What diseases would you consider (most likely first)? Include: environmental (coliform) mastitis; hypocalcaemia; acute septic metritis; other infectious conditions causing toxaemia/endotoxaemia; trauma at parturition resulting in a ruptured uterus; salmonellosis; botulism.

2 Which disease(s) is most likely? Coliform mastitis causing endotoxic shock is the probable cause of this clinical appearance. It may prove difficult to rule out the possible contribution of hypocalcaemia and many clinicians may elect to administer 400 ml of 40% calcium borogluconate slowly by the IV route while monitoring the cow's heart rate. Constipation is more likely in hypocalcaemia than diarrhoea.

3 What treatments would you administer? Treatment of endotoxic shock (coliform mastitis) includes IV injection of a NSAID, repeated 12 hours later. Hypertonic saline (7.2%) infusion (5 ml/kg; 3 litres for a 600 kg [1,320 lb] cow) within 5–7 minutes is achieved through a 13 gauge/4 inch jugular catheter. Access to 30–60 litres of warm water, which may contain electrolytes, must be provided, although not all cows drink. Some clinicians recommend stomach-tubing volumes up to 30–40 litres if the cow does not drink immediately. This cow made a full recovery. Mastitis caused by *Streptococcus uberis* can present with many of the clinical features of coliform mastitis and it may prove prudent to administer a broad-spectrum antibiotic both parenterally and by intramammary infusion.

4 What control measures could be adopted? Control measures include proper hygiene in the calving accommodation (**1.27b**). Use teat sealants at drying-off. Consider use of J5 *E. coli* core antigen vaccine. Include pre-milking teat dipping in the parlour routine. Keep cows standing for 30 minutes after milking by offering fresh feed to enable complete teat sphincter contraction before lying down. Sand-bedded cubicles perform better than those bedded with sawdust. Ensure ventilation in the cubicle shed and a maximum occupancy of 90%.

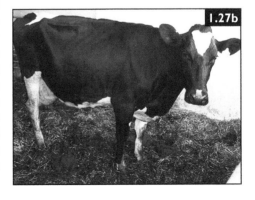

1.27b

CASE 1.28

1 What area of the brain could be involved? The clinical signs are suggestive of a cerebellar lesion. The calf has shown clinical signs since birth, therefore a congenital rather than a developmental lesion would be suspected.

2 What conditions would you consider? Cerebellar aplasia/hypoplasia; cerebellar abscess/focal meningitis; cerebellar abiotrophy; hydranencephaly. Cerebellar hypoplasia was considered to be the most likely diagnosis. The possible involvement of BVDV during fetal development could not be further examined because of the presence of maternally-derived antibody in the calf (unless the dam was a persistently infected BVD animal herself and therefore seronegative). Congenital BVDV infection is a common cause of cerebellar hypoplasia in calves with clinical

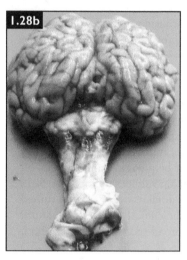

signs apparent from birth. Doming of the head caused by hypertensive hydrocephalus is an uncommon finding associated with congenital BVDV infection.

A lumbar CSF sample was collected under local anaesthesia. The sample was clear and colourless and laboratory examination revealed a normal protein concentration and white cell concentration. There was no evidence of infection of the central nervous system, therefore antibiotics were not indicated.

3 What action would you take? BVDV was subsequently isolated from a peripheral blood sample from this calf. Necropsy revealed gross evidence of cerebellar hypoplasia (**1.28b**).

CASE 1.29

1 What conditions would you consider? Congenital pseudomyotonia; cerebellar abiotrophy/abscess; otitis media; muscular dystrophy (white muscle disease); tetanus; Schmallenburg virus infection.

2 What tests could be undertaken? Brody's disease is a rare human congenital disorder associated with exercise-induced impairment of muscle relaxation. The underlying cause for this condition has been determined to be a mutation of the *ATP2A1* gene resulting in disturbed calcium reuptake into the sarcoplasmic reticulum at the end of the contractile phase. Recently, diseases associated with different /ATP2A1/ gene mutations have been described in the Chianina and Belgian Blue breeds and termed pseudomyotonia and congenital muscular dystonia 1, respectively. Analysis of the collected Chianina pedigree data suggested that congenital pseudomyotonia has monogenic autosomal recessive inheritance.

3 What action would you take? A further two calves were affected out of 40 calves born alive. All three affected calves were the progeny of a recently purchased Charolais bull. This bull was culled because of the hereditary component of this disease; no affected calves were born in the following four breeding seasons.

CASE 1.30

1 What conditions would you consider (most likely first)? Malnutrition/poor dam milk yield; parasitic gastroenteritis; coccidiosis; copper deficiency. A trace element deficiency problem would be expected to affect the majority/all of the growing animals in the group and in this herd only several of 30 calves are affected, suggesting that poor dam milk yield/nutrition could be a contributing factor. A thin, dry, sparse hair coat should not be confused with delayed shedding of winter coat (see **1.30**). Faecal worm eggs were negative; ostertagiosis is not usually a problem until much later in the grazing season.

2 What samples could you collect? Plasma or serum copper levels are suitable for the diagnosis of clinical disease, but not for the estimation of body copper reserves. A group of seven to 10 cattle should be sampled to establish a diagnosis. Liver biopsy samples from three to four animals give an indication of body copper reserves, and can be used to monitor copper supplementation. Response to treatment is perhaps the most important indicator of copper deficiency; randomly treat 15 calves in this group and leave 15 calves unsupplemented. Injectable copper compounds vary in respect to their speed of absorption from the injection site and duration of activity, but a growth response, if present, would be detected within 6–8 weeks.

3 What advice would you offer? Where the cause of poor growth is caused by poor dam milk supply, provision of creep feed should improve calf growth rates. As the protein content of spring grass is likely to be adequate, barley or another cereal would suffice.

CASE 1.31

1 How would you collect a lumbar CSF sample? It is necessary to puncture the subarachnoid space at the lumbosacral site. Collection of lumbar CSF is facilitated if the animal can be positioned in sternal recumbency with the hips flexed and the hind legs extended alongside the abdomen (this case); samples can also be collected when the animal is standing restrained in cattle stocks. The site for lumbar CSF collection is the midpoint of the lumbosacral space identified as the midline depression between the last palpable dorsal lumbar spine (L6) and the first palpable sacral dorsal spine (S2). The site must be clipped, surgically prepared and between 1 and 2 ml of local anaesthetic injected SC. The needle (see below for a guide to needle length and gauge) is slowly advanced (over 10 seconds) at a right angle to the plane of the vertebral column or with the hub directed 5–10° caudally. It is essential to appreciate the changes in tissue resistance as the needle point passes sequentially through the subcutaneous tissue and interarcuate ligament, then the

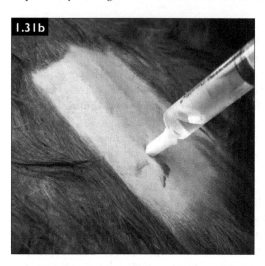

sudden 'pop' due to the loss of resistance as the needle point exits the ligamentum flavum into the extradural space. Once the needle point has penetrated the dorsal subarachnoid space, CSF will well up into the needle hub within 2–3 seconds. Between 1 and 2 ml of CSF is sufficient for laboratory analysis and while the sample can be collected by free flow over 1–2 minutes, it is more convenient to employ very gentle syringe aspiration over 10–20 seconds (**1.31b**).

- Calves <100 kg 1 inch, 19 gauge
- Calves 100–250 kg 2 inch, 19 gauge
- Cattle >250 kg 4 inch, 18 gauge + internal stylet

The normal range of CSF protein concentration quoted for cattle is <0.3 g/l (<30 mg/dl). Normal CSF contains <10 cells/ml, which are predominantly lymphocytes with an occasional neutrophil. In cattle with a lesion causing thoracolumbar cord compression, thereby preventing equilibration of CSF protein concentration within the lateral ventricles, the lumbar CSF protein concentration is 3–10 times normal.

CASE 1.32

1 What conditions would you consider (most likely first)? Chronic suppurative pulmonary disease (CSPD); pleural abscesses; liver abscessation/hepatocaval thrombosis; endocarditis; parasitic bronchitis.

2 How could you confirm your provisional diagnosis? Auscultation of the chest is an unreliable method to assess the extent of lung pathology, and confirmation of the diagnosis of CSPD (bronchiectasis) necessitates real-time B-mode ultrasonographic examination of the chest with a 5 MHz sector/linear scanner. The bright linear echo formed by normal visceral pleura is present in the dorsal lung field but is replaced ventrally (18 cm above the point of the elbow on the left side and 12 cm on the right side; fifth and sixth intercostal spaces) by hypoechoic areas extending up to 4–8 cm into the lung parenchyma (**1.32b**), consistent with extensive lung consolidation.

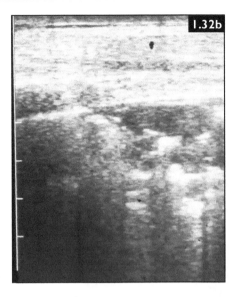

3 What treatment would you recommend? *Trueperella pyogenes* is most commonly isolated from such cases with bronchiectasis. The most effective treatment is 22,000 IU/kg procaine penicillin administered IM daily for up to 6 weeks, with a good treatment response within 2–3 days. Marbofloxacin is indicated for acute respiratory disease typically involving *Pasteurellae* spp., and is wholly ineffective in treating chronic suppurative pneumonia.

4 What is the prognosis for this heifer? This heifer made a good recovery but the farmer was advised not to breed from her again because of the likelihood of relapse after the next calving. As a guide, the prognosis is reasonable if the extent of the lung pathology, measured in a vertical plane from the point of the elbow on both sides of the chest, totals less than 40 cm.

CASE 1.33

1 What condition is the farmer talking about? An ovarian cyst is defined as a thin-walled anechoic (fluid-filled) structure >2.5 cm in diameter present for more than 10 days on one or both ovaries in the absence of a corpus luteum (**1.33b**). Cysts can be classified either as follicular, which are thin-walled, non-progesterone-producing structures (plasma P <2 ng/ml), or luteinised or luteal, which are thicker-walled (>3 mm) and produce progesterone (plasma P >2 ng/ml). Many normal corpora lutea have fluid-filled centres (lacunae) visible on ultrasound scan and must not be mistaken for luteal cysts.

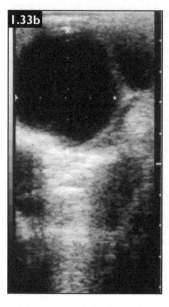

2 What causes the abnormal oestrous behaviour?
Follicular cysts develop due to either failure of the luteinising hormone (LH) surge around the time of normal ovulation, or failure of the follicle to respond to LH. The follicle fails to ovulate and, instead of undergoing atresia, continues to grow to form a cyst. Cystic follicles initially produce oestradiol (this cow), which suppresses further follicular development in the ovaries. They then enter an oestrogen-inactive phase, which can persist for many weeks. Many cysts that form during the early postpartum period (<30 days) regress spontaneously without treatment. Some follicular cysts become luteinised and persist as luteal cysts.

3 What treatment would you administer?
Gonadotrophin-releasing hormone (GnRH) analogues (e.g. buserelin, gonadorelin). GnRH induces an LH surge effecting luteinisation (not ovulation) of the follicular cyst and possibly ovulation or luteinisation of any mature follicles present in the ovaries.

Injection of human chorionic gonadotrophin (hCG), which is an LH agonist, can be used to treat follicular cysts, with the mode of action as described for GnRH. Return to oestrus is variable but within 20–30 days post treatment.

Progesterone treatment (PRID™ or CIDR™). The PRID/CIDR device is inserted into the vagina for 10–12 days. Oestrus normally occurs within 2–3 days of PRID/CIDR removal, along with ovulation of a new dominant follicle.

Manual rupture of ovarian cysts is not recommended because of possible trauma/haemorrhage within the ovary and its bursa.

4 What advice would you offer? At present, the best advice to reduce incidence of cystic ovarian disease in dairy cows is to manage cows to minimise negative energy balance and metabolic and management stress in early lactation, as these factors have been associated with higher incidence of disease.

CASE 1.34

1 While this barbaric practice is not now as common as 20–30 years ago, what analgesic protocol would you adopt? Subcornual block using 10 ml of 2% lidocaine SC (perineural) immediately below the frontal ridge using a 1 inch/18 gauge hypodermic needle. This blocks the cornual branch of the lacrimal nerve (a branch of the ophthalmic nerve arising from the trigeminal nerve). After inserting the needle, draw back on the syringe plunger to check for blood, which would indicate accidental puncture of a branch of the internal maxillary artery. Accidental intra-arterial injection produces instant collapse and possible seizure activity and must be avoided by redirecting the needle, drawing back and injecting when no blood is aspirated into the syringe.

Sedation with xylazine (0.05 mg/kg IM) in addition to local infiltration with lidocaine is used for surgical castration and disbudding/dehorning by many practitioners. As well as sedation, xylazine will provide some analgesia, but injection of a NSAID before the procedure may be a much more effective analgesic strategy, although considerably more expensive. For convenience, xylazine can be added to the local anaesthetic solution (approximately 4 ml of 2% xylazine added to 100 ml of 2% lidocaine; for dehorning a 300 kg (660 lb) animal receives 2 injections of 10 ml lidocaine containing a total of 16 mg of xylazine, equivalent to 0.05 mg/kg). The volume of local anaesthetic solution is reduced pro-rata for a calf weighing 150 kg (330 lb), when 5 ml of the combined solution is injected at each site.

Following diffusion of anaesthetic from the injection site, drooping of the upper eyelids is observed in many calves after injection (blocking of the auriculopalpebral branch of the facial nerve) and is a useful indicator that the block has been successful (**1.34b**).

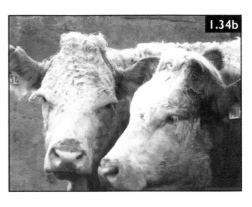

Lidocaine is not licensed for use in food-producing animals in the EU; however, procaine is only licensed for minor surgical procedures; dehorning is not a minor surgical procedure. From an animal welfare perspective, lidocaine and xylazine plus a NSAID injection is perhaps the best compromise in this unfortunate situation. However, disbudding within the first few weeks of life causes much less tissue damage and must be undertaken unless there is very good reason to postpone this mutilation.

CASE 1.35

1 Comment on the significant radiographic abnormalities. There is marked soft tissue swelling over the abaxial aspect of the coronary band and widening of the interdigital space. There is marked widening of the articular space of the distal interphalangeal joint with extensive erosion of articular cartilage. There is marked osteophytosis of the second phalanx.

2 What is the likely cause(s) of this condition? Puncture wound of the distal interphalangeal joint, although none is visible. Ascending infection from a sole ulcer is the more common aetiology in dairy cattle.

3 What is the likely duration of this condition? The development of these bony lesions would likely have taken a minimum of 3–4 months, during which time the cow would have been severely lame. It is likely that the history of 4 weeks' lameness is a gross underestimate of this cow's suffering. The chronicity of such lesions is clearly demonstrated by radiographic changes (**1.35b**).

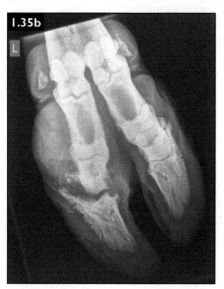

4 Has this cow received appropriate treatment and care? Interdigital necrobacillosis (foul of the foot) is a common cause of severe lameness in cattle at pasture and responds rapidly to antibiotic therapy provided there is no penetrating foreign body in the interdigital space. It is unreasonable to wait (at least) 3 weeks without improvement before requesting veterinary assistance.

5 How can this problem be resolved? Digit amputation under IVRA. Flunixin meglumine (or other NSAID) is injected IV before surgery. A robust tourniquet is placed below the hock. Thirty ml of 2% lidocaine solution is injected into the superficial vein running on the craniolateral aspect of the third metatarsal bone; analgesia is effective within 2 minutes. The affected digit is removed using embryotomy (Gigli) wire through distal P1. A pressure bandage is applied to limit haemorrhage, removed after 3–4 days and a light dressing applied for a further 3–4 days.

CASE 1.36

1 Describe the important features shown. There is marked soft tissue swelling and considerable lysis around the root of the third permanent molar tooth of the left mandible, with localised bone remodelling.

2 What conditions would you consider (most likely first)? Tooth root abscess; actinomycosis; bone neoplasia. The bone lesion appears to be too focal for *Actinomyces bovis* infection, which typically causes a more extensive pyogranulomatous osteitis/osteomyelitis in the maxilla and mandible of adult cattle.

3 **What treatment would you recommend?** The response is likely to be poor even with prolonged antibiotic therapy. Extraction of the tooth was attempted *per os* but it could not be removed; more excessive force could have caused mandibular fracture. Discussions with the insurers resulted in an agreed plan to treat the bull for 2 weeks with a penicillin and streptomycin combination and re-evaluate after that treatment period. Initially, there was improvement with an increase in the bull's appetite, but this situation lasted only a few days. The bull started quidding again and the decision was taken to euthanase the bull for welfare reasons; the meat withdrawal period dictated by the antibiotic treatment was considered too long for the bull's welfare so there was no carcass value. Radiographs in this case provided an accurate assessment of the lesion, which aided discussions with the insurance company's expert assessors.

CASE 1.37

1 **Describe the sonogram.** There is loss of the bright linear echo formed by normal visceral pleura, replaced by a hypoechoic area containing numerous 1.5–2.0 cm well-encapsulated circular anechoic areas containing multiple hyperechoic dots typical of abscesses. This sonogram is typical of chronic suppurative pneumonia; the demonstration of bronchiectasis requires postmortem examination, but such pathology is typical in such cases.

2 **What conditions would you consider?** Chronic suppurative pulmonary disease (CSPD) and bronchiectasis.

3 **What treatment would you recommend?** *Trueperella pyogenes* is most commonly isolated from such cases with lung abscessation and bronchiectasis and typically follows incomplete/inappropriate antibiotic treatment for acute respiratory disease, often caused by *Mannheimia haemolytica*. The most effective treatment is 22,000 IU/kg procaine penicillin (IM daily for up to 6 weeks), with a good treatment response within 2–3 days. This heifer responded well to treatment, but a rescan of her lungs showed little change after 6 weeks treatment (**1.37b**). The animal improved because infection was cleared from the airways (bronchiectasis); lung abscesses remain unaffected.

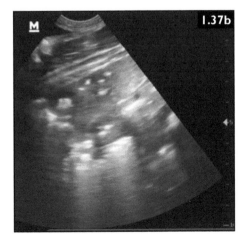

4 **What is the prognosis for this heifer?** The response rate for CSPD

largely depends on the extent of pathology, which can be determined ultrasonographically. As a guide, the prognosis is reasonable if the extent of the lung pathology, measured in a vertical plane from the point of the elbow on both sides of the chest, totals less than 40 cm in a mature cow; scale down to ca. 25 cm in a bulling heifer (guideline only). The extent and chronicity of these lung lesions were severe and the farmer was advised not to breed this heifer and cull her for beef when she reached a marketable weight.

CASE 1.38

1 What is the definition of a downer cow? A cow that has been sternally recumbent for more than 24 hours, is not suffering from hypocalcaemia and has no obvious condition (e.g. mastitis, toxaemia or injury).

2 What is the likely cause? Downer cow syndrome has a multifactorial primary aetiology mostly related to dystocia and milk fever. Unless the initial cause of recumbency is promptly treated, lying in one position for more than 6 hours results in muscle damage and ischaemic necrosis, which may become irreversible after 12 hours' recumbency in the same position.

3 What treatment would you administer? Move to a dry, clean comfortable lying area, either a deep-bedded straw pen or outside into a sheltered grass paddock. The cow must be turned every 3 hours to prevent pressure damage to muscles and nerves. Ensure provision of *ad-libitum* good quality food and fresh water. A NSAID or corticosteroid injection reduces pain and tissue damage, as well as improving demeanour and appetite. Assist the cow in attempting to stand using cow nets, supportive harness, inflatable bags and water flotation tanks. Hip clamps (Bagshaw hoist) may be used once to assist diagnosis; however, repeated application may cause severe muscle damage.

4 What is the prognosis for this cow? Cows that cannot maintain sternal recumbency and fall into lateral recumbency, and are depressed or hyperaesthetic, have a poor prognosis. Cows that make repeated attempts to rise and can move themselves about are often called 'creepers' or 'crawlers'. Such cows are usually bright and alert, and have a good prognosis.

CASE 1.39

1 What conditions would you consider (most likely first)? Include: bacterial endocarditis; chronic suppurative pulmonary disease; pleural effusion/abscess; traumatic reticuloperitonitis; septic pericarditis; myocarditis.

Surprisingly, despite the sometimes large vegetative lesions present on heart valves, heart murmurs are inaudible in most cases of endocarditis. Transthoracic ultrasonographic examination of heart valves requires a sector scanner. Transthoracic ultrasonography revealed no evidence of lung pathology on either side of the chest. There was no peritoneal effusion ruling out traumatic reticuloperitonitis.

2 What treatment would you recommend? The organisms most commonly isolated from endocarditis lesions, including streptococci, are sensitive to penicillin. Treatment with 22,000 IU/kg procaine penicillin administered daily was commenced and a single injection of dexamethasone given IM (cow not pregnant).

3 What is the prognosis? The prognosis for endocarditis cases is hopeless but it is difficult to establish a definitive diagnosis; therefore, antibiotic therapy is often administered in case another treatable condition has been overlooked (unlikely in this cow as all other possibilities had been excluded from the differential diagnosis list). This cow failed to respond to treatment and was euthanased. At necropsy a large vegetative lesion was present on the tricuspid valve (**1.39b**). The liver was enlarged as a consequence of chronic venous congestion and the cut surface had the typical 'nutmeg appearance'. There were numerous infarcts in the kidney. No primary septic focus was found but this is not unusual.

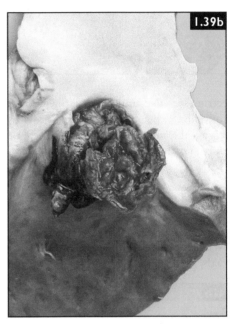

CASE 1.40

1 What conditions would you consider (most likely first)? Pharyngeal abscesses/enlarged retropharyngeal lymph nodes; oral and laryngeal lesions caused by *Fusobacterium necrophorum*; actinobacillosis of retropharyngeal lymph nodes.

Pharyngeal abscesses/enlarged retropharyngeal lymph nodes in cattle result from penetration wounds, most commonly caused by incorrect drenching/bolus administration. It is not always possible to distinguish the deep-seated retropharyngeal lymph nodes even when they are grossly enlarged.

2 How would you confirm you diagnosis? Diagnosis is not simple, especially when the infection has tracked along fascial planes and may erupt distant to the entry site in the pharynx. History of recent drenching/bolusing provides strong circumstantial evidence of pharyngeal trauma. Poor appetite resulting from enlarged

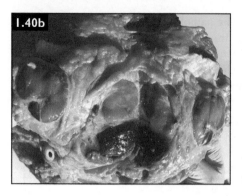

retropharyngeal lymph nodes (**1.40b**) or an abscess can prove difficult to diagnose. Radiography to illustrate soft tissue swellings, and possibly a fluid line should a large abscess be present, can prove very helpful but such facilities are not readily used in practice. Endoscopy and ultrasound-guided needle aspiration are also possible diagnostic techniques.

3 What treatment(s) would you administer? Response to broad-spectrum systemic antibiotic treatment for 10–14 days (e.g. clavulanate potentiated amoxycillin or penicillin/streptomycin) will be variable depending on the extent of pharyngeal trauma/abscessation. Surgical drainage of retropharyngeal abscesses is possible via the oral cavity or using a lateral approach, but is not without risk.

CASE 1.41

1 What conditions would you consider (most likely first)? Epididymitis; orchitis; photosensitisation; inguinal hernia.

2 What further investigations would you undertake? Ultrasonography (**1.41b**) reveals marked swelling of the tail of the epididymis (5 MHz linear scanner,

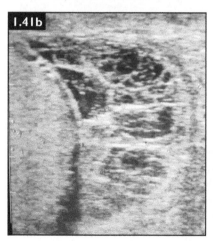

ventral pole of testicle to the left side with the tail of the epididymis to the right, there is marked thickening [oedema] of the scrotal skin). These findings are consistent with a diagnosis of epididymitis. Rectal examination reveals enlarged seminal vesicles. There is no evidence of orchitis. This bull is intended for fattening; semen collection would be indicated after a further 3 months to assess semen quality in potential breeding bulls but is not indicated in this case. Repeat ultrasonography would be helpful to monitor treatment.

3 What is the likely cause? Numerous bacteria including *Trueperella pyogenes*, *E. coli*, *Histophilus somni* and *Staphylococcus* spp. have been isolated from cases of orchitis and epididymitis.

4 What treatment would you administer? The bull was treated with florfenicol and was much improved the following day. The florfenicol treatment was repeated on day 3. The bull was normal by day 4 and was slaughtered 3 months later; no repeat ultrasound examination was considered necessary.

CASE 1.42

1 What conditions would you consider (most likely first)? Nervous acetonaemia/ketosis and LDA. Excessive loss of body condition may have led to development of a severely fatty liver and other parenchymatous organs.

2 How could you confirm your diagnosis? Diagnosis of ketosis is based on clinical examination and confirmed by a positive cow-side Rothera's reagent test or laboratory demonstration of a 3-OH butyrate concentration in excess of 4.0 mmol/l. Various liver enzymes can be assayed to determine liver dysfunction caused by fat infiltration of the liver, but they tend to underestimate the severity of the problem. The LDA can be confirmed at corrective surgery (right omentopexy).

3 What treatment would you administer? Treatment included dexamethasone and 400 ml 50% dextrose IV. Propylene glycol was given orally along with 40–60 litres of warm water. Surgery to correct the LDA was postponed until the following day. The cow deteriorated overnight and was recumbent and unable to stand. The prognosis was hopeless and the cow was euthanased for welfare reasons. The highly friable and very fatty liver was evident at necropsy (1.42a, b). It can prove difficult to predict the extent of fatty infiltration of the liver even with an array of liver enzyme test results; liver biopsy is rarely undertaken in general practice. It is highly likely that this cow had been ill for much longer than the stated 24 hours.

4 How could this condition be prevented? A review of the far-off and close-up dry cow rations is necessary. Increased plasma NEFA concentrations are a good indicator of excessive fat mobilisation in the close-up dry period. Cows should enter the dry period in BCS 3/5 and maintain this value until calving. Excessive conditioning (BCS >4) is often the result of extended dry periods due to poor fertility.

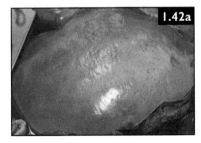
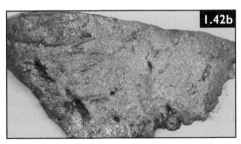

CASE 1.43

1 What conditions would you consider? Femoral fracture; femoral nerve paralysis; sciatic nerve damage.

2 How could you confirm your diagnosis? Fracture through the distal femoral growth plate is demonstrated by radiography (**1.43a, b**).

3 What is the prognosis? Repair of the fracture was not possible and the calf was euthanased for welfare reasons.

4 How could this situation have been prevented? Excessive force using a calving jack to deliver oversized beef calves is not uncommon. Wherever possible, the cow should be haltered and released from the cattle stocks and allowed to assume lateral recumbency before pulling the calf. A caesarean operation was clearly indicated in this case.

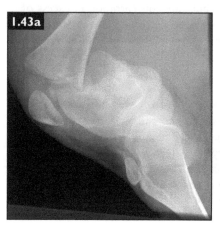
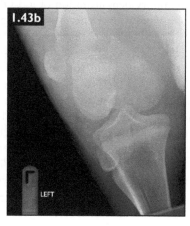

CASE 1.44

1 Age at first calving. According to the English Beef and Lamb Executive (EBLEX), the age at calving in beef heifers is approximately 34 months. The target of calving beef heifers is 2 years old. While management and nutrition will be important factors, the extent to which disease contributes to poor liveweight gain and delayed breeding is not known.

2 Calving period. In England surveys show calving periods in the range of 20–22 weeks for 2010/11. Calving periods for beef suckler herds in Scotland were 14–16 weeks for 2010. The average calving intervals for suckler cows calving in England and Wales in 2010 were broadly similar, ranging from 440 to 446 days. Producers should be aiming for a compact calving period of 9 weeks. This suggests that 21% more calves are possible from the same number of cows by improving herd fertility and reducing the calving interval to an average of 365 days for all cows in the herd.

3 Barren rate. Data from enterprise costing surveys show barren cow rates in the range of 6.3 to 8.1 barren cows per 100 cows exposed to the bull in 2010. The industry benchmark for barren rate is less than 5% of females exposed to the bull.
4 Bull infertility. Up to 40% of bulls are subfertile. Bull fertility assessments are more often undertaken after detection of a high barren rate during a pregnancy diagnosis test or following an extended calving period. These fertility parameters are invaluable to those veterinary practitioners with a proactive approach to convincing their farming clients of the financial value of bull breeding soundness assessments ahead of the service period rather than after a problem has arisen. Whether semen collection using electroejaculation and microscopic analysis is a better assessment than palpation and ultrasound examination of scrotal content is another matter. The former assessment has proven popular with veterinary practitioners but there are few convincing published data to support this practice in UK beef herds.

CASE 1.45
1 **What conditions would you consider (most likely first)?** Liver fluke. Inadequate nutrition also presents as a whole group/herd problem of poor production and weight loss, but diarrhoea would be an uncommon finding.
2 **How would you confirm your diagnosis?** Undosed beef cattle grazing potentially infected pastures should either be treated or checked for the presence of fluke eggs in faeces (**1.45b**). Metacercariae ingested from pasture will be mature patent flukes by late winter (3-month pre-patent period). Liver enzymes, particularly GLDH and GGT, reflect liver and bile duct damage, respectively, but are not specific for liver fluke infection. Serology indicates past liver fluke infection but this may not be current. The coproantigen ELISA test detects digestive enzymes that are released into the bile by migrating (late immature) and adult flukes and detected in faeces. Active fluke infection can be detected 3–4 weeks after infection but more reliably after 6–9 weeks, approximately 3–6 weeks before eggs can be detected in faeces.

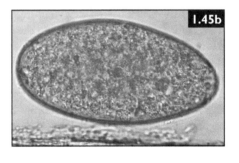

3 **What treatment would you administer?** Triclabendazole is effective against developing flukes from several days old but is not necessary and should not be used for mature flukes. Closantel and nitroxynil are very effective against immature flukes from around 7 weeks post infection and can be used for the treatment of chronic fasciolosis.

Albendazole and oxyclosanide are effective from 10–14 weeks post infection and such treatment is recommended to remove adult flukes in late spring.

4 What advice would you give to the farmer? Slaughterhouse data reveal that more than 25% of bovine livers are condemned because of liver fluke damage. The farmer should discuss such positive liver fluke results with their veterinary surgeon and develop an appropriate control programme.

CASE 1.46

1 What conditions would you consider (most likely first)? Femoral paralysis (the predominantly unilateral paralysis allows differentiation from a spinal lesion caudal to T2); congenital sarcocystosis; unilateral femoral nerve paralysis (should be differentiated from femoral fracture(s) [particularly through the proximal epiphysis], dislocated hip, pelvic fracture and infection of hip/stifle joints). Fractures of long bones following dystocia are rare and would be detected on careful clinical examination with radiography where appropriate.

2 What treatment would you administer? A single injection of dexamethasone may be useful (unproven) to reduce perineural swelling if the injury has just occurred (e.g. during calving [not this case]). NSAIDs could be administered but, as with the use of dexamethasone, there is no published evidence for their use in this situation. Calves with bilateral femoral nerve paralysis have a grave prognosis; unilateral injuries may take 6 months to fully recover. Careful examination of the calf is necessary to check for evidence of septicaemia and focal infections such as meningitis, polyarthritis, hypopyon, and omphlophlebitis, as these are more likely to result if there has been a delay/failure of passive antibody transfer due to the calf's recumbency and inability to find the cow's udder unaided.

3 How could this problem have been prevented? When a calf presents in anterior longitudinal presentation, two people pulling should be able to extend both fore leg fetlock joints one hand's breadth beyond the cow's vulva (indicates extension of the elbows into the pelvis) within 10 minutes. Any greater traction to achieve such progress forewarns of potential hip-lock and its consequences. This simple guideline is frequently ignored by farmers, when too much traction can also cause obturator and sciatic nerve damage to the cow; uterine prolapse is also not uncommon after prolonged dystocia and excessive traction.

CASE 1.47

1 What is the likely cause? Granulosa cell tumour; mastitis.

2 How would confirm your diagnosis? Transrectal ultrasonography (**1.47b**) reveals a multi-loculated mass, approximately 6 cm deep and 12 cm long, just beyond the pubis, consistent with a granulosa cell tumour.

3 What action could be taken? The tumour could be removed via a high right flank laparotomy under paravertebral anaesthesia, although there may be problems with exteriorisation of the tumour and effective ligation of its blood supply in the broad ligament. Access via a ventral midline approach under general anaesthesia may give better surgical access but is not without risk. The future breeding of the heifer is very difficult to predict because few such surgeries have been undertaken. Unless the genetic merit of the heifer is unique (which is seldom the case) the best financial option may be to cull the heifer for beef.

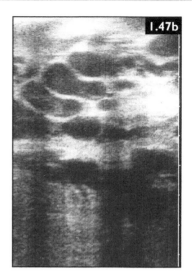

CASE 1.48

1 Describe the abnormal radiographic findings. There is marked soft tissue swelling and widening of the distal tibial growth plate. There is no evidence of significant bone lysis suggestive of infection.

2 What is the likely cause? Fracture involving the distal tibial growth plate.

3 What action should have been taken at the first veterinary examination? The animal was euthanased for welfare reasons after examination of the radiographs and the diagnosis confirmed at necropsy (**1.48c**). This type of fracture will not heal with casting the leg. The animal could not be slaughtered on-farm for human consumption because of prior antibiotic therapy.

Care must be taken when reaching a provisional diagnosis in cattle with sudden-onset severe lameness. If there is no evidence of infection, do not administer antibiotics. Sudden-onset severe lameness is most commonly caused by fracture of a long bone or joint trauma leading to marked effusion. Lameness caused by foot lesions and growth plate infections is more gradual in onset. NSAID injection is not an aid to diagnosis and is no excuse for an incomplete clinical examination – where doubt exists ask a colleague for a second opinion immediately.

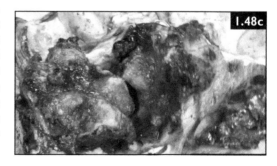

CASE 1.49

1 What is this lesion? An extensive organised haematoma extending >30 cm from the probe head.

2 What is the likely cause? Trauma; a bulling injury would be possible in this age group. A coagulopathy may have been present at that time but was not investigated because only one animal was affected and there was no history of a similar problem on the farm.

3 What action should be taken? The mass has not reduced in size over 2 months and the animal has difficulty rising, therefore the heifer should be euthanased for

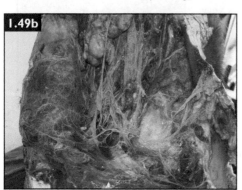

welfare reasons. Necropsy (**1.49b**) reveals that resorption of this haematoma has not occurred over 2 months and may not occur at all. The size and organised nature of the haematoma, which is firmly adherent to adjacent tissues, mean that attempted drainage would not have been possible and would simply have allowed infection to enter, with the development of a massive subcutaneous abscess.

CASE 1.50

1 Describe the important features of the sonogram obtained using a 5 MHz sector scanner in the sixth intercostal space approximately half way up the chest wall (1.50a). Ultrasound examination shows the absence of the hyperechoic line representing the visceral pleural (lung surface). There is approximately 5–6 cm of fluid (anechoic area) separating the chest wall and the pericardial sac, which

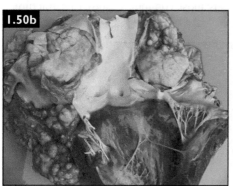

itself is distended to 5–8 cm. There is a large 5–10 cm hyperechoic mass firmly attached to the epicardium.

2 What conditions would you consider (most likely first)? These findings are consistent with a heart base tumour (**1.50b**). It is unusual to find significant pleural transudate in cattle with septic pericarditis. Furthermore, the fluid within the pericardial sac is uniformly anechoic and not purulent (absence of multiple hyperechoic dots), therefore it is not consistent with septic pericarditis. This case clearly demonstrates the clinical application of ultrasonography because the most likely cause on clinical examination would be septic pericarditis. At necropsy there was a large amount of blood within the pericardial sac from the tumour.

3 What treatment would you administer? There is no effective treatment and the cow should be euthanased immediately for welfare reasons. Indeed, this cow should have been euthanased several weeks ago and not allowed to deteriorate to this state.

CASE 1.51

1 What conditions would you consider (most likely first)? Hepatocaval thrombosis; chronic suppurative pulmonary disease.

2 What tests could be undertaken to confirm your provisional diagnosis? A diagnosis of hepatocaval thrombosis is very difficult to confirm on clinical examination and is based on exclusion, where possible, of more common/ likely conditions. Epistaxis is the cardinal clinical sign of advanced hepatocaval thrombosis and indicates a hopeless prognosis such that affected cattle should be culled for welfare reasons. Often there is a minor bleed followed several days later by a fatal episode. Ultrasonographic examination of the chest would rule out chronic suppurative pulmonary disease; haematogenous spread from the thrombus gives a more caudodorsal distribution deeper within the lung parencyma. Ultrasonographic demonstration of the thrombus present in the caudal vena cava can be achieved in some cases, but such examination requires a sector scanner and is not commonly undertaken in general practice. Hepatomegaly, with rounded liver margins, would also be present, although not easily identified. A lesion involving a nasal passage would be unilateral.

3 What treatment would you administer? Effective treatment is limited by the difficulties inherent in early diagnosis of this problem. Theoretically, procaine penicillin injected daily for at least 6 weeks may overcome the bacteraemia but will not remove the massive thrombus, with the result that further bacterial shedding is likely. This cow could be sent for slaughter. Chronic venous congestion leads to hepatomegaly and a 'nutmeg appearance' (**1.51b**). Evidence of significant bacteraemia with liver, kidney and lung involvement may

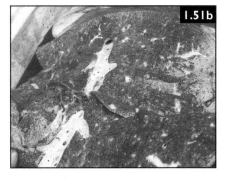

result in carcass condemnation. There is no effective treatment in cattle with significant pulmonary haemorrhage and these animals should be euthanased for welfare reasons.

4 What control measures would you recommend? The role of subacute ruminal acidosis is proposed in the aetiology of this condition, therefore reducing risk factors for this condition may help, although there are no specific control measures.

CASE 1.52

1 What is the prognosis for this calf? The prognosis is guarded because there is already considerable damage to the gut and omentum in the 30 minutes it takes for you to attend. It is also impossible to render the omentum and serosal surface of the intestines sterile before returning them to the abdomen.

2 What action would you take, including details of your anaesthetic approach? Inject flunixin (or other NSAID) IV. Inject antibiotics IM – there are no specific recommendations, but amoxicillin/clavulaninic acid combination is often used. Protect the prolapsed intestines in a sterile plastic drape until replacement (see **1.52**). There are a number of anaesthetic options but xylazine sedation followed by ketamine is the most commonly used. Xylazine is given IM (0.05–0.07 mg/kg) and the animal left for approximately 10 minutes. Induction of anaesthesia is then achieved by administering ketamine (3–5 mg/kg IV), which produces 10–20 minutes of surgical anaesthesia. Anaesthesia can be extended with incremental doses of ketamine (2–3 mg/kg IV), which give a further 10 minutes of surgical anaesthesia. Alphaxane (4.4 mg/kg IV) is very safe in young calves and gives 10 minutes of surgical anaesthesia. Propofol (4–6.5 mg/kg IV) can also be used.

Once surgical anaesthesia has been achieved, place the calf in dorsal recumbency and extend the hernial ring cranially with scissors taking great care not to damage the intestines present within the ring. Remove gross contamination and replace the prolapsed intestines while flushing all surfaces with sterile saline. Suture the incision and the hernial ring. The benefits of intra-abdominal antibiotics are debatable. Stomach tube with 3 litres of colostrum. Monitor carefully and continue antibiotics and NSAIDs for the next 2 days. The major risk is peritonitis, which will be manifest as reluctance to suck but with a distended abdomen due to static fluid-filled intestines and possible accumulation of exudate, dullness and colic.

3 How can this problem be prevented? This problem occurs sporadically, often caused by an overzealous dam with vigourous licking of the calf and the umbilical remnant. Some farmers maintain that application of iodine to the umbilicus aggravates this behaviour.

CASE 1.53

1 Describe the radiographic findings. A grid would have improved the quality of the ventrodorsal radiograph shown because of the large amount of muscle in this area. However, there is evidence of a shallow acetabulum and flattening of the femoral head affecting both hip joints.

2 What conditions would you consider? Include: hip dysplasia; osteochondrosis dissecans; rickets (would be unusual in this natural rearing system).

3 What action would you take? There is no treatment and the calf should be euthanased for welfare reasons. The

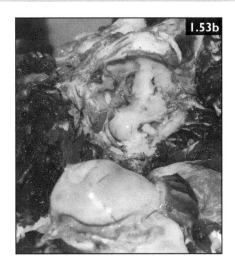

severity of the hip lesion is evident at necropsy (**1.53b**). Portable x-ray facilities are available in most large animal practices but are rarely used in cattle, mainly because of cost. However, the animal welfare implications of this case must be very carefully considered because this calf has been lame for 3 months without decisive action. Attempting to fatten the animal will not be successful because the animal is already poorly grown and spends much of its time lying down; isolation will reduce competition for feed but will not necessarily increase intake. While radiography may be seen as an unnecessary expense by the farmer, the veterinary surgeon's constant endeavour is the health and welfare of animals committed to his/her care, not the farm's profitability. No other calves were affected and the cause of the hip dysplasia was not determined.

CASE 1.54

1 Why would the farmer apply hobbles? Obturator nerve and sciatic nerve injuries (L6) result in adductor paresis in newly calved animals. Hip-lock during anterior presentation of the calf is the most common cause of adductor paresis. Severe abduction ('doing the splits') can also occur when the cow loses her footing on wet slippery surfaces. Hobbles are a crude but effective means of restricting abduction for a short period of time. Husbandry measures are also essential such as non-slip walking surfaces (**1.54b**, where the cow is bedded on deep straw), housing the animal in a small group to reduce competition at the feed bunk and milking at the end to prevent bullying.

2 Are the hobbles fitted correctly? Hobbles should be placed just above the cow's fetlock joints (**1.54b**) and checked regularly for skin abrasions. Inflatable cushions, webbing nets and swim tanks can all be used in the animal's rehabilitation, but the

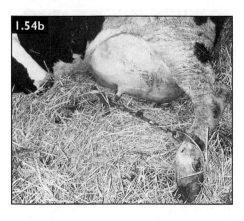

amount of time on busy commercial dairy farms is rarely adequate for such individual animal care.

3 How long should hobbles remain in place? Hobbles should only be necessary for 7–10 days and should not be left on for as long as 2 months, as was the case in this heifer.

4 How could the risk of this problem be reduced? Avoid excessive traction during calf delivery. Avoid sharp corners and wet slippery walking surfaces, especially for recently calved cows.

CASE 1.55

1 What conditions would you consider (most likely first)? Cerebral abscess; congenital abnormality such as hydanencephaly or hydrocephalus; polioencephalomalacia; vitamin A deficiency; lead poisoning; closantel toxicity.

2 What tests would you undertake? A provisional diagnosis of cerebral abscess is based on chronicity of the condition, insidious onset and lack of other clinical signs suggestive of particular toxicities. A lumbar CSF sample collected in the standing animal under local anaesthesia failed to reveal any abnormality; however, this is not an unusual finding in cerebral abscess cases and a normal sample should not rule out this possibility.

3 What treatment would you administer? The calf was treated daily with procaine penicillin for 3 weeks without improvement. The decision was taken to euthanase the calf due to the 3 months' duration of altered behaviour and failure

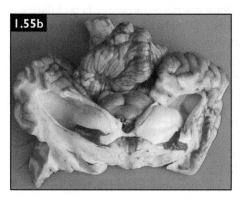

to respond to treatment; necropsy revealed hydrocephalus (**1.55b**). The cause of the hydrocephalus was not determined but clinical signs would probably have been present from birth (congenital lesion) and not been noted by the farmer. It is possible that the hydrocephalus resulted from a developmental lesion, but this could not be determined. No similar cases had occurred on this farm nor were there any in the following 3 years.

CASE 1.56

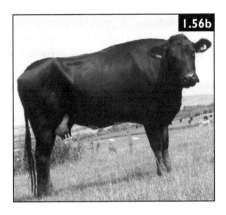

1 What conditions would you consider (most likely first)? Hypomagnesaemia; lead poisoning; urea/nitrate poisoning.

2 What treatment would you administer immediately? While unlicensed for use in cattle, 8 ml of 20% pentobarbitone sodium solution injected IV as a bolus controls seizure activity a great deal more effectively than either diazepam or xylazine. Within 30 seconds the seizure activity is controlled and 50 ml of 25% magnesium sulphate added to a bottle of 400 ml of 40% calcium borogluconate solution is given by slow IV injection over 10 minutes. The remaining 350 ml of the bottle of 25% magnesium sulphate solution is given SC in two divided sites immediately behind the shoulder. The cow was able to maintain sternal recumbency when pulled upright after all the treatments had been administered and walked off to find its calf after a further 20 minutes.

3 What samples would you collect to confirm your diagnosis? A serum sample for magnesium concentration was collected before treatment but was not analysed because of the good response (**1.56b**).

4 What control measures could be adopted for the rest of the herd? It is unusual to encounter hypomagnesaemia during the summer months (absence of stormy weather and no lush pasture). It is possible that bulling behaviour had interrupted grazing patterns and reduced feed intake over the previous 12–24 hours. General recommendations are to feed at-risk cattle up to 2 kg per head per day of high magnesium concentrates and good quality barley straw, but it unlikely cattle would eat these feeds when there is a good supply of grass. No management changes were adopted and no further cases occurred during the remainder of the grazing season. *Ad-libitum* minerals are often provided to cows at pasture but there is no convincing evidence that this measure prevents hypomagnesaemia.

CASE 1.57

1 What conditions would you consider (most likely first)? Infectious bovine keratoconjunctivitis (IBK); foreign body (e.g. grass awns) within the conjunctival sac; bovine iritis; infectious bovine rhinotracheitis. With IBK, spontaneous recovery starts in mild cases 3–5 days after clinical signs are first observed, and is complete 2 weeks later. In severe cases, ulceration may progress to corneal perforation and panophthalmitis but this is uncommon.

2 What treatment would you administer? Topical ophthalmic antibiotic cream containing cloxacillin is commonly used by farmers. Antibiotic injection (penicillin, oxytetracycline or ceftiofur) into the dorsal bulbar conjunctiva is the best treatment but can be difficult to achieve in fractious adult cattle and requires good restraint. Injection into the upper palpebral conjunctiva is commonly used, but it should be noted that this technique will not give residual antibiotic levels in the eye and relies on leakage onto the cornea from the injection site. This technique has no advantage over systemic injection, except for the much lower cost because of the smaller antibiotic dose. When subconjunctival or topical treatment is not practical, single dose long-acting oxytetracycline, florfenicol, tilmicosin or tulathromycin have all been reported to be effective.

Metaphylactic injection of all at-risk cattle with a single IM injection of long-acting oxytetracycline or tilmicosin could be considered in severe epidemics, but there are no supporting field data.

3 What action would you take? Outbreaks of IBK may occur after the introduction of purchased stock, therefore whenever possible, all new stock should be managed separately as one group away from the main herd. Fly control can be attempted using impregnated ear tags and pour-on insecticides, but these are often of short duration and repeated treatments can prove relatively expensive. Development of immunity following infection is variable and recurrence is common.

CASE 1.58

1 What conditions would you consider (most likely first)? Include: infectious bovine rhinotracheitis (IBR); pasteurellosis; recrudescence of chronic suppurative pneumonia.

2 How would you confirm your diagnosis? Ocular swabs (vigorous action to obtain cellular material) for a FAT and PCR for IBR. Paired serology would involve 2 weeks' delay but could be undertaken because the bull was from an IBR-accredited herd and had not been vaccinated.

3 What treatment(s) would you recommend? The farmer was advised to vaccinate all cattle immediately with an intranasal IBR vaccine. The bull was treated with procaine penicillin (44,000 IU/kg IM for 3 consecutive days) and was much improved the following day.

4 What control measures could be adopted for future years? IBR vaccination (and possibly BVD and leptospirosis vaccination) on arrival on the farm is very effective and introduced cattle should be quarantined for at least 2–4 weeks after arrival.

CASE 1.59

1 What conditions would you consider (most likely first)? Include: inhalation pneumonia; septic pericarditis; chronic suppurative respiratory disease exacerbated after calving; pleurisy; hepatocaval thrombosis; endocarditis.

2 What tests would you undertake? Real-time B-mode ultrasonographic examination of the right chest with a 5 MHz sector scanner reveals normal lung surface and no distension of the pericardium. On the left side there is normal lung in the dorsal third of the chest replaced ventrally by an extensive anechoic area containing multiple hyperechoic dots typical of a pleural abscess/pyothorax extending at least 12 cm from the chest wall. These sonographic findings, in addition to the tinkling/splashing sounds, are consistent with a diagnosis of unilateral inhalation/necrotising pneumonia progressing to pyothorax. The unilateral nature of the lesion, presumably because the cow was recumbent on that side, would explain how the cow was still alive.

3 What treatment would you recommend? The extensive nature of the pyothorax lesion (**1.59b**) and destruction of the left lung (**1.59c**) means that treatment would be ineffective and the cow was euthanased for welfare reasons. Drainage of the pyothorax could be attempted in addition to an extended treatment regime of penicillin (and metronidazole where licensed), but this would be a salvage procedure only and cannot be justified for welfare reasons.

4 How could this condition have been prevented? Prevention of the hypocalcaemia by calculating the dry cow ration based on dietary cation anion balance, together with prompt treatment, would have prevented this case occurring. Other causes of inhalation pneumonia include incorrect drenching technique, especially in hypocalcaemic cows with temporary loss of the swallow reflex.

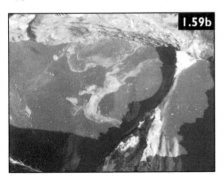

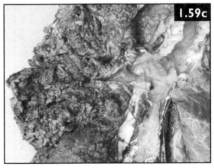

CASE 1.60

1 What conditions would cause weight loss and diarrhoea (most likely first)? Include: Johne's disease (*Mycobacterium avium var paratuberculosis;* MAP); chronic fasciolosis; chronic salmonellosis; chronic bacterial infection leading to debility.

2 What further tests could be undertaken? The ELISA test specificity is 97% but the sensitivity of this test is low until the latter stages of disease. If the clinical signs are suggestive of Johne's disease but the first sample proves negative, quarantine the animal and retest in 4–6 weeks. PCR testing of faeces is generally undertaken where serology is positive but the cow shows no clinical signs. Culture of MAP from faeces takes 4–6 weeks. At necropsy, acid-fast bacteria can be demonstrated both within the gut wall and ileocaecal lymph nodes in cattle with Johne's disease. Cattle with patent fasciolosis pass eggs in the faeces, although numbers may be low due to the host's immune reaction.

3 Why is the calf much smaller than other calves in the group? The calf suffered from chronic intrauterine growth retardation as a consequence of poor dam protein status caused by leakage across the diseased intestines (protein-losing enteropathy).

4 What is the prognosis for the calf? The calf is highly likely to have already been infected with MAP from transplacental infection, via contaminated colostrum and milk, and a highly contaminated environment considering the dam is in the advanced clinical stage of disease and has profuse diarrhoea. While the incubation period for clinical disease is typically 4–5 years, clinical disease leading to emaciation is not uncommon in cattle as young as 15–18 months (**1.60b**). It is generally assumed that such early mainfestation of clinical signs is a consequence of massive challenge,

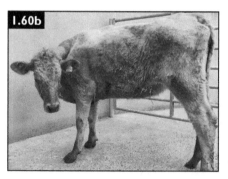

usually from a dam in the agonal stage of disease (this case). Against veterinary advice, the farmer fostered this calf onto another cow whose calf had died. This action will simply lead to environmental contamination and greater risk of disease dissemination and the possibility that the animal will succumb to clinical disease before reaching slaughter weight at 15–18 months.

CASE 1.61

1 What is your diagnosis? LDA. The LDA occupies the craniodorsal area of the left side of the abdominal cavity where auscultation and succussion reveal high-pitched 'tinkling' sounds. There is also evidence of (secondary) ketosis.

2 What other conditions could cause tympany in this area? Rumen void, which refers to the gap caused by the shrunken rumen falling away from the left abdominal wall; gas cap in the rumen associated with ruminal atony, acidosis, grain overload, etc.; pneumoperitoneum is rare.

3 What action would you take? There are numerous treatment options:

- Rolling the cow to correct the LDA has been practised but requires three people, is as time consuming (therefore as costly) as surgery, and less than 40% successful.
- A Grymer/Sterner blind toggle suture is not without risk if the operator is inexperienced in this technique.
- Corrective surgery is best performed in the standing cow under distal paravertebral analgesia. A right laparotomy incision is made and the abomasum deflated using a 14 gauge needle connected to a flutter valve. On release of gas, the abomasum slowly sinks towards the ventral midline, pulled by its liquid contents. The greater omentum is grasped by the surgeon's right hand and carefully pulled around to the ventral margin of the right laparotomy incision. An omentopexy (**1.61b**) or pyloropexy is performed whereby a continuous suture taking four 4–5 cm bites of omentum or pylorus is continued to close the peritoneum and internal oblique muscle layer. The laparotomy wound is closed routinely.

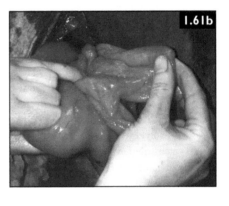

4 What treatment(s) would you administer? Treatment for the secondary acetonaemia comprises an IM injection of dexamethasone and 400 ml of 50% dextrose administered IV. Propylene glycol can be administered orally.

CASE 1.62

1 What conditions would you consider? Lice (pediculosis); forage mites; sarcoptic mange; chorioptic mange; bovine besnoitiosis, a vector-transmitted disease caused by the protozoan parasite *Besnoitia besnoiti*, is not present in the UK.

2 What further tests could be undertaken? Inspection of the skin reveals extensive louse infestation. Microscopic examination of skin scrapings reveal numerous chewing (round mouthparts; *Damalinia bovis*) and sucking lice (narrow and more pointed mouthparts; *Linognathus vituli.*).

3 What actions/treatments would you recommend? Treatment options include pour-on pyrethroid (e.g. cypermethrin) compounds that effect rapid improvement but may require repeat treatment in 2–4 weeks. All in-contact cattle must be treated. Injectable group 3 anthelmintics (macrocyclic lactones, including avermectins and milbemycins) are not always wholly effective against chewing lice and pour-on formulations should be used; however, this is an expensive option because anthelmintic treatment is not necessary. Furthermore, use of a group 3 anthelmintic may increase the selection pressure for resistant parasite strains, including gastrointestinal parasites.

Pediculosis is widespread in all beef herds and routine treatment is recommended at housing. Interestingly, bulls are invariably more severely affected than cows.

4 Are there any consequences of this problem? Disruption to grazing/feeding may cause reduced liveweight gain/loss of body condition in severe infestations, although very heavy burdens are more often a consequence rather than the cause of debility. Anaemia as a consequence of severe louse infestations is rare.

CASE 1.63

1 Describe the sonogram. There is a well-encapsulated 2 cm diameter abscess immediately beneath the capsule with adherent small intestine wall. There are five more 3–8 cm diameter abscesses detected throughout the liver (not shown).

2 What conditions would you consider (most likely first)? Include: liver abscessation; liver abscessation and localised adhesions involving small intestine.

3 What treatment would you recommend? The liver abscesses appear well-encapsulated and are not sufficient in size or number to cause a significant effect, although it is not possible to examine all of the liver, particularly where

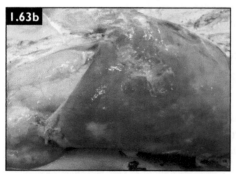

it is in contact with the diaphragm. Continue the course of penicillin for a further 10 days.

The cow failed to improve despite treatment and was culled. Necropsy revealed focal peritonitis with adhesions between the liver capsule and small intestine (**1.63b**), where there is considerable fibrin deposition on the liver surface.

CASE 1.64

1 What conditions would you consider (most likely first)? Lungworm (*Dictyocaulus viviparus*) challenge; fog fever; IBR; BRSV; influenza A; bluetongue.

2 What laboratory tests could be undertaken to confirm your provisional diagnosis? Larval challenge in susceptible adult cattle results in clinical signs typical of lungworm infection, but the challenge may not yet be patent (Baermann technique – negative).

3 What treatment would you administer? Remove cattle from the contaminated pastures. Prompt anthelmintic treatment is essential. Some cattle may have a protracted convalescence.

4 What control measures would you recommend? Vaccination of calves before their first grazing season confers life-long immunity in most situations unless severely challenged as adults. Avoid grazing cattle on potentially heavily contaminated pastures. Alternate annual grazing with sheep where possible.

CASE 1.65

1 What conditions would you consider (most likely first)? Malignant catarrhal fever (MCF); mucosal disease; severe IBR; listerial iritis; bluetongue; foot and mouth disease.

2 How could you confirm your suspicions? Diagnosis is based on clinical signs and confirmed by demonstration of MCF virus by PCR, antibodies in serum and/or characteristic postmortem findings. Only one animal affected in the group would exclude many diseases (e.g. IBR, bluetongue and foot and mouth disease).

3 What treatment would you administer? There is no treatment for MCF and affected cattle must be euthanased immediately for welfare reasons. High doses of corticosteroids given systemically may give temporary improvement of clinical signs in a small number of mild cases, but these recovered cattle never thrive.

4 List any preventive/control measures. MCF is caused by ovine herpesvirus-2. Contact with periparturient sheep or goats appears necessary for transmission to cattle and deer, although several months may elapse between such contact and overt disease (2 months in this case). A sheep flock may have a high seroprevalence but the method of transmission to cattle remains unknown. Cattle do not transmit MCF. Control relies on avoiding contact with sheep, but such management is not possible on most mixed stock farms.

CASE 1.66

1 **What conditions would you consider?** Bacterial meningoencephalitis; septicaemia.
2 **How could you confirm your diagnosis?** Diagnosis of meningoencephalitis follows lumbar CSF collection under local anaesthesia using a 20 gauge 1 inch hypodermic needle. Samples are usually collected with the calf positioned in sternal recumbency, but can easily be collected when the calf is in lateral recumbency (this case). The collected sample is turbid, caused by the influx of

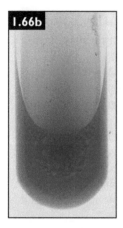

white cells, and has a frothy appearance visible after sample agitation due to the increased protein concentration (**1.66b**). Laboratory analysis reveals a total protein concentration of 1.9 g/l (19 mg/dl) (normal <0.3 g/l [3 mg/dl] with a white cell concentration of 1.9×10^9/l (1,900/µl) (normal <0.012 $\times 10^9$/l [120/µl]) comprised almost entirely of neutrophils (neutrophilic pleocytosis). The total plasma protein of 49 g/l (4.9 g/dl) indicates failure of passive antibody transfer (normal value for beef calves that have sucked colostrum; should be >60–65 g/l [6.0–6.5 g/dl] after 24 hours but values >55 g/l [5.5 g/dl] are often quoted).
3 **What is the likely cause?** *Escherichia coli* is the most common isolate from septicaemic calves but *Pasteurella* spp., *Staphylococcus pyogenes* and *Trueperella pyogenes* have been isolated from clinical cases of meningoencephalitis.
4 **What treatment(s) would you administer?** The calf was treated with IV marbofloxacin and soluble corticosteroid (dexamethasone, 1.0 mg/kg) but failed to improve and was euthansed for welfare reasons 6 hours later.
5 **What recommendations would you offer?** This condition arose due to failure of antibody transfer plus a contaminated calving pen. The calving was assisted late at night and the calf unsupervised until morning. In this situation either the farmer milks colostrum from the cow immediately or uses stored frozen then thawed colostrum from another cow (3-2-1: 3 litres, first 2 hours of life, first milk).

CASE 1.67

1 **How could effective analgesia be achieved?** The calf is injected with flunixin meglumine or other NSAID IV. Effective analgesia after lumbosacral extradural injection of 3 mg/kg of 2% lidocaine solution allows a detailed and pain-free clinical examination of hind leg joint lesions and fractures, and presents a cheap and readily available alternative to general anaesthesia. Injectable general anaesthetic drugs such as alphaxalane or propofol may be considered prohibitively expensive. Administration of xylazine (0.1 mg/kg IM) followed by administration of ketamine (2–3 mg/kg IV) is commonly used in practice.

2 What action would you take? Reduce the fracture under extradural block and apply a fibreglass cast.

3 What is the likely prognosis? The prognosis for metatarsal fracture is generally good. The cast was removed after 5 weeks when the fracture had healed well and the calf was not lame.

CASE 1.68

1 What conditions would you consider (most likely first)? Squamous cell carcinoma of the nasal cavity; ethmoid carcinoma; nasal lymphosarcoma; nasal osteosarcoma; osteomyelitis of the hard palate; advanced erosive fungal sinusitis.

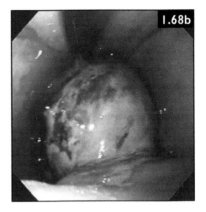

2 What further tests could be undertaken? Rhinoscopy reveals a large >5 cm mass occupying the ventral meatus (**1.68b**).

3 What action would you take? There is no evidence of metastasis to the drainage submandibular lymph nodes and squamous cell carcinomas do not usually spread beyond the local drainage lymph nodes. Immediate slaughter for human consumption is the best course of action in this case. Surgical removal is possible but unrealistic and not in the animal's best interest.

CASE 1.69

1 What conditions would you consider (most likely first)? Necrotic enteritis; mucosal disease; salmonellosis; coccidiosis.

2 How could you confirm your suspicions? Diagnosis is based on exclusion of other diseases and confirmed at necropsy, as the prognosis is grave. Mucosal disease is possible but unlikely in such a young calf. Coccidiosis, caused by *Eimeria alabamensis*, is usually a group problem. Typical, although non-diagnostic, haematological findings in this disease are anaemia (variable in its severity) and leucopenia caused by a severe non-regenerative neutropenia. Many affected calves have high blood urea concentrations associated with kidney pathology.

3 What necropsy findings would confirm your suspicions? Ulcers often overlain by necrotic debris and secondary fungal infection may occur in the larynx, rumen, abomasum and small and large intestines, extending as far as the rectum. The ulcerative lesions vary from small discrete punctate lesions to large linear diphtheritic plaques overlying Peyer's patches (**1.69b**). The ulcers may be full thickness, leading to areas

113

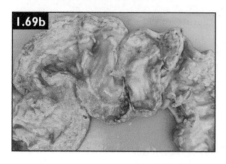

of localised peritonitis on the serosal surface with adhesions to adjacent gut. The kidneys often appear swollen and pale with infarcts. Inhalation pneumonia is often seen in association with severe pharyngeal and laryngeal diphtheresis.

4 List any preventive/control measures. As the cause remains unknown, there are no specific control measures.

CASE 1.70

1 Describe the sonogram. There is evidence of the right kidney, extending from the abdominal wall for 2–3 cm only, containing several small anechoic areas, possibly part of the renal pelvis, but this structure is poorly defined. Distal to this structure is a 5–6 cm diameter, well-encapsulated uniform mass.

2 What could this structure represent? Nephroblastoma; perirenal abscess.

3 What action would you take? No other reason for poor growth in this calf was

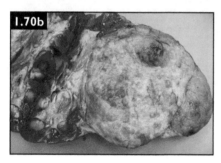

found on clinical examination. The calf was too small to attempt to palpate/image the left kidney per rectum. Due to the poor prognosis the calf was euthanased for welfare reasons and the diagnosis of nephroblastoma confirmed at necropsy (**1.70b**). The left kidney was normal; it was not possible to explain why the nephroblastoma caused poor growth or whether it was simply a coincidental finding.

CASE 1.71

1 What conditions would you consider? Osteochondrosis is caused by abnormal differentiation of cells in growing cartilage and can progress to osteochondritis dissecans, with impaired vascularisation of articular cartilage leading to necrosis and fragmentation of cartilage. Some degree of joint effusion of the hock joint is very common in many beef bulls. It may be due to a mild osteochondrosis lesion that never progresses to osteochondritis dissecans and thus causes little or no lameness.

2 Is this bull fit for sale as a breeding bull? Diagnosis of osteochondritis dissecans is based on the presence of considerable joint effusion in association with chronic mild to moderate lameness. Radiography may confirm the presence of calcified flaps free within the joint ('joint mice'), but such identification is not easy. Diagnosis is confirmed at necropsy in bulls that remain so lame as to prevent natural service (**1.71b**).

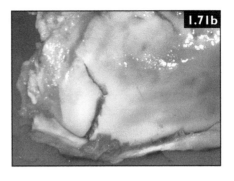

3 How could this problem be reduced/prevented? Less emphasis should be placed on achieving maximum growth rate to sale in beef bulls, but this parameter features highly in estimated breeding values. Start breeding when the bull is fully mature at around 2 years old.

CASE 1.72

1 What are the important sonographic features seen in the sonogram? There is a thick-walled (1–1.5 cm) umbilical abscess (anechoic area containing multiple hyperechoic dots), extending to 4 cm diameter, to the right of the sonogram. In the centre there is a poorly defined 4 cm diameter anaechoic area containing fine hyperechoic lines. This area represents localised accumulation of peritoneal fluid with fibrin tags (exudate), consistent with localised peritonitis. Normal intestine is visible distal to this accumulation of exudate and to the left side of the image. The ultrasound findings are suggestive of a focal peritonitis associated with an umbilical abscess.

2 What action would you take? The cause of the abscess and associated peritonitis was thought to be *Trueperella pyogenes*, but no samples were taken for culture. The calf was treated with a 14-day course of daily penicillin injections (time-dependent action) and made an uneventful recovery. Amoxycillin/clavulanic acid combination could also have been used but is considerably more expensive. The abscess was not lanced at the initial veterinary visit because of its thick wall and adjacent, and possibly adherent, intestine. Furthermore, the well-encapsulated abscess was considered to be much less significant than the peritonitis. The good response to antibiotic therapy was surprising because peritonitis lesions from umbilical infections in young calves can form adhesions between loops of intestines, blocking flow of digesta (**1.72b**) and leading

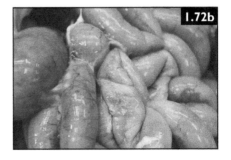

to severe consequences of collapse, toxaemia and death. The diagnosis of focal fibrinous peritonitis was based on the ultrasound examination; had this scanning not be undertaken then the full extent of the problem would not have been identified. The examination took less than 5 minutes, but allowed a more accurate diagnosis.

CASE 1.73

1 What conditions would you consider (most likely first)? Include: type I ostertagiosis; copper deficiency; poor pasture management; transient BVDV infection (persistently infected animal added to naïve group).

2 What further tests could be undertaken? Modified McMaster technique for strongyle eggs. Either count 4–6 individual samples or pool together. Examination revealed individual counts from 800 to 1,400 strongyle eggs per gram of faeces in four animals. Low serum copper concentrations samples from 4–6 calves would indicate depletion of liver copper reserves – normal values were recorded in this investigation.

3 What treatment(s) should be administered? Treatment with an injectable avermectin anthelmintic effected a good response (cessation of diarrhoea within a few days) and provided protection against reinfestation for the remainder of the summer grazing period (cattle housed 3 weeks later).

4 Could this problem(s) be prevented next year? Parasitic gastroenteritis control on contaminated pasture requires strategic anthelmintic treatment including intraruminal pulse release boluses (benzimidazole every 3 weeks), ivermectin injections 3, 8 and 13 weeks after turnout, doramectin injections at turnout and 8 weeks later, or doramectin slow release injection at turnout. Where there is a known risk, lungworm is best prevented by vaccination 2 and 6 weeks before exposure.

CASE 1.74

1 What are the potential benefits and risks?
Benefits:
- Much reduced environmental pathogen challenge, provided good weather and a sufficiently large field, which should reduce cryptosporidiosis problem but requires good handling facilities nearby.
- Easier to identify first stage labour – cow isolates herself from the group.
- Reduced bedding and medicine costs.

Risks:
- Time-consuming to check all cows in a large field, especially during the 9–10 hours of darkness.
- May prove difficult to attend to calving problems and get cow into handling facilities, especially at night.

- May prove difficult to treat the calf's umbilicus soon after birth, although far fewer problems are encountered when calving outdoors.
- May encounter problems with catching and tagging calves, especially if aggressive dam.
- Hypothermia of newborn calves during severe weather.

CASE 1.75

1 Describe the abnormal radiographic findings. There is a fracture of P1.

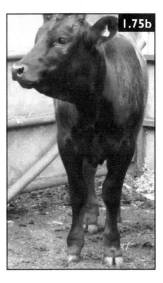

2 What action should be taken? The calf was sedated with xylazine and short duration general anaesthesia induced with 3 mg/kg ketamine IV. The fracture was reduced by realigning the lateral deviation of the distal leg (see **1.75a**) and a fibreglass cast applied. The calf was sound after a few days and the cast removed after 1 month. The calf made an uneventful recovery and is shown 6 months later (**1.75b**). Fracture of P1 presumably resulted from torsional forces applied to the sole remaining digit of that foot. This author has seen only one other case of P1 fracture following digit amputation in the same foot in 37 years of farm animal practice.

Other causes of lameness after digit amputation include cellulitis involving the incision site and osteomyelitis of the P1 stump.

CASE 1.76

1 What conditions would cause such weight loss and diarrhoea (most likely first)? Include: Johne's disease (*Mycobacterium avium paratuberculosis*; MAP); chronic salmonellosis; chronic bacterial infection leading to debility/amyloidosis.

2 What further tests could be undertaken? The cow tested positive on ELISA for paratuberculosis. The ELISA test specificity is 97%, but the sensitivity of this test is low until the latter stages of disease. If the clinical signs are suggestive of Johne's disease but the first sample proves negative, quarantine the animal and retest in 4–6 weeks. PCR testing of faeces is generally undertaken where serology is positive but the cow shows no clinical signs. Culture of MAP from faeces takes 4–6 weeks. At necropsy, acid-fast bacteria can be demonstrated both within the corrugated small intestine (**1.76b**, left side; normal gut on right side) and ileocaecal lymph nodes in cattle with Johne's disease.

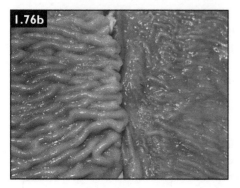

3 **What control measures could be adopted?** A test and cull policy could be adopted after a whole herd screen to determine the true prevalence of paratuberculosis. If the seroprevalence is high, then whole herd slaughter and restocking may be the most cost-effective programme, but few beef farmers are able to embark on such a strategy. There are no guidelines for a whole herd culling policy but a seroprevalence of >15–20% would warrant serious consideration. There are several problems with the test and cull policy, not least the cost of annual testing, but also the low test sensitivity and less than 100% specificity (see above).

Vaccination against Johne's disease prevents overt disease but is not an option for many beef farmers because replacement heifers are typically bought as either yearlings or in-calf heifers, while vaccination has to be undertaken within the first 2 weeks of life. Disadvantages of a vaccination policy include a granulomatous reaction at the injection site, cost, interference with the comparative intradermal tuberculin test and trade/export restrictions.

CASE 1.77

1 **What conditions would you consider (most likely first)?** Proximal duodenal obstruction; retroflexed caecum; intestinal torsion; peritonitis; intussusception.

2 **What further tests would you undertake?** Ultrasonography provides immediate results of the peritoneum and viscera to the depth of 20 cm from the abdominal wall for most 5 MHz sector scanners (10 cm for 5 MHz linear scanners). Particular attention should be paid to fluid distension (>5–7 cm) of lengths of intestines, with reduced peristalsis suggestive of an obstruction. This fluid also appears more uniformly anechoic rather than containing multiple hyperechoic dots typical of normal digesta.

Abdominocentesis should be guided by ultrasound findings. Demonstration of an inflammatory exudate with a high protein concentration and an increased white cell count with predominance of leucocytes is indicative of peritonitis. However, peritonitis localised by the omentum is not a simple diagnosis because infection can be contained within the omentum and therefore cannot always be sampled by abdominocentesis.

3 **What action would you take?** In this case, fluid-filled intestines (duodenum) were identified ultrasonographically in the lower right cranial quadrant, suggestive of a duodenal obstruction. At surgery a thin 'thread-like' taut fibrinous band was

found on the serosal surface, constricting the duodenum. As this constriction was at arm's length from the right flank laparotomy site, it was snapped between the surgeon's fingers. The bull made a full recovery. The cause of the constricting fibrinous band was not identified.

CASE 1.78

1 What conditions would you consider (most likely first)? Hepatocaval thrombosis; chronic suppurative pulmonary disease; nasal tumour; sinusitis; endocarditis.

2 How can you confirm your provisional diagnosis? Epistaxis is considered to be the cardinal clinical sign of advanced hepatocaval thrombosis. Diagnosis of hepatocaval thrombosis is very difficult and is often based on exclusion of more common/likely conditions. Ultrasonographic demonstration of a thrombus present in the caudal vena cava can be achieved in some cases, but such examination is rarely undertaken in general practice. Ultrasonographic examination of the chest would rule out chronic suppurative pneumonia. Bacteraemic spread from the thrombus often forms foci deep within the lung parenchyma, which do not involve the visceral pleura and therefore cannot be imaged. Endocarditis cases often have an increased and irregular heart rate (>100 beats per minute) but normal heart sounds without an audible murmur.

3 What treatment would you administer? Once arterial bleeding occurs there is damage to the wall of a major blood vessel, which cannot be repaired. Theoretically, procaine penicillin injected daily for at least 6 weeks may overcome the bacteraemia, but will not remove the massive thrombus within the vena cava such that further bacterial shedding is likely.

4 What action would you recommend? Emergency slaughter on farm is likely to be ill-advised because the cow is in poor condition and there is likely to be foci in the liver, lungs and kidneys, which may result in carcass condemnation. Necropsy findings typically include chronic venous congestion leading to hepatomegaly and a 'nutmeg appearance'. The cow should not be transported to a slaughter plant because it may bleed out at any time. The best action is to shoot the animal for welfare reasons. At necropsy, liver abscesses are common adjacent to the vena cava and extending into the lumen (**1.78b**), seeding the lungs and other organs.

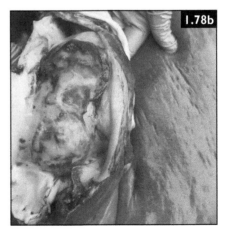

1.78b

CASE 1.79

1 What conditions would you consider (most likely first)? Pedal bone fracture extending to involve the articular surface. Careful examination of the foot has eliminated other more common causes of lameness including white line abscess.

2 What action would you take? A wooden block applied to the sound claw relieves lameness and the prognosis is very good where the fracture does not involve the articular surface. However, the prognosis in this bull is guarded. Unfortunately, no follow up is available for this bull.

CASE 1.80

1 Describe the important features of the sonogram obtained at the sixth intercostal space using a 5 MHz sector scanner (1.80a). Ultrasound examination reveals purulent material (5–6 cm anechoic area with multiple hyperechoic dots) distending the pericardial sac. There is fibrin deposition on the epicardium (broad irregular hyperechoic band) and oedema of the myocardium (narrow anechoic band underlying the fibrin deposits). These findings are consistent with a diagnosis of septic pericarditis (1.80b).

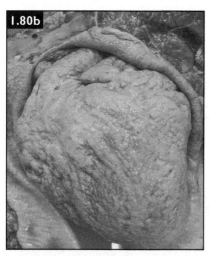

2 What treatment would you administer? There is no effective treatment and the cow should be euthanased immediately for welfare reasons. While 'pericardial strips' have been described, it is clear from the necropsy image that removing the pericardium will not be successful due to the large amounts of fibrin deposited on the epicardium. Such surgery is rarely, if ever, justified.

3 Could this situation have been prevented? Septic pericarditis occurs in some cases of traumatic reticulitis following penetration of the pericardial sac by a sharp metal object. Prompt detection of traumatic reticulitis cases would permit removal of the wire, but sometimes the wire passes through to the pericardium very quickly, as evidenced by the lack of significant peritoneal reaction. Routine administration of magnets to lodge within the reticulum is practised in herds with a history of 'hardware disease' to attract and bind ingested metal objects.

CASE 1.81

1 Describe the important sonographic findings. Transabdominal ultrasonographic examination reveals fluid distension of loops of the caecum (estimated to be approximately 20 cm in diameter), with large amounts of fibrin on the serosal surfaces. The caecal wall appears oedematous.

2 What further tests might you undertake? Ultrasound-guided abdominocentesis could be undertaken but the peritoneal fluid is an inflammatory exudate, as evidenced by the large amounts of fibrin.

3 What action would you take? There is severe localised peritonitis involving the wall of the caecum, with fibrinous adhesions between adjacent loops. The prognosis is hopeless and the cow was euthanased immediately. Necropsy confirmed the severe localised fibrinous peritonitis (**1.81b**).

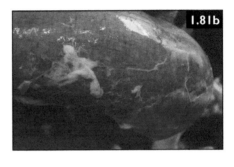

4 Comment on the value of an exploratory laparotomy in this case. There was no indication for an exploratory laparotomy in this case because transabdominal ultrasonography had clearly indicated the severity of the fibrinous peritonitis (see **1.81a**). The cost and, more importantly, the unnecessary surgery cannot be justified in this case. A more thorough investigative approach obviates the need for 'heroic' last ditch exploratory surgery, which is rarely, if ever, successful.

CASE 1.82

1 What conditions you would consider (most likely first)? Septic pericarditis; dilated cardiomyopathy; pleural effusion associated with either thymic lymphosarcoma or end-stage farmer's lung.

Ultrasonography revealed massive distension of the pericardial sac extending half way up the chest wall on both sides and containing fibrinous exudate.

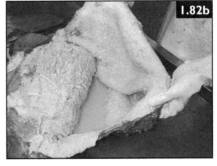

2 What treatment would you recommend? There is no effective treatment and the cow was euthanased for welfare reasons. The extent of the pathology was revealed at necropsy (**1.82b**).

3 What recommendations would you make? Attention to storage of car tyres used on top of silage sheets. Use of prophylactic magnets in the cow's reticulum. Bonfire sites can be a source of sharp metallic objects.

Septic pericarditis is a common sequela to traumatic reticuloperitonitis. While surgery to remove sharp metallic objects from the reticulum was common in veterinary practice 30 years ago, these cases are no longer detected at an early stage and have progressed to septic pericarditis before veterinary attention is requested on farm. As a consequence, septic pericarditis is a common cause of culling/ fatality on both beef and dairy farms. One explanation may be that farmers delay requesting veterinary attention until the next routine visit (often every 1–2 weeks). Some large farms have standard operating procedures with respect to treatments for various clinical presentations; this further delays veterinary examination and surgery to remove the wire while it is still within the reticular wall. Traumatic reticuloperitonitis is one of the few conditions that results in a dramatic reduction in milk yield and appetite; farmers must present such cases that day and not delay, otherwise the consequences are usually fatal.

CASE 1.83

1 What conditions would you consider (most likely first)? Localised peritonitis; endocarditis; pleurisy; recrudescence of chronic suppurative pulmonary disease; liver abscessation.

2 What furthers tests would you undertake? Diagnosis of localised peritonitis can be made following abdominocentesis and demonstration of an inflammatory exudate with a high protein concentration and an increased white cell count with a predominance of leucocytes. However, localised peritonitis is not a simple diagnosis because infection can be contained within the omentum and therefore cannot always be identified by abdominocentesis. In addition, the needle point may enter fibrin deposited on serosal surfaces in many cases. A positive belly tap

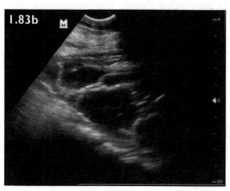

result is diagnostic, but remember the limitations if no sample or indeed a normal transudate is obtained.

Transabdominal ultrasonography provides immediate results of the peritoneum and viscera to the depth of 20 cm for most 5 MHz sector scanners and is most useful for examination of the anterior abdomen. An inflammatory exudate with extensive fibrin tags is shown (**1.83b**) in the right cranial abdomen and therefore probably involves the abomasum rather than the reticulum. Five MHz linear scanners are also extremely useful – do not be distracted by their 10 cm range, as 7 cm of exudate is significant (3 cm depth of body wall). Once again, be aware of omental bursitis, which cannot be identified by transabdominal ultrasonography because the infection is enveloped by the omentum and cannot be imaged.

3 What treatment would you administer? Parenteral antibiotic therapy is hopeless in all but very localised cases of peritonitis and is often undertaken in those situations where there has been only limited investigation with the expectation that the animal is suffering from another infectious disease.

4 What action would you take? Because antibiotic therapy is rarely successful in diffuse peritonitis cases, the animal should be euthanased for welfare reasons.

CASE 1.84

1 What conditions would you consider (most likely first)? Primary photosensitisation and dermatophilosis.

2 What are the possible causes? Primary photosensitisation occurs when preformed photodynamic agents are absorbed from the gut. Hepatogenous (secondary) photosensitisation results from liver disease and the inability to excrete phylloerythrin, a metabolite of chlorophyll. Liver disease and secondary photosensitisation can be caused by the ingestion of mouldy feed containing aflatoxins and from chronic liver fluke infection (there was no history of liver fluke on this farm and faecal sedimentation results were negative).

3 What advice would you offer? The cow should be housed to protect it from direct sunlight. Systemic corticosteroids may be indicated in the acute erythematous stage of photosensitisation to prevent extensive inflammation and necrosis, but this stage had long passed and the cow was 6 months pregnant (risk of abortion). Topical emollients and antibiotics may help soften and protect the skin but are not commonly used.

CASE 1.85

1 List four important observations. (1) The cow has an arched back consistent with severe lameness. (2) The cow has an extreme plantigrade stance of both hind feet (right hind foot more obvious with the accessory claws almost touching the ground). There is considerable swelling around the right hind fetlock joint. (3) The cow is in very poor body condition (BCS <1.5/5). (4) The cow has poor abdominal fill due to poor appetite.

2 What conditions would you consider (most likely first)? Prior sciatic nerve damage; 'wear and tear' coupled with neglect of the cow's welfare; deep digital flexor tendon rupture (but the toe is in contact with the ground).

3 What other tests could you employ? Detailed radiographic and ultrasonographic examinations are unnecessary because this cow must be culled for welfare reasons irrespective of further findings.

4 What treatment would you administer? Analgesics may afford some very temporary reduction in lameness (3–5 days), but this cow's stance and gait will not be improved with analgesics.

5 What action would you take? It can prove difficult to determine whether such cattle are fit to be transported to a slaughterhouse; the best plan is that the cow is slaughtered on farm, but this will not happen because of loss of cull slaughter value.

CASE 1.86

1 Describe the sonogram and the likely cause. There is a large >13 cm diameter abscess extending from the chest wall. The lesion could be present within the pleural space (more likely) or within the lung.

2 What treatment(s) would you administer? *Trueperella pyogenes* is most commonly isolated from lung abscesses/bronchiectasis lesions. An effective treatment is procaine penicillin (22,000 IU/kg IM daily for up to 6 weeks). Procaine penicillin is inexpensive. Marbofloxacin is indicated for acute respiratory disease, typically involving *Pateurella* spp.

3 What changes would you expect with successful treatment? The response rate for chronic suppurative pulmonary disease is about 50% depending on severity (extent of pathology determined ultrasonographically) and interval to effective treatment, taking into account delays caused by previous (ineffective) treatments. There are no published detailed studies on the treatment of pleural/lung abscesses. This heifer was rescanned at the end of the treatment course when the lesion was

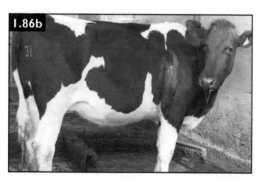

reduced to <9 cm diameter. The heifer was much brighter (**1.86b**) and the daily milk yield had increased to 24 litres/day. While drainage and lavage of large pleural abscesses has been described in horses, with a good response, such a treatment protocol would be cost-prohibitive in cattle and several previous attempts by this author have proven unsuccessful. It is possible that antibiotic therapy treated other pyogenic foci and not just the pleural/lung abscess visualised, because antibiotic therapy alone would not be expected to reduce the size of a well-encapsulated abscess. Several other similar cases have responded well but further studies are necessary before any conclusions can be drawn from a small number of cases, but this treatment response is encouraging.

CASE 1.87

1 What conditions would you consider (most likely first)? Pregnancy toxaemia; severe chronic fasciolosis; metritis; hypocalcaemia.

Pregnancy toxaemia can occur during the last month of gestation in cows carrying twin calves fed a very low energy diet such as straw without supplementary feeding. This situation can occur in beef cows under severe drought/starvation conditions. Occasionally, fatty liver disease/pregnancy toxaemia results when farmers elect to drastically reduce feeding to over-conditioned pregnant beef cows after several dystocia cases in the group, mistakenly believing this regimen will reduce calving difficulties in the remainder; such abrupt energy reduction/starvation occurred in this case.

2 What tests would you undertake? Elevated serum ketone bodies (3-OH butyrate) and low plasma glucose concentrations support the clinical diagnosis. Markedly increased serum concentrations of liver enzymes, such as GLDH and GGT, and hypoalbuminaemia would reflect significant liver damage. Transabdominal ultrasound examination would reveal hepatomegaly (extending well beyond the costal arch). Further interpretation of liver ultrasound appearance is difficult because severe fatty change simply results in loss of normal liver architecture and can be difficult to differentiate from poor image quality.

3 What treatments would you administer? Recumbent cattle with pregnancy toxaemia (this case) should be destroyed for welfare reasons because the liver damage is so severe that recovery is not possible (**1.87b**). Less severely affected cattle could be treated symptomatically with oral fluids containing propylene glycol, IV multivitamin preparations, IV glucose, dexamethasone and antibiotics to treat septic metritis.

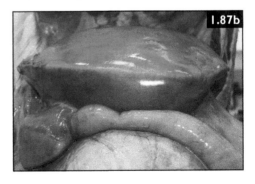

4 What control measures would you recommend? Provide adequate dietary energy (60–80 MJ/day) during late gestation with an extra 20 MJ/day for twin-bearing cows and those in low body condition. Regular condition scoring of cows will detect weight loss. Ultrasound scanning during early pregnancy (weeks 5–14 after bull removed in a 9-week breeding season) identifies twin pregnancies, allowing grouping of these cows and correct nutrition.

CASE 1.88

1 What is the likely cause of such mortality? An 8–11% pre-weaning mortality rate has been quoted in several published surveys undertaken in the UK and the USA. The most likely cause of death is septicaemia and bacteraemic conditions, such as meningitis and polyarthritis, resulting from failure of passive antibody transfer. Umbilical infection leading to peritonitis is also a possible contributing factor. Losses due to septicaemia usually occur within the first 3–5 days; diarrhoea is an agonal finding.

2 How would you investigate this problem? Several methods can be used to determine passive antibody transfer; collection of plasma samples and measure of total protein concentration using a refractometer is by far the cheapest and allows a meaningful number of calves to be sampled as part of ongoing monitoring. Failure of passive transfer has been defined as a <10 g/l (1 g/dl) increase in total plasma protein after 24–48 hours. Typically, a concentration of 40–45 g/l (4.0–4.5 g/dl) at birth increasing to >55 g/l (5.5 g/dl) by 24 hours after ingestion indicates adequate colostrum ingestion. Necropsy of septicaemic calves may reveal only widespread petechial haemorrhages on serosal surfaces. A lumbar CSF tap is the best method to confirm meningitis, otherwise histopathology is required, as the gross appearance of congested blood vessels covering the brain is difficult to interpret.

3 What simple practical recommendations would you make? In simple practical terms, all calves must receive 3 litres of colostrum (first milking) within 2 hours of birth. Calves born within a large communal area may not find their dam and removal from the cow at birth to an individual pen and feeding colostrum by oesophageal feeder is the better option in a busy farm situation. There is debate whether a bottle and teat results in more effective antibody transfer, but this is overcome by feeding 3 litres. Feeding this volume also overcomes the problem of varying immunoglobulin concentrations in colostrum; estimating specific gravity using a 'colostrometer' can be helpful but is not essential. Feeding pooled colostrum depends on the herd paratuberculosis status because of the transmission risk for this disease, which is reaching endemic proportions in the UK and other countries. This potential problem can be overcome by installing a pasteurisation facility on the farm. The umbilicus of all calves should be immersed in strong veterinary iodine as soon as possible after birth of the calf.

CASE 1.89

1 What conditions would you consider (most likely first)? Puerperal metritis; toxic mastitis; salmonellosis; grain overload; concurrent LDA.

Puerperal metritis commonly affects cows after unhygienic manual interference to correct fetal malpresentation/malposture, after delivery of twins or a dead calf, and following infectious causes of abortion. In most of these situations, there is retention of some, or all, of the fetal membranes. Cows suffering hypocalcaemia during second stage labour have an increased incidence of retained fetal membranes and metritis. Bacterial entry and multiplication within the uterus produces toxins that are absorbed across the damaged endometrium. The likelihood of metritis increases in proportion to the duration of manual intervention in dystocia cases. The provisional diagnosis is based on history, clinical findings and elimination of other common diseases. Vaginal examination often stimulates discomfort and vigorous straining, and reveals copious amounts of red–brown foetid fluid.

2 What treatments would you administer? IV oxytetracycline and flunixin meglumine or a similar NSAID with IM oxytetracycline for the following 2–4 days. In toxic cows, rapid IV infusion of 3 litres of 7.2% hypertonic saline is indicated, with clean drinking water readily available. Thirty to 60 litres of warm water containing a variety of electrolytes, rumen stimulants and propylene glycol are often administered by stomach pump.

Retained fetal membranes should only be removed if they come away with gentle traction. Uterine lavage with several litres of warm sterile saline administered through the cervix using an orogastric tube has been suggested, with fluid and uterine detritus siphoned off by lowering the end of the tube to about the level of the udder. Care must be taken when attempting uterine lavage, as this technique may further damage a compromised uterine lining and promote further toxin absorption.

3 What follow-up treatment would you recommend? Observe closely as metritis/twins are risk factors for LDA. The farmer is advised to present the cow for a pre-breeding check 21–28 days post calving when clinical endometritis, if present, can be treated with antibiotic wash-out or prostaglandin injection.

CASE 1.90

1 What conditions would you consider (most likely first)? Include: cystitis/pyelonephritis; bladder tumour; chronic peritonitis.

2 How could you confirm your provisional diagnosis? Urinalysis reveals a strong positive result for protein, blood and white blood cells consistent with cystitis/pyelonephritis. A direct smear of mid-stream urine sediment yields gram-positive rods. The BUN concentration is 14.9 mmol/l (41.8 mg/dl) (normal range 2–6 [5.6–16.8]). There is a slight leucocytosis (10.4 × 10^9/l [10.4 × 10^3/μl), resulting from a marginal neutrophilia. There is a marked hypoalbuminaemia and elevated globulin concentration (18.8 g/l [1.88 g/dl] and 61.3 g/l [6.13 g/dl], respectively), consistent with chronic bacterial infection.

Bacteriological culture of a urine sample yields a pure growth of *Corynebacterium renale*.

Transrectal ultrasonography using a linear scanner typically reveals a markedly thickened bladder wall (>1 cm). Transabdominal ultrasonography of the right kidney using a 5 MHz scanner reveals almost complete loss of normal kidney structure

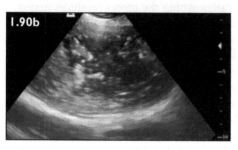

replaced by an irregular 6 cm diameter anechoic area containing hyperechoic dots consistent with a large abscess (**1.90b**). This appearance is consistent with pyelonephritis, with almost complete loss of normal kidney structure.

3 What is the prognosis? The prognosis for pyelonephritis is very poor due to the extent of kidney destruction despite prolonged penicillin therapy. Some clinical improvement can be achieved in the short term in less severely affected cattle, which may allow slaughter.

4 What treatment would you recommend? Penicillin is excreted in the urine and is very effective against *C. renale*. Treatment should be administered IM once daily for 3–6 weeks. Unilateral nephrectomy has been described, but should be carefully considered; rarely does infection involve only one kidney and flank analgesia is wholly inadequate for such surgery.

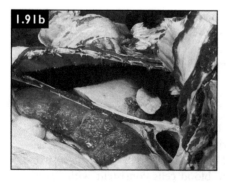

CASE 1.91

1 Describe the important sonographic and necropsy findings. There is an extensive pleural effusion occupying the ventral half of the chest extending to 15 cm (**1.91a**). There is dorsal displacement of the lung with consolidation of its ventral margin caused by the amount of fluid within the chest (**1.91b**). There is no evidence of fibrin suggestive of an inflammatory exudate.

2 What are the possible causes? The most likely conditions to consider would include: (Holstein) dilated cardiomyopathy; right-sided heart failure caused by a space-occupying mass in the thorax (e.g. thymic lymphosarcoma or large mediastinal abscess); myocarditis.

There is no sonographic evidence of a distended pericardial sac suggestive of pericarditis. The lung surface appears normal with no evidence of chronic suppurative pneumonia or pleuritis. Hypoproteinaemia can result in peripheral oedema, but such an extensive pleural effusion would be rare.

3 What action would you take? Thoracocentesis could be undertaken to measure protein concentration and white cell concentration to confirm the fluid as a transudate. The heifer should be euthanased for welfare reasons. Holstein dilated cardiomyopathy affects 2–4-year-old animals where an inherited aetiology has been suggested. Diagnosis is based on exclusion of other possible aetiologies of right-sided heart failure, although an increased heart rate and dysrhythmia are common findings.

CASE 1.92

1 How would you correct this problem? The vaginal prolapse is replaced after sacrococcygeal extradural injection of 5 ml of 2% lidocaine (procaine is not licensed for extradural injection). (**Note:** The needle should be advanced at 45° to the (horizontal) vertebral column.) The

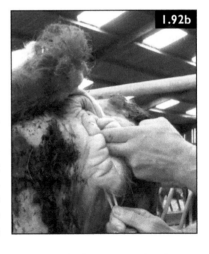

prolapsed tissues are thoroughly cleaned in warm dilute antiseptic solution but it may not be possible to remove all faecal material. After waiting for 5 minutes after extradural injection, steady pressure is applied to the prolapsed tissues and they are easily replaced. A Buhner suture of 5 mm umbilical tape is placed in the subcutaneous tissue surrounding the vulva to retain the prolapse and pulled tight to approximately two fingers (**1.92b**). Antibiotic therapy may be advisable because of the faecal contamination of the vaginal mucosa, but there are no guidelines based on field studies.

2 What is your advice regarding the management of this cow? The farmer is advised of the high probability of recurrence and the cow should be culled after she has reared her calf this year. Note that in natural mating systems cows can become pregnant despite the Buhner retention suture *in situ*. Should this happen, the suture must be slackened before the expected calving date. The suture can be retied after calving and passage of the fetal membranes. Vaginal prolapse is more commonly encountered 1–3 months after calving, often during oestrus when the cow mounts another cow.

CASE 1.93

1 What conditions would you consider (most likely first)? Include: radial nerve paralysis following trauma in the mid/distal humeral region; trauma of the shoulder/elbow joints; penetration wound causing cellulitis/joint infection; severe foot lesion (foot abscess, septic pedal arthritis).

2 What treatment(s) would you administer? Clinical examination failed to reveal any evidence of a fracture and there are no joint swellings. The injury occurred 2 weeks ago, therefore corticosteroid injection to reduce any associated soft tissue swelling would be unlikely to have much beneficial effect. The cow was isolated with her calf in a small paddock.

3 What is the prognosis for this cow? The cow showed signs of improvement after 3 months and was fully recovered after 6 months. Such protracted convalescence is normal for radial nerve damage.

CASE 1.94

1 Identify the potentially toxic plant present in the field? *Senecio jacobaea* (ragwort). This plant is uncommon in the UK but can occur in many countries worldwide, especially under extensive grazing conditions. *Senecio* spp. contain pyrrolizidine alkaloids. Poisoning usually occurs following ingestion of the wilted plant in conserved forage such as hay or silage.

2 What clinical signs might be expected? Clinical signs are caused by chronic liver damage and include chronic weight loss, diarrhoea, jaundice and peripheral oedema, with possible ascites caused by hypoproteinaemia. Affected cattle are often dull and even obtunded. There may be evidence of tenesmus with resultant rectal prolapse. The important differential diagnoses include chronic liver fluke infestation and lead poisoning.

3 How is the diagnosis confirmed? Diagnosis is based on clinical evidence of a hepatopathy with exposure to ragwort (check silage/hay). Elevated liver enzyme concentrations reflect the hepatic insult. Diagnosis is confirmed following liver biopsy or necropsy.

4 What treatment and control measures could be adopted? There is no effective treatment once clinical signs appear. Remove contaminated feed. Control ragwort on pasture by use of selective herbicides. Wilted ragwort is more palatable to cattle, therefore it must not be topped if cattle remain in the field. Ragwort is not a problem in mixed grazing system with sheep.

CASE 1.95

1 What conditions would you consider (most likely first)? Rickets, osteochondrosis dissecans.

Lack of mineralisation of a cereal-based ration along with vitamin D deficiency can lead to gradual osteomalacia of growing bones and spontaneous long bone fractures. Fractures involving the cervical vertebrae lead to recumbency, with evidence of cervical pain. This situation arises due to inadequate calcium supplementation with excess dietary phosphorus typically present in a cereal-based ration. Less severely affected calves show widening of the metaphyses, particularly of the proximal third metacarpal and third metatarsal bones, causing moderate lameness.

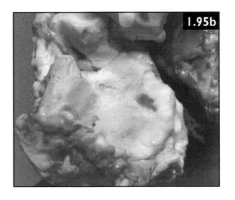

1.95b

2 What further examinations could you undertake to confirm your diagnosis? Radiography reveals poor mineralisation and flaring of the distal metaphyses. In some cases there may be erosion of articular cartilage and exposure of subchondral bone (**1.95b**) with accompanying joint effusion and severe lameness. Diagnosis is based on a cluster of spontaneous long bone fractures and review of the diet, with detailed investigation of its mineral supplementation including vitamin expiry date.

3 What treatment would you administer? There is no specific treatment for the lame bulls in the group. Depending on the degree of lameness, these animals should be reared in isolation and slaughtered as early as possible on farm, as they are unlikely to be fit for transport to a slaughterhouse. Immediate correction of the mineral content of the ration with appropriate vitamin D supplementation is necessary.

Problems have occurred when farms have changed to organic rearing systems and it is essential to ensure that diets contain the correct vitamin and mineral supplementation.

CASE 1.96

1 What conditions would you consider (most likely first)? Include: ringworm (*Trichophyton* spp. infection); sarcoptic mange; lice (pediculosis); chorioptic mange.

2 What further tests could be undertaken? Microscopic examination of hair/skin scrapings from the periphery of the lesions reveals fungal hyphae typical of *Trichophyton* spp. infection. Culture examination can be undertaken on special media.

3 What actions/treatments would you recommend? There are no specific treatments in many EU countries, although in-feed griseofulvin medication for 10–14 days is still available in some countries. Most farmers elect to do nothing, as lesions eventually regress over 3–6 months, but in the interim the cattle do not look well and there is the risk of transmission to other livestock. Unless buildings are thoroughly cleaned when depopulated, infection may remain and clinical signs appear in the next batch of cattle.

An attentuated ringworm vaccine strain of *T. verrucosum* is routinely used in many dairy herds but rarely in beef cattle.

4 Are there any special concerns? There is a zoonotic risk following contact with the calves or their environment.

CASE 1.97

1 Describe the abnormal findings in the sonogram. The walls of the right ventricle are clearly visible at 7 and 13 cm from the probe head. There is an increased amount of fluid (transudate) within the pleural space (anechoic areas). There are 5–6 almost spherical hypoechoic 'nodules' present within the pleural space, several of which appear adherent to the pericardium; there are several 'nodules' that are adherent to the parietal pleura. As the probe head is moved dorsally there is an increased depth of pleural effusion extending to 10 cm deep. Examination of the lungs fails to reveal any abnormality of the visceral pleura.

2 What is this lesion? The masses are consistent with a tumour. The absence of inflammatory exudate (fibrin within the anaechoic pleural fluid) would suggest that infection is unlikely. Furthermore, the 'nodules' do not have the appearance of abscesses.

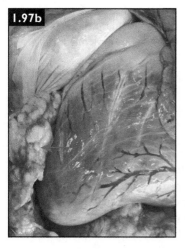

3 What is the likely cause? Enzootic bovine leucosis (EBL) must be considered a possible cause of a tumour in countries where this virus is endemic in the cattle population. The suspected tumour masses are outwith the pericardial sac, therefore a heart base tumour is unlikely.

4 What action should be taken? The cow should be culled for welfare reasons. Where appropriate, blood samples should be collected for EBL testing. In some countries regulatory authorities should be informed about the suspicion of a tumour in an adult bovine animal. Necropsy of this cow revealed the nature of the tumour mass (**1.97b**, arrow) with metastases to the mediastinal lymph nodes. EBL testing was negative; the nature of the tumour was not identified because of cost.

CASE 1.98

List five biosecurity measures and five biocontainment measures that will reduce the risk of *Salmonella dublin* infection in a dairy herd.

Biosecurity:
- Avoid introducing potentially infected animals by maintaining a closed herd. Quarantine all introduced stock for at least 4 weeks.
- Source new stock from other farms with high health status and not from markets.
- Avoid communal grazing.
- Maintain good fences to prevent straying of neighbouring stock.
- Insist visitors have clean boots and disinfect before entering and leaving the farm premises.

Biocontainment:
- Consider herd vaccination.
- Isolate sick animals in dedicated isolation boxes and not calving boxes.
- Clean and disinfect buildings between occupancies. Provide good drainage and waste removal.
- Protect all feed stores from vermin
- Only spread slurry on arable land wherever possible. Leave all grazing land at least 3 weeks after spreading slurry.

CASE 1.99

1 What conditions would you consider (most likely first)? Septicaemic colibacillosis; enterotoxigenic *Escherichia coli*; peritonitis from ascending umbilical infection.

2 What is the cause of this problem? Two factors are critical in the development of septicaemic colibacillosis:
- Inadequate passive immunity from colostral immunoglobulins.
- Exposure and invasion via the nasal, oropharyngeal mucous membranes, tonsil, upper respiratory tract, or intestine of an *E. coli* serotype able to produce an overwhelming septicaemia, endotoxaemia and death. The umbilicus is not the major portal of entry for bacteria causing septicaemia. A dirty calving environment with high bacterial challenge increases the risk of disease.

3 What treatment would you administer, and what is the prognosis? Florfenicol is a good antibiotic choice for septicaemic calves, but the prognosis is hopeless if the calf shows seizure activity and there is early evidence of polyarthritis

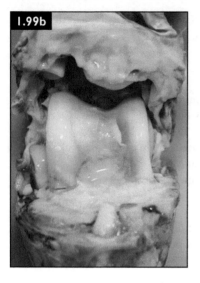

(slight fluid distension of several joints; see necropsy findings in **1.99b**; note that joint infection and accumulation of exudate can be severe even at 3 days old). Supportive therapy includes IV NSAID injection. A high dose of soluble corticosteroid (1.0 mg/kg dexamethasone) reduces cerebral oedema but remains controversial in the treatment of bacterial meningoencephalitis, which is part of the septicaemic condition.

4 What control measures would you implement? Septicaemia is best prevented by ingestion of 7–10% of the calf's body weight of colostrum (3 litres minimum is recommended) within the first 6 hours of the calf's life. Stored colostrum can be used if there is insufficient dam supply, but note the potential risk for paratuberculosis transmission. Hygiene in calving boxes should be improved as should calf accommodation. Numerous methods can be used to assess passive antibody transfer, but total plasma protein determination using a refractometer is the cheapest and can be readily undertaken in the practice laboratory. Pre-colostral values of 40–45 g/l (4.0–4.5 g/dl) rise to >55–65 g/l (5.5–6.5 g/dl) from 24 hours after appropriate colostrum ingestion.

CASE 1.100

1 What action would you take? A large volume, low extradural lidocaine block (3 mg/kg) is administered to paralyse the hind legs and allow pain-free examination of the distal left hind leg. The bull is then heavily sedated with IV xylazine. (**Note:** Sedation should be given after extradural injection of the standing animal because paresis and sedation take effect at much the same time with the animal quietly and safely assuming sternal recumbency.) Flunixin is then injected IV. Careful paring of both claws of the left hind foot fails to reveal any sole abnormality and there are no discharging sinuses at the coronary band nor widening of the interdigital space typical of septic pedal arthritis.

A dorsoplantar radiograph of the right fetlock region is shown (**1.100b**). There is considerable sidebone of the lateral claw but no evidence of infection of either distal interphalangeal joint.

Further examination of the fetlock region was suggestive of thickening of the joint capsule but this interpretation was limited by the surrounding subcutaneous oedema. There was no indication to amputate a digit and the severity and duration

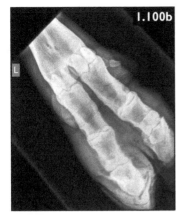

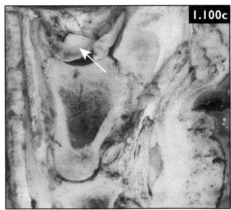

of lameness therefore dictated that the bull be euthanased for welfare reasons. The provisional diagnosis of septic fetlock was confirmed at necropsy, which revealed the fetlock joint to be filled with a pannus (**1.100c**, arrow). Arthrocentesis would have failed to yield a sample; arthrotomy would have been unsuccessful and only further prolonged suffering. The cause of the septic fetlock joint was not determined.

CASE 1.101

1 Describe the abnormalities present. There is marked erosion of the articular surface of the third metacarpal bone.

2 What action would you take? The prognosis is hopeless and the calf must be euthanased for welfare reasons. The extent of joint pathology is clearly evident (**1.101b**). There is extensive pannus within the joint. Marked joint effusion is uncommon in septic arthritis in cattle in all but neonatal calves.

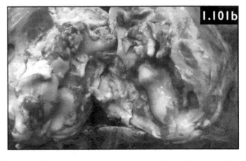

In the absence of significant radiographic changes (or indeed radiographic examination in most practice situations), the decision to euthanase this calf should be based on the chronicity of the severe lameness, which is refractory to antibiotic therapy. Antibiotic therapy, and possibly joint lavage, for septic arthritis is rarely successful in calves more than several weeks old. It can prove difficult to convince a farmer that an animal with a septic joint will not respond to a 'stronger' antibiotic, but the welfare of the animal is paramount.

3 **Are there any specific control measures?** The cause of the joint infection in this case was not determined but presumed to be haematogenous in origin. It is not uncommon to find a single septic joint in growing ruminants where there is no obvious primary lesion.

CASE 1.102

1 **What conditions would you consider (most likely first)?** Spastic paresis; dislocated hip. Dorsal patellar luxation is rare in cattle.

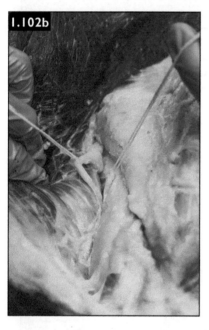

2 **What options would you consider?** Many calves are euthanased for welfare reasons following clinical examination because of the prohibitive cost of surgery and only 75% success rate in early cases; calves showing signs for several months, or affecting both hind legs, have a poor outcome.

Tenotomy of the gastrocnemius muscle is rarely undertaken because of frequent recurrence. Partial or total tibial neurectomy is performed under xylazine sedation and large volume extradural block (3 mg/kg lidocaine at the sacrocoggyceal space) with the affected leg uppermost for surgery. Blunt dissection between the two heads of the biceps femoris muscle in the lateral thigh reveals the tibial and peroneal nerves, which are isolated and stimulated with forceps (nerves shown in **1.102b** in a prepared necropsy specimen). Stimulation of the tibial nerve causes flexion of the digits and fetlock; once identified, a 5 cm portion of nerve is sectioned and removed.

3 **What control measures could be implemented?** The cause is not known but a hereditary component is likely. The condition is more common in the Belgian Blue breed. There are no specific control measures in this particular herd with crossbred cattle and no Belgian Blue genetics.

CASE 1.103

1 What conditions would you consider (most likely first)? Squamous cell carcinoma of the hard palate or nasal cavity; ethmoid carcinoma; nasal lymphosarcoma; nasal osteosarcoma; osteomyelitis of the hard palate; advanced erosive fungal sinusitis.

2 What further tests could be undertaken? Mediolateral radiographs of the muzzle revealed a soft tissue opacity extending from the level of the first molar to the zygomatic arch and dorsal nasal conchae (**1.103b**). The opacity had ill-defined edges and protruded into the pharyngeal region and along sinus contours.

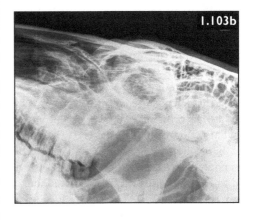

Rhinoscopy revealed the ventral and common meati of both nostrils to be filled with impacted ingesta, which prevented advancement of the rhinoscope beyond the level of the oral lesion.

3 What action would you take? There is suspicion of metastasis in the enlarged submandibular lymph nodes, but squamous cell carcinoma does not usually spread beyond the local drainage lymph nodes. Immediate slaughter for human consumption is prevented by the farmer's antibiotic administration and the interval to salvage is considered too long, therefore the cow was euthanased for welfare reasons. Histopathology confirmed the diagnosis of squamous cell carcinoma.

CASE 1.104

1 What conditions would you consider (most likely first)? Osteoarthritis of the stifle caused by repeated trauma with variable rupture of the cruciate ligaments; osteoarthritis of the hip.

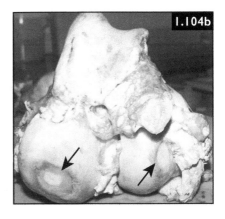

Repeated joint trauma (possibly caused by bulling injuries) results in joint instability with proliferation of fibrous tissue within the joint capsule, degeneration and loss of articular cartilage, exposure and eburnation of subchondral bone, and peripheral osteophyte formation (**1.104b**, arrows).

Crepitus is difficult to appreciate because it can be difficult to distinguish from 'clunking' of the normal hip joint. Few cows are so neglected that there is subchondral bone grating against subchondral bone to produce crepitus. Many beef bulls can reach 1.0–1.1 tonnes compared with cow liveweights of 600–700 kg (1,320–1,540 lb).

2 What other tests could you employ? Detailed radiographic and ultrasonographic examinations are rarely employed because after several months' moderate lameness and severe muscle wastage the cow must be culled for welfare reasons irrespective of further findings.

3 What treatment would you administer? Analgesics may afford temporary reduction in lameness for 3–5 days, but affected cattle should be culled because of chronic pain and they will also not be productive. It can prove difficult to be certain that such cattle are fit to transport to a slaughterhouse; the nearest plant must always be used.

4 What action would you take? There are no specific control measures. Extreme beef bulls should be avoided and their condition limited to fit not obese, as commonly purchased at breeding sales. Review underfoot conditions that could lead to slips and falls if cattle are bred indoors. Cull early to avoid chronic pain (see **1.104b**).

CASE 1.105

1 Describe the abnormalities present. There are no appreciable abnormalities visible on the radiograph.

2 What action would you take? The calf is heavily sedated with xylazine (stage 4; 0.3 mg/kg IM). The calf is left undisturbed and after 10 minutes it is found in sternal recumbency. Flunixin is injected IV. A low extradural block of lidocaine (3 mg/kg) is administered to paralyse the hind legs and allow pain-free

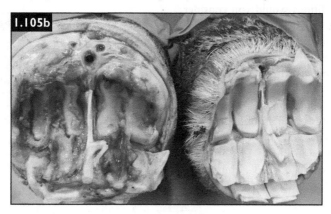

examination of the fetlock joint. A 14 gauge needle is inserted into the fetlock joint at two sites and the joint flushed with Hartmann's solution, but no foreign material is displaced. The joint is then prepped for an arthrotomy because the material in the joint is thought to be a pannus (fibrin firmly adherent to the joint surface, bacteria and inflammatory cells), which cannot be flushed through needles. The arthrotomy yields large plaques of pannus. The prognosis is hopeless and the calf is euthanased for welfare reasons. The extent of joint pathology is clearly evident (**1.105b**) and it proves impossible to remove all the pannus even via an arthrotomy.

3 Are there any specific control measures? The farmer had suspected a cellulitis lesion and treated the calf himself. It is debatable whether joint lavage/arthrotomy would have been successful at the first signs of lameness. Joint lavage is most useful in neonatal calves rather than in growing calves/adult cattle. Radiography is of little clinical help during the early stages of joint sepsis and may mislead the clinician into thinking that there is no significant joint pathology present. In some cases there is widening of the articular space, but the contralateral normal joint should be radiographed for comparison; even then, angulation of the beam can affect this measurement. Arthrocentesis is often negative as the joint contains a pannus rather than more fluid exudate.

CASE 1.106

1 What is the likely cause? Localised infection/cellulitis caused by non-sterile subcutaneous injection following treatment with calcium borogluonate or dextrose injection; subcutaneous abscess; haematoma.

2 What action would you take? No action is necessary at the moment. There is no evidence that the swelling is developing into a large abscess and about to discharge. Ultrasound examination would identify whether the swelling is a haematoma or abscess; it may prove difficult to differentiate subcutaneous accumulation of fluid that has not been absorbed from cellulitis.

3 How can this problem be prevented? Use a sterilised flutter valve and new hypodermic needle for all subcutaneous injections. Too often, the farmer's flutter valve is rinsed through with hot water and left hung up in the milk bulk tank room with the needle still attached until used again. The value of subcutaneous injection of calcium borogluconate is probably overrated because it is often poorly absorbed and is irritant and painful. The extent of subcutaneous reaction is evident at necropsy of any recently calved cow treated by this route. Calcium chloride gels are more effective as supportive treatment for milk fever, but care is needed in cattle without a proper swallow reflex. On a herd basis, high milk fever prevalence is greatly reduced by feeding a diet with a high dietary cation/anion balance in consultation with the farm's nutritionist.

CASE 1.107

1 What conditions would you consider (most likely first)? Include: summer mastitis; bacterial endocarditis; polyarthritis; other chronic bacterial infections; redwater (babesiosis).

2 What is the cause? Primary invasion of the mammary gland, with either the anaerobic organism *Peptococcus indolicus* or *Streptococcus dysgalactiae*, is followed by *Trueperella pyogenes* infection to cause summer mastitis. There is circumstantial evidence only to link the sheep headfly *Hydrotaea irritans* with disease transmission.

3 What treatments would you administer? The right forequarter will not recover normal lactogenesis. Intramammary antibiotic infusion is ineffective due to the chronicity/extent of the infection, although parenteral antibiotics, typically penicillin, are administered. Frequent stripping of the affected quarter every 2–4 hours is necessary to remove toxins and cellular debris, but is not a simple procedure because of the painful oedematous teat. Lancing the teat in the vertical plane, thereby reducing the risk of haemorrhage associated with teat amputation, to facilitate drainage often produces disappointing results. NSAIDs, such as flunixin meglumine or ketoprofen, provide pain relief and stimulate appetite. Corticosteroids reduce joint effusions and reduce inflammation, although they will cause abortion if administered to cattle later than the first trimester of pregnancy, although this is not a concern in this non-pregnant cow.

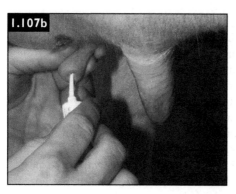

4 What control measures would you recommend? Dry cow therapy/teat sealants (**1.107b**; operator should be wearing gloves) remain the most effective means of preventing summer mastitis. Fly repellants, whether in the form of pour-on, spray-on or impregnated ear tag, provide useful protection against nuisance flies.

CASE 1.108

1 What conditions would you consider (most likely first)? Infection of the proximal interphalangeal (P1/P2) joint; septic pedal arthritis; penetration wound and associated cellulitis.

2 What action would you take? Amputate the digit through distal P1 under IVRA after first injecting flunixin IV. Use lidocaine as procaine is not licensed for IV use, observing meat withholding times as appropriate. It can prove difficult to judge the incision site through proximal P1 – aim to exit 2 cm proximal to the discharging sinus on the lateral aspect with your Gigli wire. The bull was not sound until 3 weeks after amputation, which is a longer convalescence period than usual. Putting a block on the sound claw and lavaging the infected joint could have been attempted, but this would have cost the same as digit amputation and likely not have achieved such a good outcome.

Farmers are reluctant to pay for radiography because clinical judgement is almost always correct in these cases. However, radiography provided some interesting findings (**1.108b**). There is loss of the articular surfaces of the proximal interphalangeal joint, consistent with chronic infection, and a large defect of the articular surface of P1, possibly arising from infection of the associated growth plate.

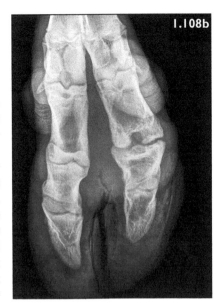

CASE 1.109

1 What is your diagnosis? Superfoul with extension of infection into both distal interphalangeal joints. Interdigital necrobacillosis with extension into both distal interphalangeal joints

Superfoul is the term often used to describe the peracute form of interdigital necrobacillosis ('foul of the foot').

2 How could you confirm your diagnosis? Radiography demonstrates extension of infection into both distal interphalangeal joints (**1.109c**). The extensive bone destruction suggests that the lesions are of more than 3 weeks' duration.

3 What action would you take? Immediate action for superfoul is essential. Under IVRA, débride the interdigital lesion and pack with 2–4 500 mg clindamycin tablets. Apply a bandage. Treat cow with tylosin (10 mg/kg IM q12h for at least 5 days). Administer a NSAID such as

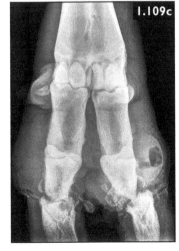

flunixin or ketoprofen for 3–5 days. Isolate the cow in a well-bedded straw pen. However, these measures are far too late for this cow and she must be euthanased immediately for welfare reasons.

Review the management of this cow and investigate whether other cattle are affected. Inspect the cattle accommodation paying particular attention to hygiene and slurry management. Advise veterinary examination of lame cows as soon as possible, especially where there is no response to antibiotic therapy of suspect 'foul of the foot' cases.

4 **List any management, prevention and control measures.** Quarantine all cattle introduced into the herd. Biosecurity is also very important for many other diseases. Reduce environmental contamination and increase bedding in cubicles. Disinfectant footbaths containing either formalin or copper sulphate are reported to provide good control. Attend to all lame cows immediately.

CASE 1.110

1 **What action would you take?** It can prove difficult to decide whether to continue with antibiotics for another day or so or to flush the joint. Previous success with early joint lavage on this farm made the farmer keen not to delay. Flunixin is

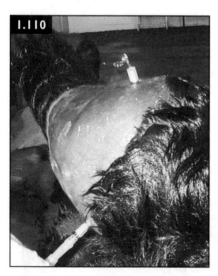

injected IV. The calf is sedated with IM xylazine. The calf is left undisturbed and after 10 minutes is positioned in sternal recumbency and a high extradural block of lidocaine (3 mg/kg) is administered to paralyse the hind legs and allow pain-free examination and lavage of the stifle joint. A 14 gauge needle is inserted into the stifle joint and a slightly turbid free-flowing (non-viscous) sample is obtained. Another needle is inserted on the other side of the joint and the joint alternately flushed through these needles with 3 litres of Hartmann's solution (**1.110**). This calf made a very good recovery and was much less lame 2 days later.

In some joint infections, large plaques of fibrin/pannus form within days of lameness being detected. The prognosis is hopeless in such cases because the material cannot be flushed out.

2 **Are there any specific control measures?** Bacteraemia with localisation within joint(s) follows management shortcomings related to failure of passive transfer

and poor environmental hygiene, allowing high bacterial challenge. Bacteraemia/septicaemia in neonatal calves is one of the few infections where a fluoroquinolone antibiotic could be considered; clinical experience shows that marbofloxacin may provide a better treatment response than florfenicol, but there are no supporting published data.

CASE 1.111

1 What conditions would you consider? Osteoarthritis of the tibiotarsal joint as a consequence of wear and tear. Some degree of joint effusion of the tibiotarsal and tarsometatarsal joints is very common in many beef bulls and proves difficult to interpret because these bulls often appear sound.

2 What assessment could you undertake? Radiography of the tarsus (**1.111b, c**) shows marked osteophytosis of the tarsometatarsal joint in particular. The extensive osteophytosis appears to contradict the history of low-grade intermittent lameness, but the tarsometatarsal joint is a low motion joint where ankylosis may not cause marked lameness.

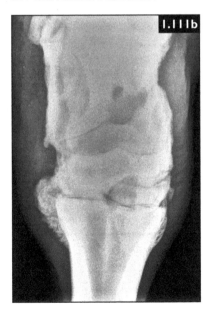 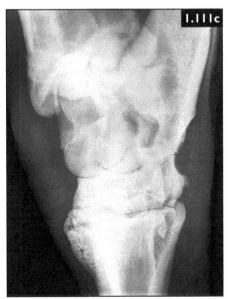

3 Is this bull fit for future breeding? Predicting future breeding of this bull is difficult based on a single examination. Repeat radiographs should be taken in 6–12 weeks to check progression of lesions, particularly those involving the more important tibiotarsal joint. In a commercial farming situation, the bull is in excellent condition and is now 6 years old; the pragmatic option may be to sell the bull for slaughter, thus generating approximately 50% of the cost of an 18-month-old replacement. An extended calving period and high barren rate as a consequence of reduced bull fertility has a major affect on beef herd profitability; farmers will often comment that their first loss is the best loss!

4 How could this problem be reduced/prevented? The osteophytosis probably resulted from joint trauma during mating and there are no obvious control measures other than appropriate underfoot conditions.

CASE 1.112

1 Comment on the significant radiographic abnormalities. There is marked soft tissue swelling over the abaxial aspect of the coronary band. There is marked widening of the articular space of the distal interphalangeal joint with extensive erosion of articular cartilage. There is extensive osteophytosis involving the distal interphalangeal joint and, to a lesser extent, the proximal interphalangeal joint. These radiographic findings are consistent with chronic infection of the distal interphalangeal joint of at least 3 months' duration and probably longer.

2 What treatment would you administer? The extensive osteophytosis will probably result in ankylosis in several weeks/months. As the cow is moderately lame, a block is fitted to the sole of the sound claw of the right hind foot and she is treated for 3 consecutive days with a NSAID. The cow was 3–4/10 lame after this treatment course. The cow continued to improve and was sound when transported for slaughter 2 months later. An alternative approach would have been to amputate the digit through distal P1, but this would have caused short-term acute pain whereas the joint was almost ankylosed and a block further reduced lameness.

3 How should this problem have been treated when the cow first presented lame? The cow should have been presented for veterinary examination soon after it failed to respond to the treatment administered by the farmer; however, several weeks/months often elapse before such examination occurs (this case). Radiographic examination greatly assisted the prognosis and management of this case and need not be expensive because only one dorsoplantar view is needed.

CASE 1.113

1 What conditions would you consider (most likely first)? Tetanus; hypomagnesaemia; lead poisoning; meningitis. The calf is too young for polioencephalomalacia.

2 What laboratory tests could be undertaken to confirm your provisional diagnosis? There is no confirmatory test for tetanus and diagnosis is based on the clinical signs and history. The elastrator ring used for castration, applied illegally to the scrotum at 6 weeks old, could be the origin of the problem (**1.113b**).

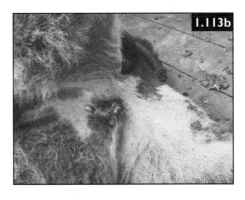

3 What treatment would you administer? There is no consensus regarding the dose rate of antitoxin; one protocol gives 50 units/kg liveweight IV followed by IM doses of the same amount as thought necessary every 12 hours. Crystalline penicillin is recommended IV at the first examination for its more rapid onset of action, followed by 44,000 units per kg of procaine penicillin IM twice daily. NSAIDs should be given daily to provide analgesia. Acetylpromazine (0.05 mg/kg q8h) should be administered to provide muscle relaxation. Local wound débridement remains controversial. Tetanus cases should be housed singly in a darkened, deep-bedded shed. None of these treatments would have produced any improvement in this case and the calf was euthanased for welfare reasons.

4 What control measures would you recommend? Efficacious vaccines are available but are not routinely used unless there is a farm history of clostridial disease (more commonly blackleg).

CASE 1.114

1 What is this defect? Horizontal fissure in the hoof horn ('thimbling').

2 What is the likely cause? Poor horn production during a severe toxaemic episode such as coliform mastitis or metritis appears as a horizontal fissure in the hoof horn of all eight digits. As this defect in the wall grows down to about two-thirds of its length 3–4 months later, it weakens and further separates from the healthy horn proximally. The corium remains intact distal to the horizontal fracture, holding the distal hoof horn attached at the toe. This fissure moves when weight is taken, tensing the corium still attached distally and causing variable pain and lameness. Foreign material can occasionally become impacted in the fissure, causing pressure, and may lead to abscesses.

3 What action would you take? Careful hoof paring is only necessary when the cow is lame in order to remove all underrun horn and impacted material. This is best achieved with hoof shears, taking note that the hoof capsule may still be attached at the toe.

4 Are there any specific control measures? There are no specific control measures except for prompt treatment of toxic conditions.

CASE 1.115

1 Describe the abnormalities present. There is extensive loss of the articular surface of the glenoid of the scapula. The articular space is greatly increased.

2 What is the likely cause? The radiographic changes are consistent with chronic septic arthritis of the right shoulder joint.

3 What action would you take? The calf should be euthanased for welfare reasons because the bony changes are now too extensive for joint lavage/arthroscopy. After several days, joint infection causes formation of a pannus, which is firmly adherent to articular cartilage and proves very difficult to remove even by arthroscopic surgery. A pannus is a membrane of granulation tissue (fibroblasts and neovascularisation) and bone marrow-derived cells (macrophages). Differentiation of fibrin deposition within a joint and a pannus proves very difficult on gross examination because a pannus is an extension of the pathological change within the joint. However, a pannus is more adherent to the synovial membrane and articular cartilage than fibrin, and is much more difficult to peel off. An example of pannus in a case of a septic stifle joint is shown (**1.115b**); the widespread and adherent nature of the pannus prevents successful treatment even by arthroscopy/arthrotomy. There are few radiographic

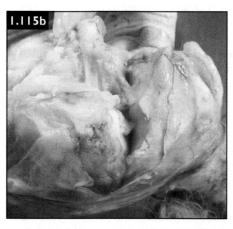

changes during the early stages of the infectious disease process except for slight widening of the articular space, which is best appreciated by comparing it with the contralateral normal joint, although projection of the beam can cause artefacts with respect to distance between articular surfaces. Arthrocentesis often fails to yield sufficient sample for analysis and must not be mistaken for the absence of pathological changes within the joint.

4 Are there any specific control measures? There was no evidence of a puncture wound over the shoulder joint and infection was assumed to have been haematogenous during the neonatal period. Review colostrum management and environmental hygiene.

CASE 1.116

1 What conditions would you consider (most likely first)? Include: thymic lymphosarcoma causing compression of the cranial vena cava and oesophagus; right-sided heart failure caused by severe interstitial pneumonia or a space-occupying mass in the thorax such as a large mediastinal abscess; dilated cardiomyopathy; septic pericarditis; chronic suppurative pneumonia/pleuritis/pleural effusion; endocarditis.

Mild bloat results from compression of the oesophagus as it passes through the mediastinum by the tumour mass.

2 How could you confirm your diagnosis? There is no confirmatory diagnostic test for thymic lymhosarcoma; however, several of the important differential diagnoses can be eliminated by transthoracic ultrasonography of the lungs, pleurae and heart; no abnormalities were found in this case. The mediastinum is separated from the chest wall by aerated lung and cannot be examined ultrasonographically.

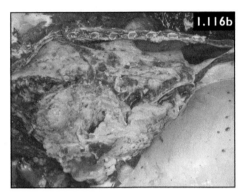

3 What action should you take? In the UK, concerns over enzootic bovine leucosis virus (EBLV) require notification of regulatory authorities. The heifer was euthanased for welfare reasons and the diagnosis of thymic lymphosarcoma confirmed at necropsy (**1.116b**). Tests for EBLV proved negative.

CASE 1.117

1 Interpret the radiographic findings (1.117a, b). Fracture through the proximal tibia involving the epiphysis.

2 What is the prognosis? Repair of the fracture is not possible and the calf was euthanased for welfare reasons.

3 How could this situation have been prevented? Excessive force using a calving jack to deliver large beef calves is not uncommon. Fractures may result when calving ropes are attached to a jack and the cow falls down, caused by the pressure exerted and the acute pain produced. Femoral nerve paralysis affecting the calf is common following 'hip-lock'. Wherever possible, after the calving problem has been assessed and the calving ropes applied, the cow should be haltered, released from the cattle stocks and allowed to assume lateral recumbency before pulling the calf. Unfortunately, this recommendation is not always possible because of insufficient farm staff, poor facilities and an uncooperative and aggressive cow. If, as a veterinary surgeon, you attempt to deliver the calf with the dam restrained in cattle stocks, always forewarn the farmer of the risks involved, otherwise you may be found liable for any adverse outcome if the cow falls down.

CASE 1.118

1 What are the possible causes (most likely first)? Sciatic nerve damage; tibial nerve damage; peroneal nerve damage.

The sciatic nerve supplies the extensor muscles of the hip and hock and the flexors of the stifle and fetlock (tibial branch), and the extensors of the fetlock (peroneal branch). Damage to the sciatic nerve proximal to the stifle (before branching) causes the hip, stifle and hock to drop and the fetlock joint is knuckled, but the leg can still take weight. Sciatic nerve injury may result from calving injury and pelvic trauma, and perineural injection.

Tibial nerve injury results in flexion of the hock and slight knuckling of the fetlock joint, but not as severe as peroneal nerve paraylsis, where the dorsal surface of the hoof may contact the ground. Peroneal nerve injury over the lateral aspect of the stifle region typically occurs following prolonged recumbency on an unyielding surface.

2 What treatment would you administer? A single injection of dexamethasone may be beneficial if the injury has just occurred (e.g. during calving), although such treatment is difficult to evaluate. Tibial and peroneal nerve damage resolves over several weeks without treatment provided the cow is ambulatory.

3 How could this problem have been avoided? Farmers must not use excessive traction during delivery of the calf. Provide deep straw bedding in calving accommodation to prevent pressure over bony prominences. Regularly turn recumbent cattle from one side to the other side. Use an aseptic technique for injection of antibiotics and other preparations.

CASE 1.119

1 Describe the important radiographic findings. There is considerable lysis of P3 and osteophytosis of the distal interphalangeal joint.

2 What is this defect, and what is the likely cause? The findings are consistent with a diagnosis of toe necrosis. The aetiology has not been determined, but spirochaetes responsible for digital dermatitis have been implicated.

3 What action would you take? The conservative approach would be to apply

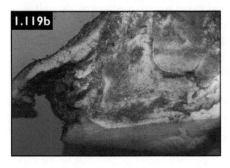

a wooden block (or equivalent) to the sound claw and pare away all underrun horn surrounding the toe necrosis lesion under IVRA, but this would create a considerable hoof defect, which is unlikely to heal. This approach would not address the osteoarthritis of the distal interphalangeal joint, as evidenced by the associated osteophytosis.

Digit amputation was undertaken under IVRA and IV injection of a NSAID. The extent of P3 lysis is shown in sagittal section (**1.119b**).

4 Are there any specific control measures? Measures should first be directed at the control of digital dermatitis; greatly improved slurry management, daily foot bathing and topical antibiotic (oxytetracycline) treatment of lesions. Be aware that spirochaete infection can be transmitted between cows by hoof knives and other equipment.

CASE 1.120

1 What conditions would you consider (most likely first)? Accidental toggling of small intestine or other viscus (not the abomasum); leakage of digesta from the toggling site and the development of diffuse peritonitis.

2 What laboratory tests could be undertaken to confirm your provisional diagnosis? Diagnosis is based on clinical signs and demonstration of an inflammatory exudate with a high protein concentration and an increased white cell count, with predominance of leucocytes, following ultrasound-guided abdominocentesis. Prior ultrasound examination is very helpful because peritonitis is not a simple diagnosis when infection has often been contained by the omentum (less likely in this case because toggling occurred just beneath the abdominal wall).

3 What treatment would you administer? Parenteral antibiotic therapy is hopeless in all but very localised cases of peritonitis, and is often undertaken in those situations where there has been limited investigation with the expectation that the animal is suffering from another infectious disease.

4 What is the prognosis? A guarded prognosis was afforded this cow; however, 3 litres of hypertonic saline was infused IV over 5 minutes followed by 30 litres of isotonic saline over the next 3 hours. Flunixin was also administered IV and florfenicol injected IM. The cow deteriorated further overnight and was euthanased for welfare reasons. Postmortem examination revealed extensive fibrinous adhesions in the cranioventral abdomen, with one toggle having torn through the wall of the small intestine.

5 What alternative surgical approach could have been undertaken? A right omentopexy undertaken in the standing unsedated cow under paravertebral anaesthesia is the more commonly adopted approach for LDA; this procedure takes longer and costs more, but results are generally better unless the surgeon is highly experienced with the toggling approach.

CASE 1.121

1 Describe the sonogram. There is a large accumulation of inflammatory exudate extending to more than 8 cm deep, with considerable fibrin deposition on the serosal surface of the reticulum and bridging the space between peritoneum and reticulum. A similar image would have been obtained using a 5 MHz linear scanner ('rectal scanner').

2 What is the prognosis for surgery? The prognosis for recovery following surgery is guarded because the fibrin deposited on the serosal surface of the reticulum and fibrinous adhesions will markedly restrict reticular contractions even if a foreign body is successfully removed.

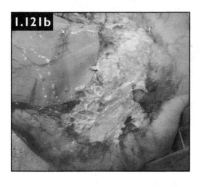

3 What action would you take? The cow should be euthanased for welfare reasons. The extensive peritonitis prevents on-farm slaughter for human consumption. This decision is proven correct by the necropsy finding (**1.121b**); note that the cow has been positioned in dorsal recumbency for postmortem examination and that the peritoneal fluid has drained, leaving only fibrin. The severity of lesions identified ultrasonographically often appears to be greater at postmortem examination.

4 What control measures could be employed? Examine farm records for history of cows culled due to unexplained poor performance (possible traumatic reticulitis and/or peritonitis cases) and any record of septic pericarditis to gauge the extent of potential problems. Check to see whether car tyres are used on silage clamps and the risk from these when fragments of decaying tyres are accidentally put into the total mixed ration wagon. Bonfire sites are another source of nails and other sharp debris. Discuss the possibility of prophylactic reticular magnets.

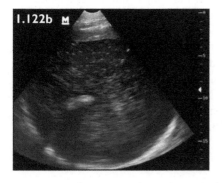

CASE 1.122

1 What is the likely cause? Large subcutaneous abscess; haematoma; umbilical hernia.

Ultrasound examination of the mass reveals a 15 cm diameter well-encapsulated anechoic area with multiple hyperechoic dots (**1.122b**) typical of an abscess.

2 What action would you take? To achieve drainage, lance the abscess at its ventral margin where the capsule is at its thinnest. Expect some bleeding from vessels in the abscess capsule wall but this will stop within 5–10 minutes.

The abscess cavity should be irrigated with very dilute povidone–iodine and repeated 2–3 days later. The incision should be packed with gauze swabs to prevent it healing. Parenteral antibiotic therapy is not necessary. While lancing the abscess is simple in a calf, a mature bull presents several risks from kicking and the bull should be confined in cattle stocks and sedated for safety reasons. While xylazine is licensed for IV use in cattle, romifine (1 mg/100 kg, off-label use) is a much better sedative.

CASE 1.123

1 What conditions would you consider (most likely first)? Include: peripheral vestibular lesion (otitis media); trauma to involve the peripheral facial nerve; listeriosis.

2 What is the likely cause? The vestibular system helps the animal maintain orientation in its environment, and the position of the eyes, trunk and legs with respect to movements and positioning of the head. Unilateral peripheral vestibular lesions are commonly associated with otitis media and ascending bacterial infection of the eustachian tube. There may be evidence of otitis externa and a purulent aural discharge in some cases, but rupture of the tympanic membrane is not a common route of infection.

3 What treatment would you administer? *Pasteurella* spp., *Streptococcus* spp. and *Trueperella pyogenes* have been isolated from infected lesions. A good treatment response is achieved with 5 consecutive days treatment with procaine penicillin, although other antibiotics including oxytetracycline and trimethoprim–sulphonamide combination are also used. *Mycoplasma bovis* is reported to be a common cause of otitis media in calves in endemically infected dairy herds. In this situation, a different antibiotic may be necessary such as a macrolide (e.g. tilmicosin, gamithromycin).

4 What is the prognosis for this case? The prognosis is very good in acute cases. The prognosis is poor in neglected cases where infection has extended into bone (empyema), but this is rare.

CASE 1.124

1 How would you correct this problem? The uterus is replaced after sacrococcygeal extradural injection of 5 ml of 2% lidocaine. Ideally, the cow should be haltered, cast and rolled onto her sternum and the hind legs positioned behind with the hips fully extended and the weight of the cow's hindquarters taken on her stifle joints, but this is not possible if there is only you and the farmer present and the cow is aggressive to humans. Instead, the cow is restrained in cattle stocks. The prolapsed uterus is cleaned in warm dilute povidone–iodine solution and any gross contamination

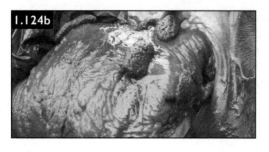

removed. The uterus is then held at the level of the vulva and replaced starting at the cervical end (**1.124b**). At first there seems to be little progress but eventually the uterine horn is replaced into the vagina and carefully returned to its normal 'comma-shaped' position. A 400 ml 'calcium' bottle (or similar) can be used to extend your reach to ensure the uterine tip is fully everted. A Buhner suture of 5 mm umbilical tape is placed subcutaneously surrounding the vulva to prevent repeat prolapse.

Very occasionally, the uterus can be inverted and would prolapse again, but it is held in place by the Buhner suture. This situation causes the cow to strain and should not be confused with the cow trying to pass the fetal membranes. Untie the Buhner suture, replace the uterus, which is often easier the second time because there is more tone in the uterine wall, and tighten the suture. The suture can be removed after 3–5 days.

2 What treatments will you administer? Oxytocin (40 iu IM). The cow is treated with parenteral oxytetracycline for 3 consecutive days to prevent metritis. There is no evidence of concurrent hypocalcaemia. The cow should be checked around 21 days after calving and treated with prostaglandin F2 alpha if there is evidence of chronic endometritis.

CASE 1.125

1 Describe the important sonographic findings. There are 5–8 very thin-walled fluid-filled structures (anechoic areas bordered by find circular white lines). There is no evidence of fibrin tags within the fluid. There is no testicular tissue or gut (small intestine) wall.

2 What conditions would you consider (most likely first)? The sonogram is consistent with a collection of very distended blood vessels forming a varicocoele. The cause of the varicocoele could not be determined but could have arisen following trauma after late Burdizzo castration, although this could not be proven. No evidence of surgical castration is noted but such scars are difficult to appreciate. There is no evidence of intestine walls, therefore a diagnosis of an inguinal hernia can be discarded. There are no visible testicles, therefore epididymitis and orchitis can be excluded.

3 What further investigations would you undertake? No further examination is necessary. You are convinced that there is no testicular tissue present in the scrotum and sign a certificate to this effect. Needle aspiration of the scrotum is contraindicated. Unfortunately, no information was available from the slaughter plant; more importantly the farmer received no complaint about this steer being a bull!

CASE 1.126

1 What conditions would you consider (most likely first)? Vitamin A deficiency; lead poisoning; polioencephalomalacia/sulphur toxicity for bore hole water supply; hepatopathy.

There is no obvious source of lead; the water is from a mains supply. The lack of a papillary light reflex would rule out polioencephalomalacia. There is no access to hepatotoxic agents/plants such as ragwort.

2 What further examinations could you undertake to confirm your diagnosis? Serum vitamin A analysis reveals concentrations consistent with deficiency.

3 What treatment would you administer? There is no effective treatment for the bulls in this group. Examination of the current supplement reveals that the minerals and vitamins are 6 months past their expiry date and included at only half the recommended rate. Immediate correction of the mineral and vitamin content of the ration is necessary for younger calves, although blindness may still result due to compression of the optic nerves as the animals grow, but the optic foramina remain the same size.

Careful loading of the blind animals and sympathetic management at the slaughter plant are essential. The affected cattle could be moved with normal cattle to guide their way. On-farm slaughter would be preferable if possible.

4 What other problems might be expected? Lack of mineralization of the cereal-based ration and vitamin D deficiency can lead to osteomalacia of growing bones and spontaneous long bone fractures. Less severely affected calves show widening of the metaphyses, particularly of the third metacarpal and third metatarsal bones, causing moderate lameness.

CASE 2.1 During autumn three of 120 7-month-old unvaccinated Suffolk-cross lambs have been found dead over the past 4 days. Some of the lambs had been noted to be very dull and depressed with foul smelling diarrhoea for 12–24 hours but died despite treatment with an antibiotic. The lambs are at pasture. Rolled barley in hoppers (**2.1**) was introduced 2 weeks ago, with the ration now available *ad libitum*.

1 What common problems could cause sudden death in these weaned unvaccinated lambs (most likely first)?
2 How could you confirm your provisional diagnosis?
3 What treatments would you consider?
4 What control measures would you recommend?

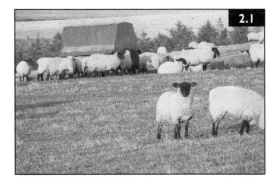

CASE 2.2 A 3-day-old Suffolk-cross male lamb presents with increasing abdominal distension, mild colic and frequent tenesmus (**2.2a**). The lamb is bright and alert but has stopped sucking its dam.

1 What conditions would you consider (most likely first)?
2 What action would you take?

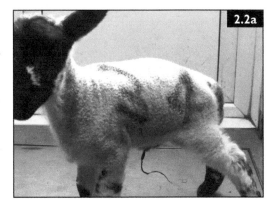

CASE 2.3 In summer, you are presented with a ewe with multiple 1–3 cm diameter subcutaneous abscesses affecting the cheeks. These abscesses are surrounding by areas of hair loss and fistulated to the skin surface (**2.3**). The submandibular lymph nodes are enlarged. The sheep has been grazing rough pasture containing gorse and other spiky plants.

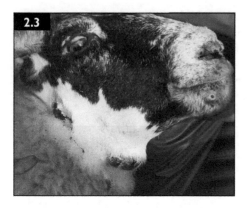

1 What common problems would you consider (most likely first)?
2 Are there any consequences to this infection?
3 How is the diagnosis confirmed?
4 What treatment(s) are necessary?

CASE 2.4 A 5-year-old ewe presents with a history of chronic weight loss (BCS 1.5/5); the remainder of sheep in the group are within a range of from 3/5 to 3.5/5. Rectal temperature is 39.0°C (102.2°F). The sheep has a reduced appetite. There is no diarrhoea. Auscultation of the chest reveals no abnormalities except for a slight increase in heart rate (96 beats per minute). There is considerable abdominal enlargement (**2.4a**, sheep on right) with an obvious fluid thrill. Ultrasonographic

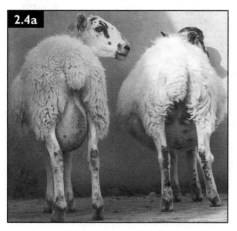

examination with a 5.0 MHz sector transducer reveals dorsal displacement of abdominal viscera by 10–12 cm of fluid; there are no visible fibrin tags.

1 What conditions would you consider?
2 What further tests would you undertake?
3 What is your diagnosis, and what treatment would you administer?
4 What is the likely cause?

CASE 2.5 During autumn, while selecting ewes to retain for the next breeding season, a client finds several young ewes to be in very poor body condition compared with normal sheep (**2.5a**; affected sheep on left, BCS 1.5/5; normal ewe on right, BCS 4/5). The fleece is also open and of poorer quality. The rectal temperature of the affected sheep is normal and there is no evidence of diarrhoea.

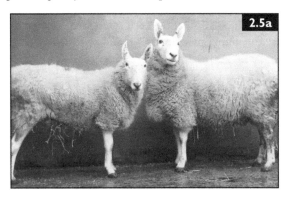

1 What is your provisional diagnosis (most likely first)?
2 What tests would you undertake?
3 What action would you recommend?
4 What control measures could be adopted?

CASE 2.6 In winter a sheep farmer receives a report of 'pneumonia' (**2.6**) affecting a batch of 20 9-month-old lambs sent to a local slaughter plant. Your client is surprised by this comment because the lambs have been growing well with no mortality in the group over the past 2 months. The lambs were housed 10 weeks ago and are fed *ad-libitum* concentrates. The lambs were vaccinated against clostridial disease at 4 and 5 months old but not against *Pasteurella* pneumonia. The lambs were last treated with an anthelmintic in September, 1 month before housing. There is a bout of coughing whenever the lambs are disturbed but they appear bright and alert.

Examination of three lambs with an elevated respiratory rate (60 breaths per minute) reveals normal rectal temperatures (39.2–39.6°C [102.6–103.3°F]). None of the lambs has a mucopurulent nasal discharge.

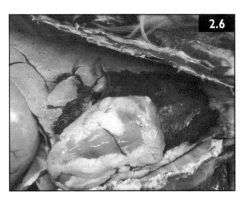

1 What conditions would you suspect (most likely first)?
2 What treatments would you administer?
3 What advice would you give?

CASE 2.7 During lambing time you are presented with a 5-day-old Texel lamb with sudden-onset tetraparesis (**2.7a**); the lamb had been normal for the first 4 days of its life. Four similarly affected lambs have died in the past week. The lamb's rectal temperature is normal. There are no palpable joint swellings and no swollen lymph nodes. There is low head carriage, evidence of cervical pain and gentle manipulation of the neck is resented. The reflex arcs are increased in all four legs. The umbilical stump is dry and brittle.

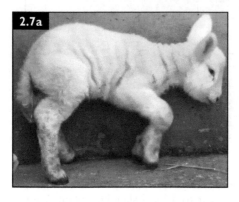

1 What is your diagnosis (most likely first)?
2 How could you confirm your diagnosis?
3 What treatments would you administer?
4 What preventive measures could be adopted?

CASE 2.8 You are presented with an emaciated 4-year-old Scottish Blackface ewe with a pendulous abdomen. The fleece is open and of poor quality. Rectal temperature is normal. The eyes appear sunken, which is thought to be largely due to the absence of intraorbital fat. Mucous membranes appear pale. There is no evidence of diarrhoea. The farmer reports that this is a common presentation on his farm and accounts for approximately 3–5% annual mortality in his flock. This sonogram (**2.8a**) is obtained on transabdominal ultrasound examination.

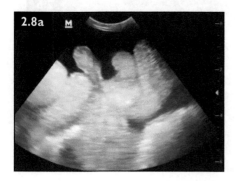

1 Interpret the important sonographic features.
2 What is your provisional diagnosis (most likely first)?
3 What further tests would you recommend?
4 What action would you take?

CASE 2.9 A new farm manager has taken over on a large Scottish highland estate and has experienced annual ewe mortality in excess of 12% in a 2,400 ewe flock, with losses occurring throughout the year. The flock is extensively managed on rough grazing most of the year (1 ewe per hectare) but housed for 10 weeks during late winter because of harsh weather. Some ewes die within 1–2 days of apparent acute respiratory disease, while others become emaciated before death. To further investigate these losses the manager consigns six non-pregnant ewes in poor condition to the veterinary laboratory without seeking your advice. Necropsy reveals one ewe with advanced ovine pulmonary adenocarcinoma (OPA) lesions, one ewe with paratuberculosis and one case of poor molar dentition. There are no significant findings in the remaining three sheep except for minor evidence of chronic fluke in two animals.

1 How would you interpret the necropsy results?
2 What advice would you offer?

CASE 2.10 You are presented with two 15-month-old Texel rams who display frequent proprioceptive deficits and stumbling on the fore legs, particularly when forced to trot (**2.10a, b**). There is obvious hindleg ataxia and weakness, and dysmetria of the fore legs. These signs were first noted 6 months ago. Hopping deficits are present in all four legs. Withdrawal reflexes are exaggerated in the hind and fore legs. Sometimes the sheep collapse when handled. When placed in lateral recumbency they have prominent extensor tone of the hindlegs. Hyperreflexia with clonus and crossed extensor reflexes are also present in the hindlegs.

1 What conditions would you consider?
2 What further tests could be undertaken?
3 What actions/treatments would you recommend?
4 What control measures could be taken?

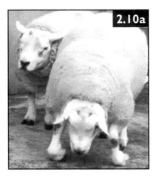
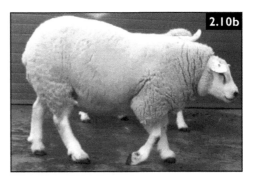

CASE 2.11 You are presented with an 8-month-old fattening lamb that shows multiple bilateral deficits of cranial nerves (CNs) III, V and VII (**2.11a**); assessment of the menace response is considered unreliable. The lamb is ataxic and has a bradycardia of 40 beats per minute. There is a bilateral mucopurulent nasal discharge.

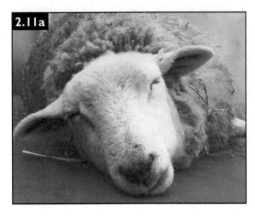

1 What conditions would you consider?
2 What is the cause of this condition?
3 What treatment would you administer?
4 What is the prognosis for this lamb?

CASE 2.12 You are presented with a 5-month-old Suffolk-cross lamb that has been unable to bear weight on the fore legs (**2.12a**) for approximately 1 week. The lamb appeared normal for the first 4 months of life. There are no foot lesions, palpable joint swellings or swollen prescapular lymph nodes. There are lower motor neuron signs to the fore legs, with reduced reflexes and flaccid paralysis. There are upper motor neuron signs to the hindlegs, with increased reflexes and spastic paralysis.

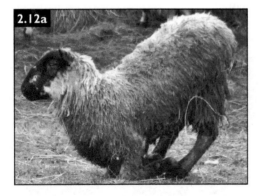

1 Where is the probable site of the lesion?
2 What type of lesion would you suspect (most likely first)?
3 What further investigations could be undertaken?
4 What prognosis would you offer?

CASE 2.13 You are presented with a dystocia where the lamb's head is presented through the vulva but both fore legs are retained alongside the chest ('hung lamb'; **2.13a**).

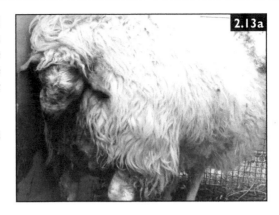

1 What action would you take?

CASE 2.14 During late winter a sheep farmer reports sudden-onset blindness affecting six of 600 ewes 4 weeks before lambing. The ewes are housed and fed *ad-libitum* grass silage and 350 g of concentrates per head per day. Four ewes are carrying twins, one ewe a singleton and one ewe is barren. The sheep are hyperaesthetic to sound and touch and are readily startled (**2.14a**). Appetite remains good. Clinical examination reveals bilateral absence of menace and pupillary light responses (**2.14b**). Ophthalmic examination reveals slightly narrowed retinal vessels and mild displacement of these vessels at the optic disc. The sheep had been treated for liver fluke 1 week previously and vaccinated against clostridial diseases.

1 What conditions would you consider?
2 What treatment would you administer?
3 What is this significance of this outbreak?

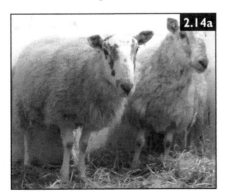
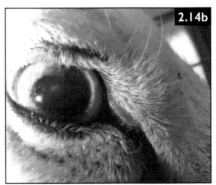

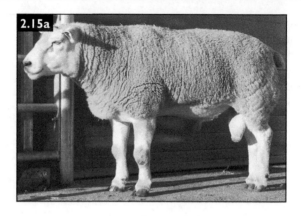

CASE 2.15 You are asked to comment on a recently purchased Texel ram that presents with large, non-painful, soft swellings over the dorsal aspect of both carpal joints (2.15a). The ram is not lame. The prescapular lymph nodes are normal sized. There is no pain on careful manipulation of the carpus. Rectal temperature is normal and the ram has a good appetite.

1 What conditions would you consider (most likely first)?
2 What further examinations would you take?
3 What advice would you offer?

CASE 2.16 A 2-crop ewe at pasture with 1-month-old twin lambs is found isolated from the remainder of the flock. The ewe appears lame and drags the right hindleg. The ewe is profoundly depressed with toxic mucous membranes. Rectal temperature is elevated (41.2°C [106.1°F]). Heart rate is increased above 130 beats per minute. Respiratory rate is increased to 45 breaths per minute. There are no ruminal sounds. Examination of the udder reveals extensive gangrenous mastitis

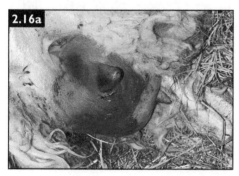

of the right gland (2.16a), with subcutaneous oedema extending along the ventral abdominal wall to the brisket.

1 What pathogens could be involved?
2 What is the prognosis?
3 What action would you take?
4 What control measures could be adopted?

CASE 2.17 An aged Suffolk ram was euthanased on a Scottish lowland farm because of poor condition. In addition to severe molar dentition problems identified at postmortem examination, a 6 cm diameter inspissated abscess was noted in the mediastinal lymph node (**2.17**).

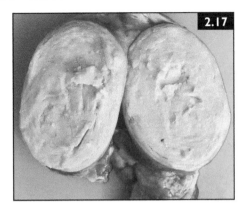

1 What is your diagnosis?
2 What action would you take?
3 What control measures should be adopted in this flock?

CASE 2.18 Two months after weaning a farmer complains of poor growth rates in 7-month-old lambs. The lambs are in poor condition with an open fleece and faecal staining of the perineum and tail (**2.18a**). The lambs have been grazing 'safe pasture' since weaning 6 weeks earlier. They were treated with monepantel (Group 4) before moving onto clean grazing; 10% of lambs were left undosed to maintain an 'in refugia' population.

1 What conditions would you consider (most likely first)?
2 How would you investigate this problem?
3 What treatment would you administer?
4 How would you prevent this problem recurring next year?

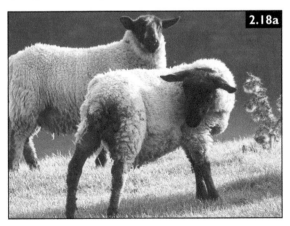

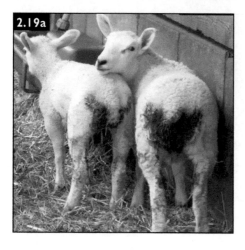

CASE 2.19 During April a client complains of diarrhoea affecting several 3–6-week-old orphan Suffolk-cross lambs (**2.19a**) reared indoors. The lambs are reared on an automatic milk dispenser with an *ad-libitum* 18% crude protein concentrate. The younger lambs are more severely affected, with considerable faecal staining of the tail and perineum. There is frequent tenesmus, with passage of small quantities of fluid faeces containing a large amount of mucus and flecks of fresh blood.

1 What common problems would you consider (most likely first)?
2 How could you confirm your provisional diagnosis?
3 What treatment would you administer?

CASE 2.20 Severe lameness is reported affecting 25 of a group of 120 6-month-old weaned lambs at pasture during late autumn. Typically, only one claw of one foot is affected, where there is separation of the hoof capsule around the entire

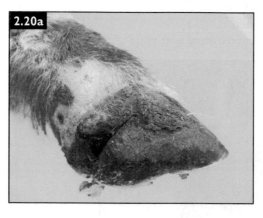

circumference of the coronary band. There is loss of hair extending for 2–3 cm proximal to the coronary band (**2.20a**).

1 What conditions would you consider?
2 What is the likely cause?
3 What action would you take?
4 How could this condition be prevented?

CASE 2.21 Describe the method you would use to collect CSF from an obtunded sheep.

CASE 2.22 During winter you are presented with an obtunded Texel ram from a group of 16 Texel and Suffolk rams. Two Texel rams have presented with similar clinical signs over the past 10 days and have died despite antibiotic treatment by the farmer. The rams have been fed *ad-libitum* silage and approximately 0.25 kg of concentrate daily for 8 weeks. Rectal temperature is 38.5°C (101.3°F). There are no cranial nerve deficits. Mucous membranes are

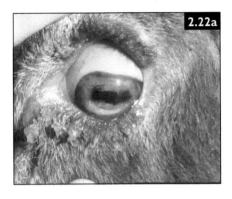

markedly jaundiced (**2.22a**). Rumen contractions are reduced and the abdomen is shrunken consistent with inappetence of several days.

1 What conditions would you consider?
2 What further tests could be undertaken?
3 What actions/treatments would you recommend?
4 What control measures could be taken?

CASE 2.23 You are presented with a 15-month-old pedigree Suffolk ram that drops its cud along with a large volume of ruminal fluid at the start of rumination (**2.23**). The farmer describes this as 'cud spilling' and it has been observed intermittently over the past 3 months. The ram is in much poorer body condition than the other yearlings in the group. The fleece of the ventral neck is stained with regurgitated ruminal contents. The ram has a poor appetite; there is no associated bloat and auscultation of the left flank reveals normal ruminal motility.

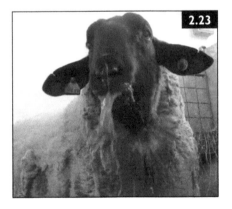

1 What is the cause of this problem (most likely first)?
2 What action would you take?
3 How could you confirm the cause?
4 Is this condition heritable?

165

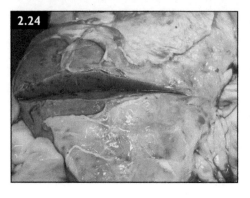

CASE 2.24 During early winter a farmer complains that some yearling sheep purchased 7 weeks ago are in very poor body condition with poor fleece quality despite abundant grazing. On arrival on the farm, the sheep received sequential full-dose treatments with 4-AD monepantel and 3-ML moxidectin. Inspection of other sheep in the group reveals lethargy and reduced grazing activity. Gathering the sheep proved difficult because they were reluctant to run. On clinical examination affected sheep show marked anaemia. One sheep has died this morning and is available for postmortem examination (**2.24**).

1 Describe the important postmortem features.
2 What is the most likely cause?
3 How could this problem be confirmed in other sheep in the group?
4 What action would you take?

CASE 2.25 During summer you are presented with a 4-year-old ewe in very poor body condition (BCS 1.5/5). There are multiple well-circumscribed 5 mm diameter

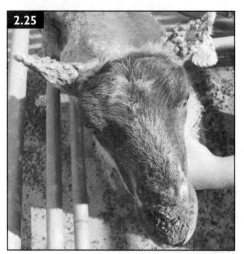

scabs (bottle-brush lesions) around the muzzle, bridge of the nose and on the margins of the ears (**2.25**), which lift off exposing ulcerated skin that bleeds readily.

1 What conditions would you consider (most likely first)?
2 What further tests could be undertaken?
3 What actions/treatments would you recommend?
4 What control measures could be taken?

CASE 2.26 A 4-year-old ewe presents in much poorer body condition (BSC 1.5/5) compared with others in the flock (BCS 3/5). The sheep has a very drawn-in abdomen and appears 'wasp-waisted' (**2.26a**). The ewe is otherwise bright and alert and has a normal appetite. The ewe is afebrile (39.6°C [103.3°F]) but tachypnoeic (48 breaths per minute), with an obvious abdominal component to her breathing. Auscultation of the chest reveals no heart or lung sounds on the right-hand side of the chest but increased heart and normal breath sounds on the left side of the chest. The heart rate, audible on the left side only, is 88 beats per minute.

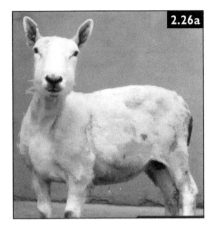

1 What conditions would you consider (most likely first)?
2 How would you investigate this problem further?
3 What treatment would you administer?
4 What is the likely cause?

CASE 2.27 You are presented with a yearling Cheviot ram with mild (3/10) lameness of the right fore leg (**2.27a**). There is considerable muscle atrophy over the scapula of the affected leg but no enlargement of the prescapular lymph node. There are no joint effusions. There is a prominent ridge of bone on the distal humerus and proximal radius of the right elbow, which is not present on the left elbow. Examination of the foot reveals no abnormality.

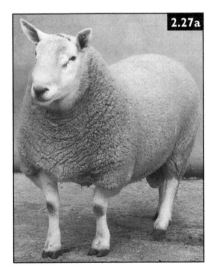

1 What conditions would you consider (most likely first)?
2 What further tests could be undertaken?
3 What actions/treatments would you recommend?
4 What control measures could be taken?

CASE 2.28 A 2-year-old ram presents off colour and inappetent for the past 2 days. The ram is noted lying around more than the other rams in the group, with occasional

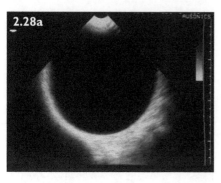

'dog sitting', and shows occasional abdominal straining, but only a few drops of blood-stained urine are voided rather than a continuous flow. Rectal temperature is normal. Heart rate is increased to 100 beats per minute. Mucous membranes are normal. Auscultation of the chest fails to reveal any abnormalities. Rumen fill and motility are reduced. Ultrasonography reveals the bladder to be 16 cm in diameter (**2.28a**).

1 What conditions would you consider (most likely first)?
2 What further investigations could be undertaken?
3 What action would you take?
4 What sequelae could result in neglected cases?
5 What control measures would you recommend?

CASE 2.29 You are presented with a Suffolk ram with a history of moderate shifting leg lameness with effusion of the fetlock joints (**2.29a**). The ram spends a lot of time in lateral recumbency. There are no obvious foot lesions. The ram has lost considerable body condition over the past 2 months. Rectal temperature is elevated (40.2°C [104.4°F]). Heart rate is elevated at 112 beats per minute and the respiratory rate is 45 breaths per minute. No abnormal sounds are heard on auscultation of the lungs and heart.

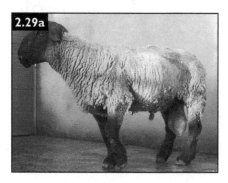

1 What conditions would you consider (most likely first)?
2 How could you confirm your diagnosis?
3 What treatment would you administer?
4 What action would you recommend?
5 What control measures would you recommend?

CASE 2.30 During lambing time a sheep farmer complains that a large number of young lambs have tear staining of the face, leading to blindness in some cases. Closer examination reveals conjunctivitis, episceral injection and corneal oedema in some lambs (**2.30a**).

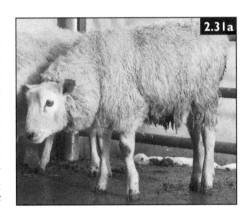

1 What conditions would you consider (most likely first)?
2 What treatments would you administer?
3 What are the consequences of no action/treatment?
4 What preventive measures could be adopted?

CASE 2.31 Four of 200 6-month-old lambs experience difficulty in raising themselves to their feet and have a stilted gait with low head carriage (**2.31a**). Lameness was first noted at 3 months old. All of the lambs have one or both stifle joints affected. Two lambs have bilateral carpal swellings with associated enlargement of the prescapular lymph nodes. There is little joint effusion but marked thickening of the joint capsule (2–3 mm), which physically restricts joint excursion.

1 What conditions would you consider?
2 What is the likely cause?
3 How would you confirm the cause?
4 What treatment would you administer?
5 What control measure(s) would you recommend?

CASE 2.32 A 7-month-old Suffolk-cross lamb presents with severe lameness (10/10) of the left hindleg and marked muscle atrophy over the hip region. There are no joint swellings from the stifle joint distally to the foot. A ventrodorsal view of the pelvis is shown (**2.32a**).

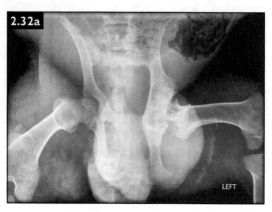

1 Describe the major radiographic changes.
2 What is the likely cause?
3 What treatment would you recommend?

CASE 2.33 A ram presents with a history of chronic weight loss (BCS 2.5/5) when the remainder of the group is within a range of from 3.5/5 to 4/5. The ram has a poor appetite and the rectal temperature is 40.0°C (104°F). At rest the ram is tachypnoeic (40 breaths per minute). Auscultation of the chest reveals no audible lung sounds on the left-hand side of the chest and much reduced heart sounds. Increased audibility of normal heart and lung sounds can be auscultated on the right-hand side of the chest.

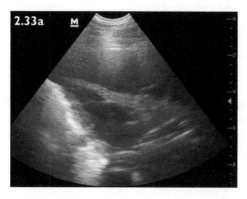

This sonogram (**2.33a**) was obtained from the 6th intercostal space, 5 cm dorsal to the point of the left elbow, using a 5.0 MHz sector transducer (longitudinal plane, dorsal to the left).

1 Describe the sonogram.
2 What is your diagnosis?
3 What treatment(s) would you administer?
4 What is the origin of this pleurisy?

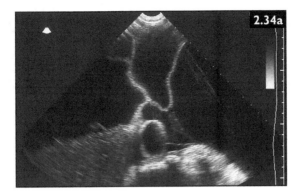

CASE 2.34 This sonogram (**2.34a**) was obtained using a 5 MHz sector scanner placed on the ventral midline immediately caudal to the xiphisternum. The ewe was presented in early winter in very poor condition, inappetent but with abdominal distension. Other recently purchased sheep in the flock were in poor body condition despite free access to good quality grass silage.

1 Describe the important sonographic findings.
2 What tests would you undertake?
3 What causes would you consider?
4 How would you confirm your diagnosis?
5 What treatment(s) would you administer?
6 Are there any control measures to recommend?

CASE 2.35 In the UK, and many other sheep-producing countries, farmers provide sheep with improved nutrition by means of access to a good grass sward for up to 6 weeks before mating (**2.35a**) and during the early breeding season ('flushing').

1 Briefly list the advantages and disadvantages of flushing.
2 List the alternatives that can achieve appropriate body condition scores at mating, and more lambs.

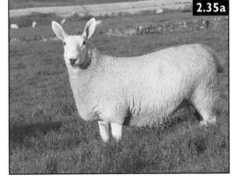

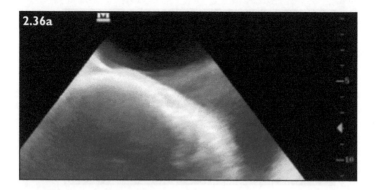

CASE 2.36 You are presented with a 3-month-old pedigree Suffolk ram lamb that has been dull and inappetent for the past 12 hours. The previous day the lamb was observed to frequently kick at its abdomen, lie down then rise again almost immediately. There was frequent bruxism and vocalisation. On clinical examination, the ram has a distended abdomen with a fluid thrill. Rectal temperature is normal. Heart rate is increased at 120 beats per minute. The lamb shows abdominal straining but only a few drops of urine rather than a continuous flow are voided when it urinates. The penis cannot be extruded in such young lambs. A sonogram of the ventral abdomen was obtained (2.36a).

1 Interpret the sonogram.
2 What is your diagnosis?
3 What other structure(s) should be checked sonographically?
4 What further tests could be undertaken?
5 What action would you recommend?

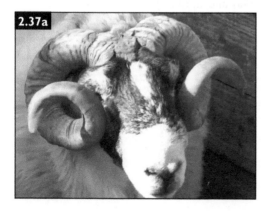

CASE 2.37 You have been asked to blood sample a group of rams for an annual visna-maedi screen. You are presented with the ram shown (2.37a).

1 What concerns you about the ram?
2 What action would you take?
3 What advice would you offer the farmer?

CASE 2.38 You arrive on a sheep farm to find the shepherd happily paring all four feet of all the rams in the flock (2.38a). He reports that foot paring is routinely undertaken every 6 months to prevent footrot.

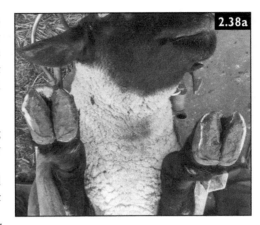

1 Does routine foot paring reduce lameness, especially footrot?
2 Are there any potential disadvantages of routine foot paring?
3 What control strategies could be suggested for footrot in this flock?

CASE 2.39 Necropsy of a 2-month-old lamb reveals lesions of the chest wall (2.39a). A radiograph was obtained at necropsy to show the extent and location of the bony lesions (2.39b).

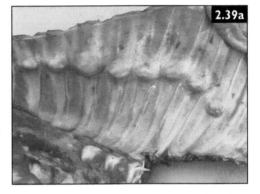

1 What are these lesions?
2 Comment on the welfare of this lamb with respect to these lesions.
3 What is the most likely cause?
4 Apart from difficulty with breathing, what other clinical signs may have been present?
5 How could this problem have been avoided?

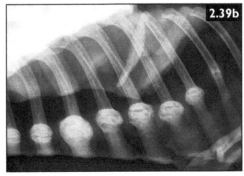

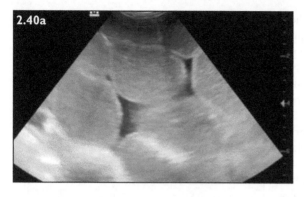

CASE 2.40 A 4-month-old twin pedigree ewe lamb presents with an arched back, distended abdomen and abdominal pain. The lamb is at pasture with its co-twin and dam with *ad-libitum* access to a creep area containing 16% crude protein concentrate. The lamb is dull and is easily caught in the field. On clinical examination, there is marked dehydration (estimated to be >7%) despite a distended abdomen. There is no evidence of diarrhoea. Gentle palpation of the distended abdomen causes pain. Rectal temperature is 39°C (102.2°F). Transabdominal ultrasound examination immediately caudal to the xiphisternum yields the sonogram shown (2.40a).

1 Describe the important sonographic findings.
2 What conditions would you consider (most likely first)?
3 What treatment would you administer?
4 How can this problem be avoided?

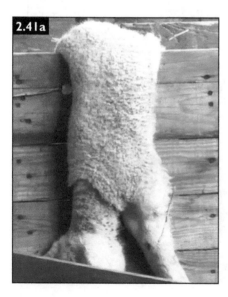

CASE 2.41 Arriving on a sheep and beef farm at lambing time you observe several dead lambs in the lambing shed.

1 What has happened in 2.41a?
2 Is this practice common?
3 What advice must be given to farm staff?
4 Are there any alternatives to this practice?

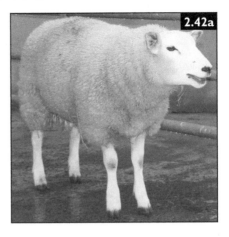

CASE 2.42 A Texel yearling ram presents in severe respiratory distress with its head lowered and the neck extended (**2.42a**). The condition was first noted 2 days ago but has deteriorated rapidly. The ram's respiratory rate is increased to 90 breaths per minute with a loud inspiratory noise (honking sound) audible 25 yards away from the animal. The ram's nostrils are flared and the mouth is held open with the tongue partially protruded and frothy saliva around the mouth and lower jaw. Rectal temperature is 40.2°C (104.4°F). Auscultation over the larynx reveals very loud crackles transferred to the whole lung field. Heart rate is increased to 120 beats per minute.

1 What conditions would you consider (most likely first)?
2 How could you confirm your diagnosis?
3 What actions/treatments would you recommend?
4 What controls measures would you recommend?

CASE 2.43 A 3-day-old 7 kg (15.4 lb) pedigree ram lamb presents with a displaced fracture of the left third metatarsal bone (**2.43a**).

1 How would you achieve effective analgesia for fracture realignment and repair?
2 How would you repair the fracture?
3 What other treatments would you recommend?

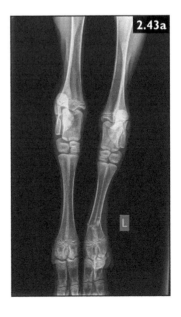

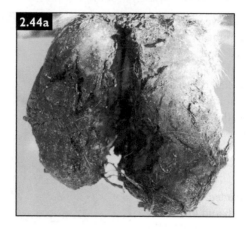

CASE 2.44 During wet and warm summer weather a sheep farmer complains of severe lameness spreading rapidly through his ewes at pasture. Examination of several sheep reveals marked hyperaemia of interdigital skin with superficial accumulations of moist, whitish, necrotic material. There is also separation of the axial hoof horn of the sole from the corium, which is swollen, hyperaemic and covered with a thick white exudate (**2.44a**). There is a characteristic smell of necrotic horn/exudate.

1 What is the likely cause (most likely first)?
2 How is the diagnosis confirmed?
3 What treatment would you administer?
4 What control measures would you include in the flock health plan?

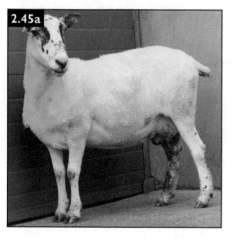

CASE 2.45 During autumn you are asked to examine a two-crop ewe with a large fibrous mass arising from the udder, which bleeds readily as evidenced by blood on the medial aspect of the hindlegs (**2.45a**). The ewe is otherwise well and in excellent body condition.

1 What is the likely cause?
2 What action would you take?
3 What control measures could be adopted?

CASE 2.46 A ewe presents with a history of chronic weight loss (BCS 1.5/5) when the remainder of the group is within a range of from 3.5/5 to 4/5. The ewe has a good appetite and a normal rectal temperature. Auscultation of the chest reveals no abnormality. Mucous membranes appear normal. During the clinical examination, the ewe urinates onto the concrete floor of the pen; the urine is blood-tinged. Urine analysis reveals protein +++ and blood +++

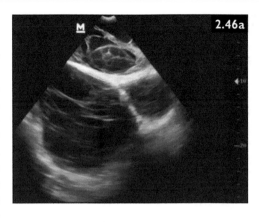

(scale 1–4). There are no flecks of blood or pus on the ewe's tail or hind quarters. A provisional diagnosis of renal neoplasia is reached during ultrasound examination of the caudal abdomen, but a separate structure (**2.46a**) was also obtained from the right inguinal region (5.0 MHz sector transducer).

1 Describe the sonogram.
2 What is this structure (most likely first)?
3 What action would you take?

CASE 2.47 A 4-year-old ewe presents in much poorer body condition (BSC 1.5/5) compared with others in the flock (BCS 3/5). The ewe is bright and alert and has a normal appetite (**2.47a**). The ewe is afebrile (39.6°C [103.3°F]) but tachypnoeic (47 breaths per minute) with an obvious abdominal component

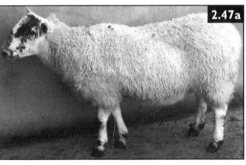

to her breathing. Auscultation of the chest reveals widespread wheezes and crackles, especially distributed anteroventrally on both sides of the chest. Heart rate is 88 beats per minute.

1 What conditions would you consider (most likely first)?
2 How would you confirm the diagnosis?
3 What treatment would you administer?
4 What control measures could be attempted in this flock?

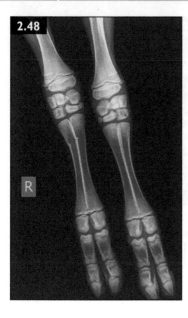

CASE 2.48 You are presented with a valuable pedigree 4-day-old lamb with sudden-onset moderate lameness of the right fore leg. There are no palpable joint swellings and the right prescapular lymph node is normal size. Pain is localised to the metacarpal region. Radiography yields the image shown (**2.48**).

1 What is the cause of the lameness?
2 What other conditions would you consider?
3 How would you correct this problem?

CASE 2.49 Driving to a farm to attend to a lame bull you observe a 4-month-old lamb abruptly stop grazing and turn its head and attempt to nibble at its tail head (**2.49a**). The lamb then suddenly trots away with frequent tail swishing before recommencing grazing. This cycle of abnormal behaviour is repeated several times. The fleece surrounding the lesion appears wet and discoloured.

1 What is the cause (most likely first)?
2 What treatment options would you consider?
3 What control measures would you recommend to the farmer?

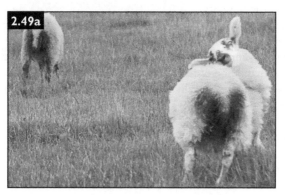

CASE 2.50 You are presented with a pedigree ram that has been dull and inappetent for the past 3 days. The ram adopts a wide stance with the hindlegs placed further back than normal and the head held lowered. There is frequent bruxism. Only a few drops of blood-tinged urine are voided when the ram urinates, rather than a 15–20 second continuous flow. Rectal temperature is normal (39.5°C [103.1°F]). The ram has a poor appetite. Heart rate is increased at 96 beats per minute.

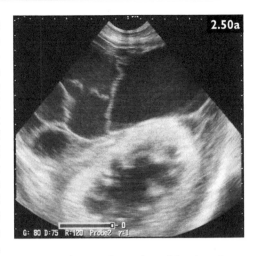

You suspect partial obstructive urolithiasis and scan the right sublumbar fossa with a 5.0 MHz sector transducer connected to a real-time, B-mode ultrasound machine (2.50a).

1 Describe the sonogram.
2 What has caused this problem?
3 What action would you take?
4 How could this problem have been prevented?

CASE 2.51 You are presented with an aged Texel ram with a 'horny' growth in the centre of the poll (2.51).

1 What is the lesion?
2 What is the likely cause?
3 What action would you take?

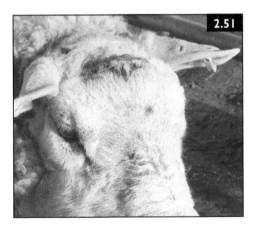

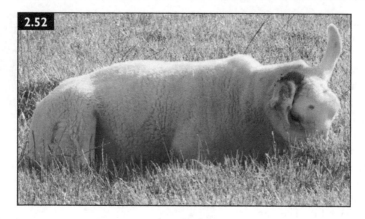

CASE 2.52 In summer a farmer complains that some ewes have lost considerable condition as a consequence of not grazing and lying around with their heads on the ground. The ewes appear distressed and frequently kick at their head with their hindfeet, causing superficial damage to the skin of the poll and ears (**2.52**).

1 What is the cause of this problem (most likely cause first)?
2 How can this problem be controlled?

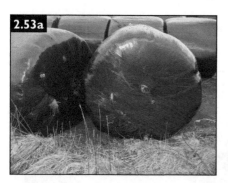

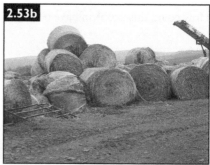

CASE 2.53 You arrive at a mixed beef and sheep farm during late winter, 2 months before lambing time, to examine a lame bull. The flock has just been housed and are bedded on straw (**2.53a**) and fed big bale silage (**2.53b**).

1 Comment on the quality of the straw and any associated disease risks to pregnant ewes.
2 Comment on the silage feeding and any associated disease risks.
3 How can these disease risks be reduced?

CASE 2.54 Having read an article in a magazine for farmers on the value of necropsy examinations in modern sheep farming, a client asks you to necropsy an ewe that died overnight following body condition loss over several months. There is no evidence of diarrhoea on the fleece. The carcass is emaciated and there is a small excess of transudate in the abdominal cavity. There is serous atrophy of fat, most noticeable in the mesentery and epicardial groove. A section of ileum is shown on the left-hand side compared with jejunum on the right side (**2.54a**).

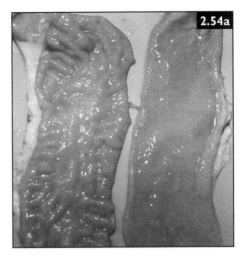

1 What is the most likely cause of this pathology?
2 What has this single necropsy revealed?
3 What advice would you offer?

CASE 2.55 A 4-year-old ewe presents with sudden severe illness (**2.55a**) 2 weeks after housing in late winter and 6 weeks before lambing commences. The ewe is very dull and reluctant to move. Rectal temperature is 41.1°C (106°F). Mucous membranes are markedly congested. The ewe is tachypnoeic (50 breaths per minute) with an obvious

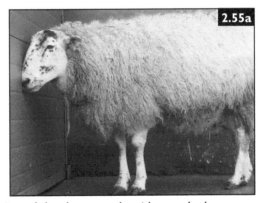

abdominal component. Auscultation of the chest reveals widespread wheezes on both sides of the chest. Heart rate is 124 beats per minute. There are no ruminal contractions.

1 What conditions would you consider?
2 What action would you take?
3 What treatment would you administer?

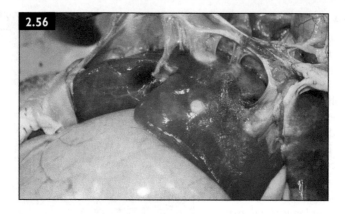

CASE 2.56 You are asked to euthanase, then necropsy, a 3-week-old lamb first noted 5–7 days ago to be dull and in much poorer condition than its co-twin. The lamb had an empty, gaunt appearance and was too easily caught in the field. Treatment with long-acting oxytetracycline has effected no improvement. The significant findings are shown (2.56).

1 What is the cause of this problem?
2 Could this problem have been diagnosed?
3 What treatment should have been given?
4 Could this problem have been prevented?

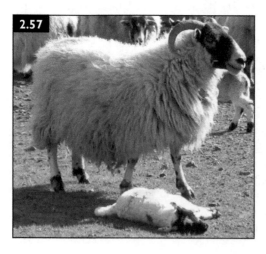

CASE 2.57 You arrive on a sheep farm in the UK in late spring and the farmer is castrating male hill lambs with rubber elastrator rings (2.57). Lambing ended 3 weeks ago.

1 What are you thoughts on this subject?

CASE 2.58 A 6-year-old ewe presents in poor body condition with a history of blindness of several weeks' duration, which was unresponsive to vitamin B_1 administered by the farmer. The ewe is dull and depressed and wanders aimlessly into the pen wall and stands there. Clinical examination reveals bilateral lack of menace response and absence of pupillary light reflexes in both eyes (**2.58a**). There are no abnormalities

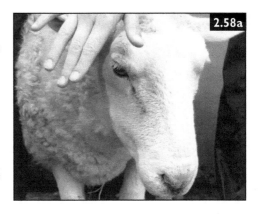

on ophthalmoscopic examination. No other cranial deficits are noted. The ewe is in very poor condition and the sublumbar fossae are very shrunken, consistent with inappetence of several days' duration.

1 What conditions would you consider?
2 What treatment would you administer?
3 What action would you take?

CASE 2.59 After severe winter weather conditions of high winds and driving snow a shepherd complains that a large number of heavily pregnant ewes on hill pastures have poor vision and some appear blind. The ewes are markedly photophobic with blepharospasm and epiphora and tear staining of the cheeks. A less severely affected sheep is shown (**2.59**). Clinical examination reveals injected scleral vessels, conjunctivitis and keratitis.

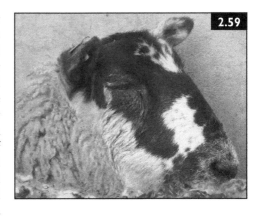

In some eyes there is also corneal ulceration, more clearly observed after fluorescein dye strips have been placed in contact with the eye.

1 What conditions would you consider?
2 What treatments would you recommend?
3 What action would you recommend?

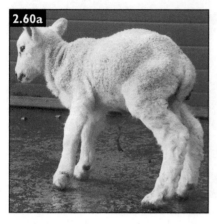

CASE 2.60 A 4-day-old twin lamb presents with an arched back and apparent abdominal pain. The lamb was turned out to pasture with its co-twin and dam at 24 hours old. It was found this morning by the shepherd sheltering behind a hedge. The lamb was dull and easily caught. On clinical examination, there is marked dehydration (estimated to be >7%) despite a distended abdomen (**2.60a**). There is no evidence of diarrhoea. Gentle palpation of the distended abdomen causes pain. Rectal temperature is 37°C (98.6°F).

1 What conditions would you consider (most likely first)?
2 What treatment would you administer?
3 What action should be taken?
4 How can this problem be avoided?

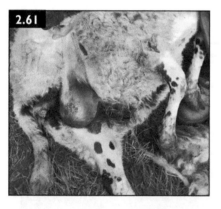

CASE 2.61 You are presented with a ewe in poor body condition (BCS 2/5) that has developed a swollen udder (**2.61**) since weaning 4 months ago. Rectal temperature is normal (39.6°C [103.3°F]). Pulse is 90 beats per minute and respiratory rate is 25 breaths per minute. There are normal ruminal sounds. Examination of the udder reveals marked swelling and hardness of the left gland. There is evidence of wool-slip.

1 What is the likely diagnosis?
2 Are there any consequences of such conditions?
3 What pathogens could be involved?
4 What is the prognosis?
5 What control measures could have been adopted?

CASE 2.62 A 5-crop ewe, scanned for twins and due to lamb in 3 weeks, is found in the corner of the shed unable to raise itself. This group of ewes was housed 3 weeks ago and fed 300 g of concentrates plus *ad-libitum* hay. The ewes were vaccinated against the clostridial diseases 2 days ago. The ewe is dull and unable to rise as you approach (**2.62a**).

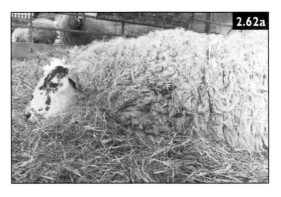

Rectal temperature is normal but the rectum is flaccid and contains a ball of firm faeces. Heart rate is 80 beats per minute. Respiratory rate is 40 breaths per minute. There are no cranial nerve deficits. There is ruminal stasis and slight bloat. The udder is well developed, there is no mastitis and there is no vulval discharge.

1 What conditions would you consider (most likely first)?
2 How could you confirm your diagnosis?
3 What treatment(s) would you administer?
4 What control measures would you recommend?

CASE 2.63 You are presented with an adult sheep that is continually rubbing against pen divisions and nibbling at her fleece overlying the dorsal midline, causing fleece damage/loss (**2.63**). The ewe is in much poorer condition than all the other sheep in the group, which do not show any signs of skin disease. The sheep is bright and alert with a normal appetite.

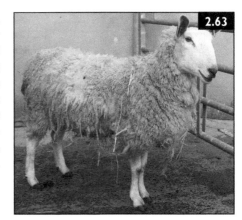

1 What conditions would you consider?
2 How would you establish a specific diagnosis?
3 What treatment would you recommend?
4 What control measures would you recommend?

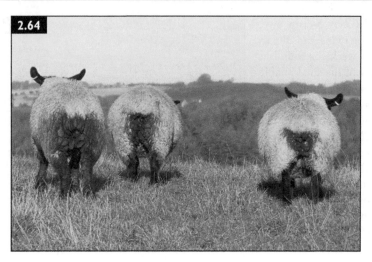

CASE 2.64 Comment on this image (2.64).

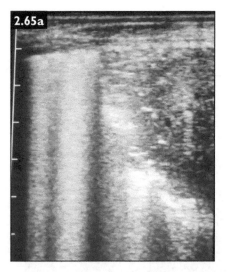

CASE 2.65 A 4-year-old ewe presents in poor body condition (BCS 1.5/5; remainder of the flock are 3.0–3.5/5; normal range 1–5/5). The ewe is bright and alert with a normal appetite. Rectal temperature is 39.6°C (103.3°F). Mucous membranes appear normal. At rest the ewe is tachypnoeic (50 breaths per minute) with an obvious abdominal component. Auscultation of the chest reveals wheezes anteroventrally on both sides of the chest. Heart rate is 96 beats per minute. No other abnormalities are detected on clinical examination. This sonogram (2.65a) was obtained at the sixth intercostal space, just above the point of the left elbow, using a 5 MHz linear scanner (dorsal to the left).

1 Describe the important ultrasound findings.
2 How could you confirm the provisional diagnosis?

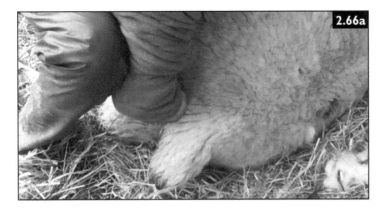

CASE 2.66 You arrive on a sheep farm during lambing time and the shepherd is assisting delivery of a lamb from an ewe experiencing difficulties (**2.66a**).

1 Comment on the hygiene approach to this common scenario.

CASE 2.67 A 3-week-old lamb shows seizure activity. The farmer reports that the lamb was observed in the field walking backwards. Rectal temperature is 40.0°C (104.0°F). The lamb now presents in lateral recumbency with the fore legs held in rigid extension, flexion of the hindlegs and dorsiflexion of the neck (**2.67**). The lamb is hyperaesthetic

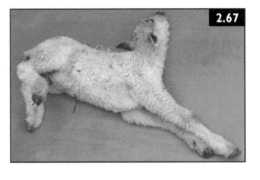

to tactile and auditory stimuli. Gentle forced movement of the neck is resisted. There is episcleral congestion and dorsomedial strabismus. The menace response is absent. There is no umbilical swelling and no joint swellings.

1 What conditions would you consider (most likely first)?
2 How could you confirm your diagnosis?
3 What treatment(s) would you administer?
4 What is the prognosis for this lamb?

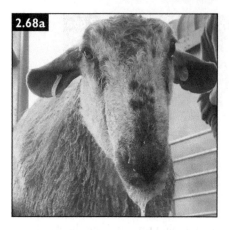

CASE 2.68 During late winter you are presented with an obtunded 2-year-old ram (**2.68a**). The sheep shows drooping of the right ear, deviated muzzle towards the left side, a flaccid right lip and a lowered right upper eyelid (ptosis). There is lack of menace response in the right eye and profuse salivation with a flaccid right cheek with impacted food material.

1 What conditions would you consider (most likely first)?
2 What laboratory tests could be undertaken to confirm your provisional diagnosis?
3 What treatments would you administer?
4 What control measures would you recommend?

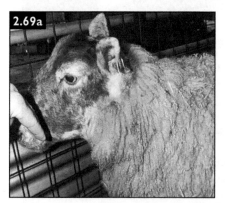

CASE 2.69 A ewe in late pregnancy is reported to be dull and not eating (**2.69a**). There is no menace response but pupillary light reflexes are normal. The ewe is hyperaesthetic to tactile and auditory stimuli. Rectal temperature is normal. The ewes are being fed *ad-libitum* average quality big bale silage plus 200 g/head/day of a 16% crude protein concentrate. The flock is due to start lambing in approximately 2 weeks. The ewe is in poorer body condition (BCS 1.5/5) compared with other sheep in the group at a similar stage of pregnancy (BCS 2.5–3.0/5).

1 What conditions would you consider (most likely first)?
2 How could you confirm your diagnosis?
3 What treatment(s) would you give?
4 What control measures could be adopted?

CASE 2.70 A ram presents with a history of chronic weight loss (BCS 2/5) when the remainder of the group is within a range of from 3.5/5 to 4/5. The ram is at the back of the group when gathered from the field. He appears to have a normal appetite and rectal temperature is 39.8°C (103.6°F). At rest, the ram is tachypnoeic (40 breaths per minute). Auscultation of the chest reveals no adventitious sounds. The heart sounds are reduced on the left hand

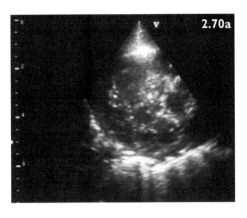

side of the chest. There are no other significant clinical findings. This sonogram (**2.70a**) was obtained from the sixth intercostal space, at the point of the left elbow, using a 5.0 MHz sector transducer (longitudinal plane, dorsal to the left). Similar but smaller lesions were identified in both lungs.

1 Describe the sonogram.
2 What is your diagnosis?
3 What treatment(s) would you administer?
4 What other imaging modality could have been used?

CASE 2.71 A 6-year-old ewe presents in very poor body condition (BCS 1.5/5) while the other sheep in the group have BSCs of 3/5 to 4/5. The ewe has a gaunt appearance and a poor fleece (**2.71a**). Rectal temperature is 39.4°C (102.9°F). Poorly masticated food is often dropped from the mouth ('quidding'). Closer examination reveals a lot of roughage impacted in the cheeks.

1 What conditions would you consider (most likely first)?
2 How would you investigate this problem?
3 What actions/treatments would you recommend?

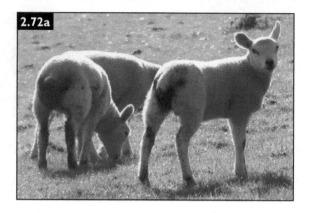

2.72a

CASE 2.72 A farmer reports diarrhoea and rapid weight loss over the past 2–3 days in a large percentage of 8-week-old lambs grazing permanent pasture (2.72a).

1 What common conditions would you consider (most likely first)?
2 What tests could be undertaken to support your provisional diagnosis?
3 What control measures would you recommend?

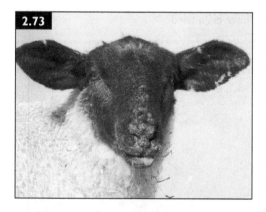

2.73

CASE 2.73 A farmer complains of skin lesions on the muzzle and lips of approximately 25% of 120 6-month-old lambs 10–14 days after movement onto pastures containing large numbers of thistles (this field is a site of special scientific interest). The skin is oedematous with excoriation of lesions where they contact the ground during grazing (2.73).

1 What conditions would you consider (most likely first)?
2 What treatment would you administer?
3 What samples would you collect to confirm your diagnosis?
4 What preventive measures could be considered for next year?

CASE 2.74 A farmer complains that 10 of 30 pedigree Texel lambs have abnormal eyes (**2.74**) and are blind. All affected lambs are thought to be the progeny of a pedigree ram used for the first time in the flock.

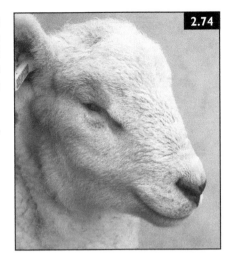

1 What is the likely cause (most likely first)?
2 What action would you take?
3 What advice would you offer?

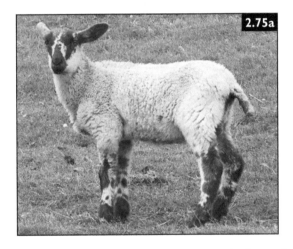

CASE 2.75 A 10-week-old lamb presents in very poor body condition with a poor fleece (**2.75a**). The lamb is depressed, dehydrated and frequently stands over the water trough. Rectal temperature is normal. Its co-twin, and other lambs in the group, appear healthy and are growing well.

1 What conditions would you consider?
2 How would you confirm your diagnosis?
3 What is the prognosis for this lamb?
4 What control measures would you recommend?

191

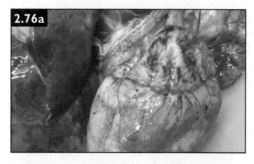

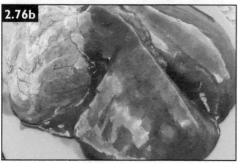

CASE 2.76 A 4-week-old lamb is found dead without premonitory signs. The lamb is in excellent body condition. The significant necropsy findings are restricted to the chest (**2.76a, b**).

1 Describe the important necropsy findings shown.
2 What is the most likely cause?
3 How could you confirm your suspicion?
4 What control measures could be adopted?

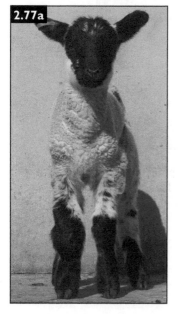

CASE 2.77 During lambing time you are presented with a 12-day-old lamb with non-weight-bearing lameness of the left fore leg of 5 days' duration (**2.77a**). This lamb, and four similarly affected lambs, have been treated with oxytetracycline by the farmer without improvement in the past week. The lamb's rectal temperature is normal. There are joint swellings of the left elbow and right carpus, with swollen prescapular lymph nodes. The umbilical stump is dry and brittle.

1 What is your diagnosis (most likely first)?
2 How would you confirm your diagnosis?
3 What treatments would you administer?
4 What preventive measures could be adopted?

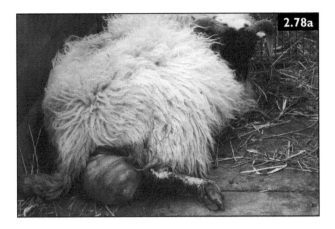

CASE 2.78 You are presented with a collapsed ewe with a vaginal prolapse 3 weeks prior to lambing (**2.78a**).

1 How will you deal with this case?
2 What is the future management of this sheep?

CASE 2.79 You are presented with a recumbent yearling sheep at pasture (**2.79a**). The previous day the farmer noted that the sheep was blind and wandered aimlessly and appeared to be 'star-gazing'. On veterinary examination, the sheep is hyperaesthetic to auditory and tactile stimuli, which precipitate seizure activity. Dorsomedial strabismus and spontaneous horizontal nystagmus are present. There is no menace response in either eye. No other abnormalities are detected on clinical examination.

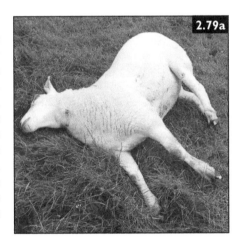

1 What conditions would you consider?
2 What treatment would you administer?
3 What is the prognosis for this case?
4 How can the diagnosis be confirmed?
5 What control measures would you recommend?

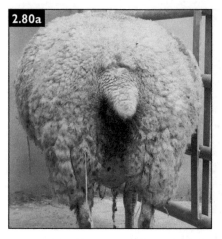

CASE 2.80 During early summer a pedigree 4-year-old ewe nursing 2-month-old twin lambs presents with an arched back and a markedly distended abdomen (**2.80a**). The ewe has been moved to lush pasture 2 days ago and is also fed 1 kg of a 16% crude protein concentrate once daily. The ewe is dull and easily restrained. On clinical examination there is marked dehydration (estimated to be >7%) with toxic mucous membranes. There is no evidence of diarrhoea. Heart rate is 124 beats per minute and the respiratory rate is shallow at a rate of 46 breaths per minute. Gentle palpation of the distended abdomen causes pain. Rectal temperature is 39.5°C (103.1°F).

1 What conditions would you consider (most likely first)?
2 What further investigations would you undertake?
3 What treatment would you administer?
4 How can this problem be avoided?

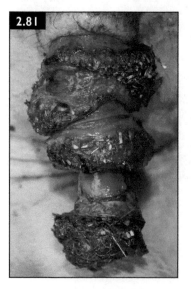

CASE 2.81 During the breeding season you are presented with a ram with paraphimosis (**2.81**) with oedematous folds on the surface of the penis and secondary bacterial infection.

1 What is the cause of this problem?
2 What action would you take?
3 What treatment would you administer?
4 What is the prognosis?

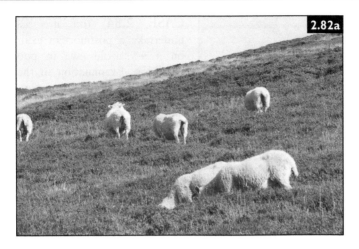

CASE 2.82 After weaning, ewes rearing lambs for meat are often turned out onto poor quality grazing (**2.82a**) or grazed at very high stocking densities.

1 What is the reasoning behind this management decision?
2 What are the alternative management strategies?

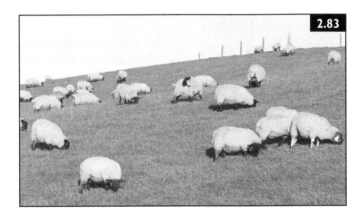

CASE 2.83 During late summer a client asks for advice regarding internal parasite control for 400 purchased store lambs that will graze silage aftermath for approximately 3 months (**2.83**). Any lambs not reaching market weights will then be housed and fattened intensively on cereals; margins are tight.

1 What advice would you give?

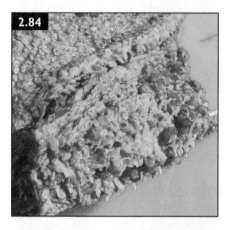

CASE 2.84 You are asked to undertake a postmortem examination on a 4-year-old ewe in poor body condition. Examination of the rumen wall identifies the structures shown (**2.84**).

1 What are these lesions?
2 Are these lesions important?
3 What action would you recommend?

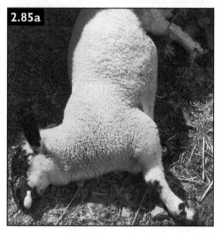

CASE 2.85 A 4-month-old ewe lamb is found dead without premonitory signs; the ewes and lambs had been checked the previous morning and no sick sheep were observed. The lamb is in excellent body condition. The only finding is the presence of frothy saliva at the mouth (**2.85a**).

1 What conditions can cause sudden death in growing lambs (most likely first)?
2 How could you confirm your suspicion?
3 What control measures could be adopted?

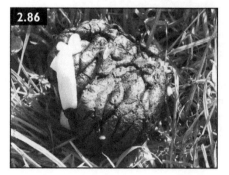

CASE 2.86 A sheep farmer comments that he has seen ribbon-like segments in the faeces of many of his 3-month-old lambs (**2.86**).

1 What are these ribbon-like segments?
2 What action is necessary?
3 What control measures would you recommend?

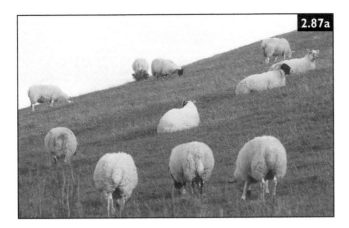

CASE 2.87 During early autumn, 1 month ahead of the breeding season, a sheep farmer asks about anthelmintic treatment of his ewes pre-tupping (**2.87a**).

1 What advice would you give?

CASE 2.88 A ewe presents with a history of chronic weight loss (BCS 1.5/5) when the remainder of the group is within a range of from 3.5/5 to 4/5. The ewe has a good appetite and a normal rectal temperature. Auscultation of the chest reveals no abnormality. During the examination, the ewe urinates onto the concrete floor of the pen; the urine is blood-tinged. Urinalysis reveals protein +++ and blood +++ (scale + to

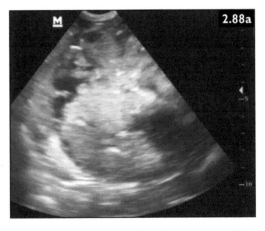

++++). There are no flecks of blood or pus on the ewe's tail or hindquarters. This sonogram (**2.88a**) was obtained from the right inguinal region with the 5.0 MHz sector transducer pointed vertically towards the tailhead of the ewe.

1 Describe the sonogram.
2 What is this structure (most likely first)?
3 What action would you take?

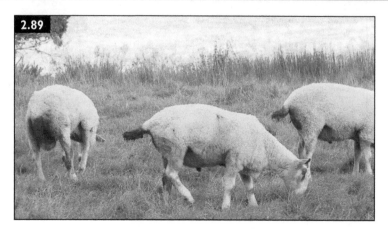

CASE 2.89 During mid-summer you are driving to a sheep and beef farm and notice that the rams are all scouring and appear to be in poor condition (**2.89**). The 20 rams graze the same 4-hectare field every year.

1 What common conditions would you consider (most likely first)?
2 What tests could be undertaken to support your provisional diagnosis?
3 What control measures would you recommend?

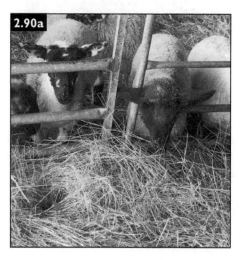

CASE 2.90 A sheep farmer houses his sheepdogs in the same building used for rearing orphan lambs. The dogs, including a litter of young puppies, frequently defecate in the hay offered to these lambs (**2.90a**, arrow).

1 Are there any risks to these young lambs?
2 What clinical signs would be expected?
3 What signs may be noted in these lambs at slaughter?
4 What simple hygiene measures would you recommend?

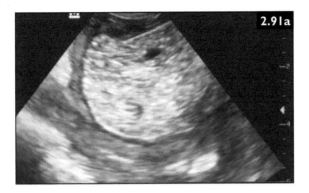

CASE 2.91 During clinical examination of an aged ewe in poor body condition two small masses can be palpated in the ventral abdomen. Ultrasound examination reveals four 3–4 cm diameter lesions (**2.91a**).

1 What is the lesion shown in the sonogram (most likely first)?
2 What is the significance of these lesions?
3 What action would you recommend?

CASE 2.92 Two weeks after weaning and turnout onto lush grazing, a 5-month-old hill lamb is found isolated from the group and appears very dull and is easily caught. The lamb is in good condition. There is frothy saliva at the mouth (**2.92a**) and the mucous membranes are congested. Rectal temperature is 40.8°C (105.4°F). Auscultation of the chest fails to reveal any adventitious sounds, although the respiratory rate is increased to 40 breaths per minute. There is evidence of recent diarrhoea, although the lambs were treated with a Group 4 anthelmintic (monepantel) when turned onto this safe grazing.

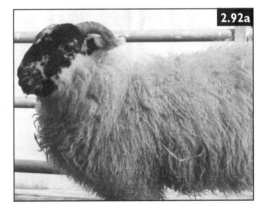

1 What conditions would you consider (most likely first)?
2 What treatment would you administer?
3 What control measures could be adopted?

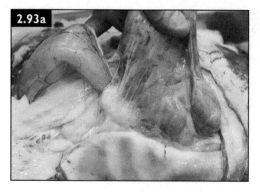

CASE 2.93 You are asked to necropsy a week-old twin lamb that was found dead in the field this morning. There is no milk in the abomasum and the lack of carcass fat is consistent with death from starvation/mismothering/ exposure. The other important findings are shown (**2.93a**).

1 What is the cause of this problem?
2 Where would you extend your necropsy examination?
3 Could this problem have been prevented?

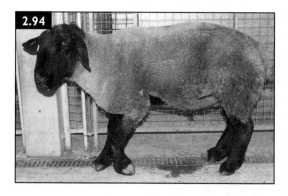

CASE 2.94 Towards the end of the breeding season a pedigree ram presents suddenly lame on the left fore leg, with weight taken on the dorsal surface of the hoof (**2.94**). The ram is at pasture with 120 ewes and two other rams. The farmer thinks that the rams have simply been fighting and elects to do nothing. One week later the ram is still unable to fully extend the left fore leg and bear weight. The ram was fitted with a keel harness, which may have been too tight, as there are pressure sores. The ram is eating normally, although it has lost considerable body condition. There is obvious loss of muscle over the scapula, with a more prominent spine than on the right side. There is a dropped elbow, flexion of the distal limb joints and scuffing of the hooves as the left leg is moved forward. The foot remains knuckled over at rest. The left prescapular lymph node is not swollen. There is no pain on careful manipulation of the leg.

1 What conditions would you consider (most likely first)?
2 What treatment(s) would you administer?
3 What is the prognosis for this ram?

CASE 2.95 While on a sheep farm in winter you are presented with a yearling sheep with no ears (**2.95a**). The sheep is in excellent condition.

1 What has happened to this sheep?
2 Could anything have been done to prevent this situation?
3 Should this sheep be kept for future breeding?

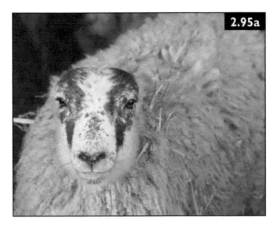

CASE 2.96 You are presented with an aged ewe with severe (10/10) lameness of the right hindleg and extensive muscle atrophy over the hip region. There is marked thickening of the joint capsule but no palpable effusion of the stifle joint; no other joint feels abnormal. Based on these clinical findings the ewe is euthanased for welfare reasons and lateral and dorsoplantar radiographs obtained of the right stifle region (**2.96a, b**).

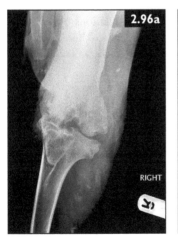

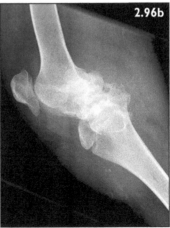

1 Comment on the radiographs.
2 Comment on the animal welfare implications of these findings.
3 What are the expected necropsy findings?
4 What advice should be given to the farmer?

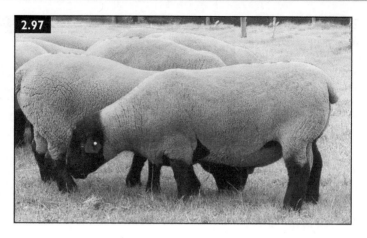

CASE 2.97 A sheep client is keen to show off his recent purchase of eight rams from prominent breeders (2.97).

1 What advice would you offer regarding flock biosecurity?

CASE 2.98 During wet warm summer weather a sheep farmer complains that many of his lambs have gone suddenly lame and are grazing on their knees. Examination of several lambs reveals superficial accumulations of moist, whitish, necrotic material on the hyperaemic interdigital skin (2.98a). There is no separation of the axial hoof horn of the sole from the corium. There are no palpable joint swellings.

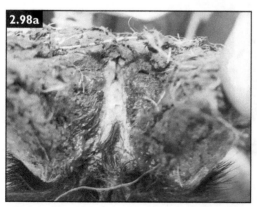

1 What is the likely cause (most likely first)?
2 What treatment would you administer?
3 What control measures would you include in the flock health plan?

CASE 2.99 You are presented with a ewe with a cervicovaginal prolapse and fetal membranes protruding through the cervix, indicating impending abortion/parturition (**2.99a**). There is no foetid vaginal discharge. The ewe is shown in right lateral recumbency and preparations are underway for surgery.

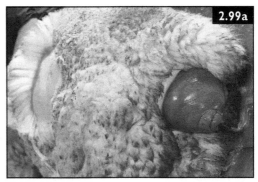

1 Do you agree with the decision to undertake a caesarean operation?
2 What anaesthetic protocol would you adopt?

CASE 2.100 A Suffolk ram presents with severe lameness (10/10) of the left hindleg and marked muscle atrophy over the hip region. The left hindfoot is swollen with marked widening of the interdigital space. There is loss of hair and thinning of the skin all around the coronary band of the medial claw, extending proximally for 1.5 cm (**2.100a**).

1 What conditions would you consider?
2 How would you confirm your diagnosis?
3 How long has this ram been lame?
4 What treatment would you recommend?

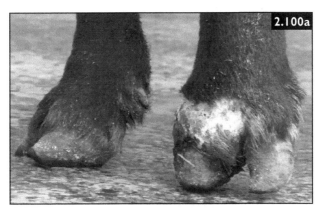

CASE 2.101 You are presented with a valuable 1-month-old ram lamb with severe (9/10) lameness of the right fore leg and extensive muscle atrophy over the scapula. There is thickening of the joint capsule of the shoulder and elbow joints but no obvious effusion. The

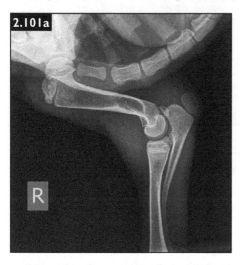

right prescapular lymph node is markedly enlarged. All other joints feel normal. The lamb has been treated for the past 5 consecutive days with penicillin injected IM. A lateral radiograph of the right fore leg is obtained (**2.101a**).

1 Comment on the radiograph.
2 What action would you take?

CASE 2.102 During winter you are presented with a group of 120 yearling sheep, many of which are very uncomfortable and nibble at their flanks and rub themselves against the pen divisions. Some ewes appear in considerable distress and kick at themselves with their hindfeet, causing fleece loss over the shoulder region (**2.102a**). The fleece is wet, sticky and yellow with serum exudation.

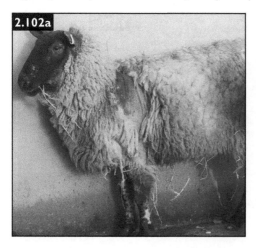

1 What conditions would you consider?
2 How would you confirm the diagnosis?
3 What treatment would you administer?
4 What control measures could be adopted?

204

CASE 2.103 During lambing time a farmer with a prolific sheep flock complains that approximately 10–15% of twin lambs are much smaller than their co-twins (**2.103**) despite adequate energy feeding during late gestation. The ewes appear to be in adequate body condition (BCS 2.5/5).

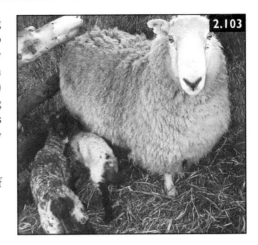

1 What are the possible causes of this problem?
2 What action can be taken?

CASE 2.104 Before the start of the breeding season you are asked to check the breeding soundness of 22 rams on a sheep farm. The rams are in excellent body condition and there is no lameness in the group. Palpating the scrotum of an aged ram reveals a bilobed structure in each side of the scrotum, with each lobe measuring approximately 5 cm in diameter. These bilobed structures are firmly adherent to vaginal tunics lining the scrotum; the skin of the scrotum is thickened and slightly oedematous. A sonogram was obtained of the distal mass of these bilobed structures (**2.104a**; proximal to the left).

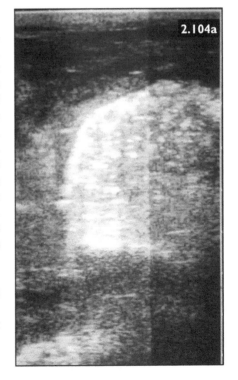

1 Describe the important features in the sonogram.
2 What conditions would you consider (most likely first)?
3 What action would you take?

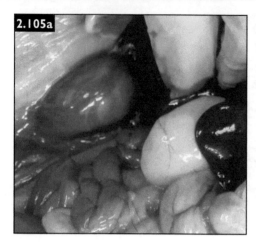

CASE 2.105 You are asked to necropsy several neonatal lambs by a sheep farmer who is experiencing losses at lambing time. A consistent finding in the necropsies is highlighted (**2.105a**).

1 What is the significant finding?
2 What other supporting evidence would you check for in the cadaver?
3 What other supporting evidence would you check for on the farm?

CASE 2.106 A farmer complains of a large proliferative skin lesion on one leg only extending proximally from the coronary band (**2.106**) and causing severe lameness in two of 120 purchased 8-month-old lambs. These lesions were first noted approximately 1 month after movement onto pastures containing large numbers of thistles. Examination of both lambs reveals that the large granulomatous mass extends 4 cm proximally from the coronary band and bleeds profusely when traumatised.

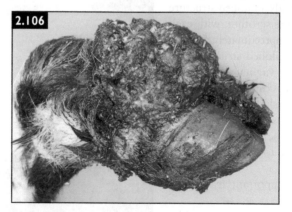

1 What conditions would you consider (most likely first)?
2 What treatments would you administer?
3 What samples would you collect?
4 What preventive measures could be considered for next year?

CASE 2.107 You are presented with a twin-bearing ewe with a vaginal prolapse 2 weeks prior to lambing. There is marked oedema of vaginal mucosa and vulva (**2.107a**).

1 How will you deal with this case?
2 What is the future management of this sheep?

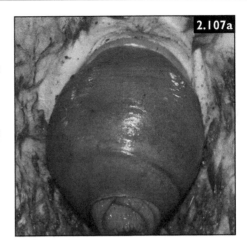

CASE 2.108 During autumn you are asked to investigate several sudden deaths in a flock over the past week. The breeding season started 6 weeks ago. The farmer suspects the losses are caused by ovine pulmonary adenocarcinoma. Unfortunately, no carcasses are available for necropsy, although one ewe is dull and depressed and is presented for examination at the veterinary surgery. Transthoracic ultrasound examination of the lungs using a 5 MHz sector scanner reveals no abnormality, but this sonogram (**2.108a**) was obtained from the right-hand side of the lower cranial abdomen.

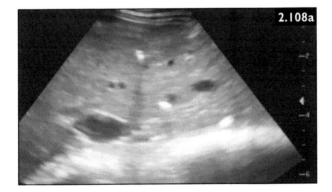

1 Describe the important sonographic findings.
2 What tests would you undertake?
3 What treatment(s) would you administer?
4 What could be a major consequence of this problem?

CASE 2.109 During early summer you are presented with a 2-month-old lamb with tetraparesis of approximately 2-weeks' duration (**2.109a**). Rectal temperature is normal. There are no joint swellings and no swollen lymph nodes. The reflex arcs are reduced in the hindlegs (**2.109b**). There is no evidence of cervical pain and no subcutaneous swelling in the neck region.

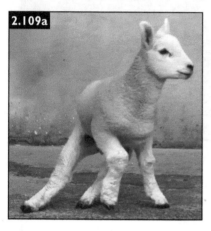

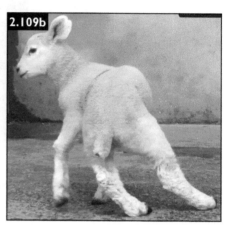

1 What is your diagnosis (most likely first)?
2 What treatments would you administer?
3 How could you confirm your diagnosis?
4 What preventive measures could be adopted?

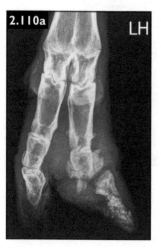

CASE 2.110 A pedigree ram presents with severe lameness (10/10) of the left hindleg, with marked muscle atrophy over the hip region. The left hindfoot is swollen, with marked widening of the interdigital space. There is loss of hair and thinning of the skin around the coronary band of the lateral claw, extending proximally for 1.5 cm. A dorsoplantar radiograph is obtained (**2.110a**).

1 Comment on the major radiographic findings.
2 What condition would you consider?
3 How long has this ram been lame?
4 What treatment would you recommend?

CASE 2.111 A potentially valuable 2-month-old pedigree ram lamb is bright and alert but unable to use its hindlegs and adopts a dog-sitting position (**2.111a**). The fore leg reflexes are normal, while there are increased reflexes in the hindlegs. The flock is intensively managed and has been housed since before lambing time. The farm dogs are kennelled in the corner of the

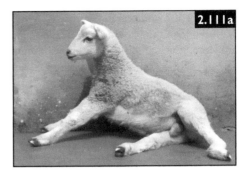

sheep shed. The lamb has exhibited no abnormalities until noted by the farmer 2 days ago; no other sheep show similar signs. The lamb has been treated with procaine penicillin but without improvement.

1 What conditions would you consider (most likely first)?
2 How would you confirm your diagnosis?
3 What action would you take?

CASE 2.112 You are asked your opinion on the skull of an aged Soay ewe (**2.112a, b**). There are no dental abnormalities.

1 What are the important features?
2 What clinical signs would this sheep have presented with?
3 What advice would you offer?

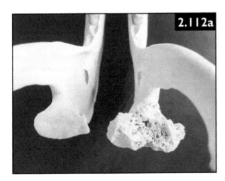

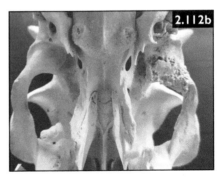

CASE 2.113 A ram presents with a 1.5 cm diameter red growth beneath the hoof horn of the toe of the lateral claw of the right fore foot (**2.113a**). The lesion is non-painful and attached to the corium by a 5 mm stalk.

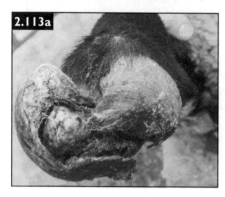

1 What might this mass be (most likely first)?
2 What factors contribute to this condition?
3 What would you do to correct this problem?
4 What advice would you offer about future control?

CASE 2.114 A ewe is found separated from the remainder of the group of lambing ewes. On clinical examination the ewe is very dull and depressed with an elevated rectal temperature (40.5°C [104.9°F]). Mucous membranes are congested. Heart rate is 130 beats per minute. The abdomen is markedly distended (**2.114a**). The udder is well developed and there is some accumulated colostrum in the glands. There is no vaginal discharge; digital examination of the posterior reproductive tract is restricted by the normal (undilated) vulva.

1 What is your differential diagnosis?
2 What further tests could be carried out?
3 What treatment/action would you consider?
4 What investigations would you undertake?

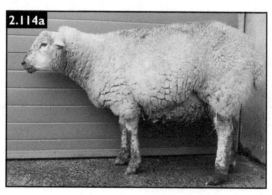

CASE 2.115 During early winter a farmer reports that a large percentage of his yearling sheep grazing permanent pasture have diarrhoea with faecal staining of the perineum (**2.115**). The sheep have lost considerable body condition over the past 4 weeks.

1 What conditions would you consider (most likely first)?
2 How would you investigate this problem?
3 What action would you take?

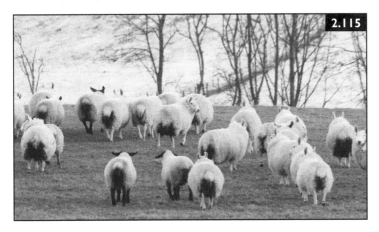

CASE 2.116 You are presented with a ewe that had an assisted lambing 2 hours ago. Severe tenesmus has caused a uterine prolapse (**2.116**).

1 How will you deal with this case?

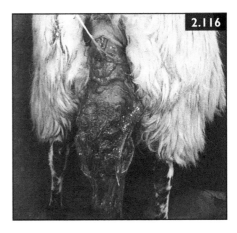

CASE 2.117 A sheep farmer asks you to prepare a vasectomised ram ahead of the breeding season.

1 List the potential advantages of management systems using a vasectomised ram.
2 What analgesia/anaesthesia would you employ?
3 How is the vas deferens identified during surgery?
4 How is successful vasectomy confirmed?
5 What is the minimal interval between vasectomy and introduction of the teaser ram to a group of ewes?

CASE 2.118 A 2-month-old twin lamb is bright and alert but unable to use its hindlegs and adopts a dog-sitting position (**2.118a**). The lamb has exhibited no abnormalities until noted by the farmer 3 days ago. The lamb has been treated for 3 consecutive days with procaine penicillin but without improvement. Examination of the lamb reveals no ticks.

1 What conditions would you consider (most likely first)?
2 What is the origin of this problem?
3 What is the significance of no ticks on the lamb?
4 What treatments would you now administer?
5 How can this condition be prevented?

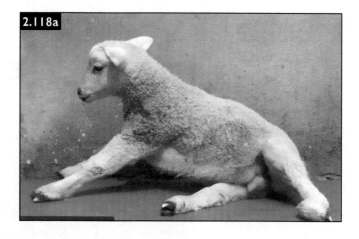

2.118a

CASE 2.119 A 3-month-old lamb presents with a head tilt towards the right side and spontaneous horizontal nystagmus, with the fast phase directed towards the left side (**2.119**). There is no circling behaviour. Ventral strabismus (eye drop) is present on the right side. Damage to the right facial nerve has resulted in drooping of the right upper eyelid and drooping of the right ear.

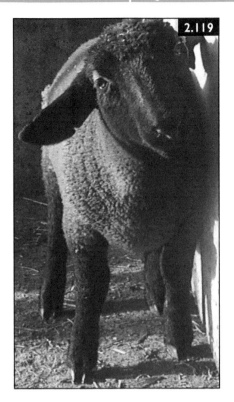

1 What conditions would you consider (most likely first)?
2 What is the likely cause?
3 What treatment would you administer?
4 What is the prognosis for this case?

CASE 2.120 Halfway through lambing time a sheep client complains of high morbidity and mortality in 24–36-hour-old lambs showing excess salivation with a wet lower jaw, cold mouth and poor suck reflex, and retained meconium (**2.120**). There is progressive abdominal distension with fluid and gas. Rectal temperature is subnormal. There is dehydration and poor peripheral perfusion, with cold extremities and a rapid weak pulse during the agonal stages.

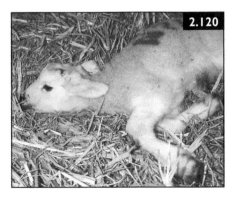

1 What conditions would you consider?
2 What treatments would you recommend?
3 What control measures would you instigate?

213

CASE 2.121 Comment on the welfare of this group of fattening lambs at the end of winter (**2.121a**).

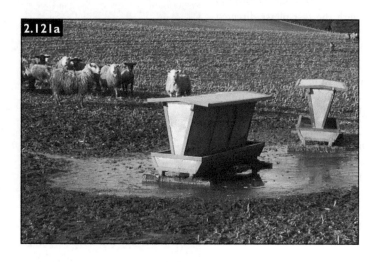

CASE 2.122 During autumn several weaned 6-month-old lambs present in very poor body condition and show depression extending to stupor (**2.122**) and aimless wandering. Many of the other lambs in the group are lethargic with a poor appetite, have poor wool quality with an open fleece, and are in very poor body condition despite adequate nutrition. Some lambs show epiphora with tear staining of the cheeks.

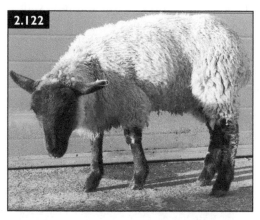

1 What conditions would you consider (most likely first)?
2 How would you investigate this problem?
3 What treatment will you administer?
4 How would you prevent this problem recurring next year?

CASE 2.123 A sheep farmer complains that several of his ewes are losing their fleece soon after lambing (**2.123**) and well before normal shearing time in 3 months time. On clinical examination, there is no inflammation of the skin, no serum exudation, no excoriation and no pruritus. No lice are visible and skin scrapings for *Psoroptes ovis* are negative.

1 What is the cause of this condition?
2 What action would you take?

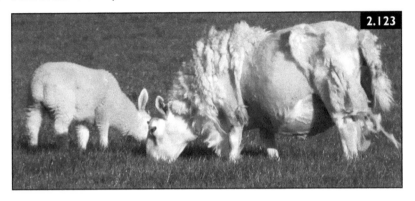

CASE 2.1

1 What common problems could cause sudden death in these weaned unvaccinated lambs (most likely first)? Include: acidosis; septicaemic pasteurellosis; pulpy kidney, struck; acute fasciolosis/black disease; parasitic gastroenteritis (especially *Trichostrongylus vitrinus*).

2 How could you confirm your provisional diagnosis? Postmortem examination of two lambs reveals rancid fluid ruminal contents ('soupy consistency') containing large amounts of barley. The rumen pH value is 5.0 (normal >6.5). The contents of the remainder of the intestines are fluid-filled. There are no significant lung/liver lesions. No glucosuria (a useful field test for pulpy kidney) is detected. Faecal worm egg counts are 100–150 epg.

3 What treatments would you consider? The relatively low economic value of fattening lambs limits treatment considerations to 3–5 consecutive days of IM penicillin injection and a single IV injection of thiamine or multivitamin preparation. Penicillin would be effective against a bacteraemia arising following rumenitis, while multivitamin preparations are believed to aid liver function. The role of bicarbonate-spiked IV fluids (5–10 mEq/kg bicarbonate in 3 litres saline over 3 hours) in recumbent (acidotic?) sheep is cost-prohibitive in most situations. Alternatively, sodium bicarbonate (10–20 g) and activated charcoal can be given by orogastric tube in 5 litres of water. The lambs must be vaccinated against clostridial disease immediately.

4 What control measures would you recommend? Options that could be considered include adding shredded beet pulp in the ration. The following suggestions are not readily applicable to hopper feeding:

- Reduce the ration to 100 g per day immediately.
- Steadily increase the concentrate feeding by 50 g/week ensuring that all feed is eaten with 10 minutes.
- Provide ration *ad libitum* once all sheep are consuming approximately 250 g/head/day.

CASE 2.2

1 What conditions would you consider (most likely first)? Include: atresia ani/coli; watery mouth disease (endotoxaemia); bladder distension after urethral constriction by an elastrator ring placed around the penis proximal to the neck of the scrotum; abomasal bloat or volvulus.

2 What action would you take? Clinical examination reveals that the lamb has no anus. A soft swelling is present under the skin where the anus should be.

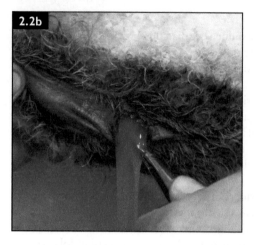

Administer a caudal block using 0.3 ml of 2% lidocaine solution at the first intercoccygeal or sacrococcygeal site using a 23 gauge 5/8 inch needle. A stab incision is made over the skin bulge with a 15T surgical blade. Incision of the skin bulge releases a large amount of mucoid material (2.2b). The farmer was advised to gently insert a thermometer into the rectum twice daily for the next 7 days to prevent stricture of the incision site. The lamb was treated with procaine penicillin (15 mg/kg IM q24h for 5 consecutive days). The lamb made an uneventful recovery.

Atresia ani is much more common in lambs than calves, whereas atresia coli is more common in calves, although it is possible that cases of atresia coli in lambs are not recognised/presented to veterinary practitioners.

CASE 2.3

1 What common problems would you consider (most likely first)? Actinobacillosis; caseous lymphadenitis (CLA).

Actinobacillosis is caused by the gram-negative rod *Actinobacillus lignieresi*. A number of cases of abscesses affecting the face may be encountered when sheep graze pastures containing spiky plants. Unlike CLA, the lesions are in the skin rather than in the parotid or submandibular lymph nodes.

2 Are there any consequences to this infection? Enlargement of the retropharyngeal lymph nodes may compress the larynx, causing stertor, but this is rare.

3 How is the diagnosis confirmed? Diagnosis is based on clinical findings and confirmed following bacterial culture.

4 What treatment(s) are necessary? When confined to the subcutaneous tissue of the face, the abscesses cause few problems. Antibiotic therapy is not necessary, nor would antibiotics penetrate the fibrous capsule of these abscesses. Lancing such abscesses is not necessary, as they will eventually discharge themselves, and is contraindicated in countries with endemic CLA in case the skin lesions are caused by CLA, with consequent environmental contamination.

Sheep with stertor caused by compression of the larynx associated with enlargement of the drainage retropharyngeal lymph nodes should be treated with a soluble corticosteroid to reduce associated swelling and procaine penicillin (15 mg/kg daily for at least 10 consecutive days) (time-dependent antibiotic).

CASE 2.4

1 What conditions would you consider? The most likely conditions to consider include: adenocarcinoma of the small intestine with transcoelomic spread impairing lymphatic drainage and causing ascites; ascites as a consequence of low serum albumin concentration (e.g. chronic paratuberculosis); ascites as a sequela to right-sided heart failure; chronic fasciolosis, but only one sheep affected; chronic peritonitis.

2 What further tests would you undertake? Serum protein analysis reveals marginally low albumin concentration (26 g/l [2.6 g/dl]) but normal globulin concentration (46 g/l [4.6 g/dl]). There is no evidence of either a protein-losing enteropathy (such as paratuberculosis) or chronic bacterial infection from these serum protein concentrations. Peritoneal fluid analysis reveals a modified transudate (protein concentration 34.8 g/l [3.48 g/dl]) with a large number of carcinoma cells on cytospin.

3 What is your diagnosis, and what treatment would you administer? Euthanasia for welfare reasons is indicated after the diagnosis of adenocarcinoma of the small intestine. Necropsy reveals a large tumour with transcoelomic spread to the omentum, abdominal wall, liver and diaphragm (**2.4b**). Blockage of lymphatic drainage led to the ascites observed in this case.

4 What is the likely cause? An association with bracken ingestion has been suggested but is unproven; this sheep had no access to bracken.

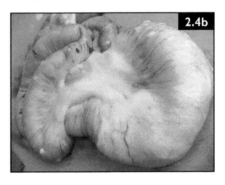

2.4b

CASE 2.5

1 What is your provisional diagnosis (most likely first)? The most likely conditions to affect individual sheep include: Johne's disease (paratuberculosis); subacute fasciolosis – these sheep may not have been drenched correctly; haemonchosis – these sheep may not have been drenched correctly; chronic suppurative pneumonia or other septic focus; poor molar dentition; intestinal tumour.

2 What tests would you undertake? Sheep with advanced Johne's disease have profound hypoalbuminaemia (serum values <15 g/l [1.5 g/dl]; normal range >30 g/l [3 g/dl]) and normal globulin concentration, but these protein concentrations may very occasionally be encountered in cases of severe chronic parasitism. Typically, in chronic fasciolosis and chronic bacterial infection there is hypoalbuminaemia (<25 g/l [2.5 g/dl]) and a marked increase in serum globulin concentration (>55 g/l [5.5 g/dl]; normal range <45 g/l 4.5 g/dl]). Serum protein values in this ewe are 12.1 and 40.1 g/l [1.21 and 4.01 g/dl], respectively, consistent with a diagnosis of paratuberculosis. A faecal sample should be checked for fluke eggs (sedimentation), although this may not yet be patent, and strongyle egg counts performed (modified McMaster technique). Be aware that sheep with Johne's disease may have disproportionately high worm egg counts and lungworm as a consequence of immune system suppression. ELISA tests have a low sensitivity during the early stages of paratuberculosis; a PCR test on a faecal sample could be undertaken but is considerably more expensive than serum protein determinations.

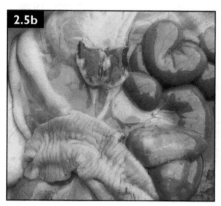

2.5b

3 What action would you recommend? The ewe in **2.5a** was euthanased for welfare reasons. Necropsy findings included an emaciated carcass with gelatinous atrophy of fat depots. The mesenteric lymph nodes were markedly enlarged (**2.5b**). There was thickening of the ileum with prominent ridging. The diagnosis was confirmed after Ziehl–Neelsen staining of gut sections and lymph nodes demonstrating acid-fast bacteria.

4 What control measures could be adopted? Vaccination has proven successful, but a positive benefit:cost results only when losses due to paratuberculosis exceed 2–3% per annum. Few farmers regularly request investigation of involuntary culls or causes of mortality to assess potential financial gain from vaccination.

CASE 2.6

1 What conditions would you suspect (most likely first)? Include: atypical pneumonia (*Mycoplasma*-type; cuffing pneumonia); *Mannheimia haemolytica* associated with viral type pneumonia (possibly parainfluenza 3 virus); lungworm.
2 What treatments would you administer? An increased respiratory rate and occasional coughing were not considered sufficient criteria to warrant immediate whole group antibiotic therapy. Faeces from the three lambs failed to reveal any

lungworm larvae (Baermann technique). The mild clinical signs and low morbidity rate indicated that there was no requirement for metaphylactic antibiotic injection. The farmer was advised to inject any inappetent lambs with a single injection of long-acting oxytetracycline (20 mg/kg IM), strictly observing meat withholding times.

3 What advice would you give? Improved ventilation and reduced stocking may reduce the extent of enzootic pneumonia, but this disease does not usually impact on health and production. Purchased stock should be housed in separate buildings wherever possible. Vaccination against pasteurellosis would be most effective if completed before weaning, when most losses caused by *Pasteurella trehalosi* (systemic pasteurellosis) typically occur.

CASE 2.7

1 What is your diagnosis (most likely first)? Include: *Streptococcus dysgalactiae* infection of the atlanto-occipital joint causing spinal cord compression; infection tracking to the cervical spinal canal from a puncture wound such as a dog/fox bite or contaminated injection site; muscular dystrophy (white muscle disease); extradural haemorrhage following trauma in the region C1-C6; polyarthritis.

2 How could you confirm your diagnosis? Radiography would be unlikely to yield conclusive evidence of joint distension. Myelography could be attempted but is not indicated. Ultrasonography of the atlanto-occipital joint to detect joint swelling could be attempted but would necessitate a 10 MHz sector probe. Compression of the spinal cord causes a 3- to 5-fold increase in lumbar CSF protein concentration (>1.0 g/l [0.1 g/dl]). Muscular dystrophy causes a >100-fold increase in serum creatine kinase concentration.

3 What treatments would you administer? There is a rapid and dramatic response to IV dexamethasone and IM procaine penicillin injections such that lambs are ambulatory 6–12 hours later (**2.7b**). Procaine penicillin remains the drug of choice for all streptococcal infections in farm animals (amoxicillin/clavulanic acid combination is not necessary). Procaine penicillin (15 mg/kg IM) should be administered for a further 5–10 consecutive days.

4 What preventive measures could be adopted? The shepherd had immersed the lambs' navels in strong veterinary iodine on three occasions within the first 6 hours of life. Hygiene measures in the lambing shed and ensuring passive antibody transfer often fail to reduce ongoing problems of *S. dysgalactiae* polyarthritis. In this situation it was suggested that the *S. dysgalactiae* bacteraemia arose from

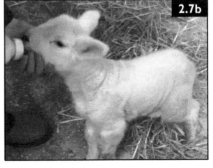

2.7b

either the lamb's upper respiratory tract or tonsils because there was no gross evidence of omphalitis. Changing the lambing accommodation is rarely possible other than turning housed ewes out to pasture, but this increases the risk from hypothermia and causes difficulty catching ewes with problems such as dystocia.

The prevalence of polyarthritis caused by *S. dysgalactiae* may become so high that it justifies metaphylactic penicillin injection when the lambs are turned out to pasture with their dam at 24–48 hours old, but this practice is not consistent with good clinical practice and responsible use of antibiotics.

CASE 2.8

1 Interpret the important sonographic features. There is a large accumulation of fluid in the abdominal cavity with dorsal displacement of viscera. There are no fibrin tags, therefore the fluid would likely be a transudate.

2 What is your provisional diagnosis (most likely first)? Include: ascites associated with Johne's disease (paratuberculosis); ascites associated with intestinal adenocarcinoma; fasciolosis; ascites associated with haemonchosis; right-sided heart failure.

It is not possible to differentiate the cause of ascites from ultrasound examination alone; ultrasound measurement of ileal wall thickness is not sufficiently accurate to diagnose paratuberculosis; identification of a 3–5 cm mass would be suggestive of an intestinal adenocarcinoma. In this situation, paratuberculosis would be the more likely diagnosis because of high annual losses from similar cases, although

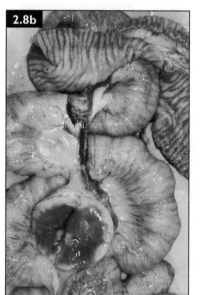

necropsy confirmation is important for future control advice.

3 What further tests would you recommend? Sheep with advanced Johne's disease have profound hypoalbuminaemia (serum values <15 g/l [1.5 g/dl]; normal range >30 g/l [3 g/dl]), but obvious ascites is unusual. Adenocarcinoma can also lead to a protein-losing enteropathy. ELISA tests for Johne's disease have a high specificity but low sensitivity; the advanced nature of lesions in this sheep would very likely lead to a positive result. Faecal PCR testing is also possible for Johne's disease but is more expensive. Necropsy reveals serous atrophy of fat, thickening of the ileal wall and enlargement of mesenteric lymph nodes (**2.8b**), consistent with Johne's disease.

4 What action would you take? Explore the potential economic benefits of vaccination; increased production and reduced mortality must be balanced against the cost of vaccination.

CASE 2.9

1 How would you interpret the necropsy results? Necropsy of six sheep is expensive and fails to give any meaningful information regarding disease prevalence in a 2,400 ewe flock.

2 What advice would you offer? A visit to the farm is essential and reveals that many of the ewes that die show vague respiratory signs of exercise intolerance and increased respiratory rate, but these observations have been largely ignored because the ewes appeared bright and alert with a normal appetite before death. Fifty-eight sheep in poorer condition were separated from the main flock at shearing time and made available for veterinary examination. Transthoracic ultrasonography takes less than 2 hours and seven of the 58 sheep are identified with OPA; examination at the slaughter plant confirms the diagnosis in all cases. (**Note:** These animals were sold for slaughter, thereby generating income for the farmer.)

The major risk for OPA is housing, with transmission spread via fomites. There is a cost involved in scanning all breeding stock, but this is offset by selling all OPA-positive cases immediately for slaughter rather than be collected later as cadavers. Culling OPA cases as early as possible greatly reduces disease transmission and mortality over the coming years compared with instituting no control measures at all.

CASE 2.10

1 What conditions would you consider? The most likely conditions to consider include: compressive cervical myelopathy (CVM); cervical vertebral empyema; cerebellar abiotrophy.

2 What further tests could be undertaken? In CVM cases, CSF specific gravity, total protein content, and cell count are within normal ranges. Radiographic examination of the cervicothoracic vertebral column fails to demonstrate any gross bony abnormalities; however, radiographic myelograms have revealed extradural lesions at the level of C6-C7, where the dorsal contrast column ends abruptly.

Postmortem examination of the two rams reveals discrete, smooth, nodular to polypoid projections of adipose tissue prolapsing through the dorsolateral intervertebral space at C6-C7, causing localised spinal cord compression. Histopathology of the nodules confirms that they are composed of well-differentiated adipocytes typical of fatty tissue. There is marked Wallerian degeneration at the site of compression, with milder changes present cranial and caudal to the lesion.

3 **What actions/treatments would you recommend?** The rams should be culled for welfare reasons.

4 **What control measures could be taken?** CVM has been recognised in Texel and Beltex sheep and is related to particular bloodlines. Affected rams must not be used for breeding in purebred flocks; there are no reports of this condition in crossbred sheep.

CASE 2.11

1 **What conditions would you consider?** Basillar empyema; listeriosis.

Listeriosis is the primary differential diagnosis because of involvement of multiple CNs, but it is unusual to find bilateral CN deficits in lambs more than 3–4 months old. A lack of menace response would be unusual in listeriosis.

2 **What is the cause of this condition?** Localised infection of the frontal sinuses is considered to be one source of haematogenous spread to the rete mirabile (a complex of blood capillaries surrounding the pituitary gland) extending into the cranial cavity and

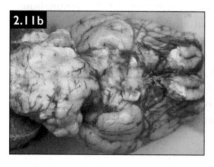

along the floor to affect CNs II–VII. Typical necropsy findings are shown (**2.11b**); note the purulent exudate on the surface of the brain in relation to the CN roots, which further explains the clinical signs. This route of infection may be supported by the mucopurulent nasal discharge. Radiography is unlikely to detect superficial infection of the frontal sinuses. The prevalence of basilar empyema is not known because it is commonly mistaken for listeriosis. Fighting injuries causing infected head wounds may explain the more common occurrence in rams. Nose rings in bulls are a common source of such infection in cattle.

3 **What treatment would you administer?** The treatment protocol comprises an extended course of procaine penicillin (15 mg/kg IM daily) and a single injection of dexamethasone (1 mg/kg) on the first day of antibiotic therapy.

4 **What is the prognosis for this lamb?** The advanced pathology at presentation, and lack of drainage from within the cranium, suggests a guarded prognosis. The lamb should be euthanased for welfare reasons if there is no dramatic improvement within 2–3 days.

CASE 2.12

1 **Where is the probable site of the lesion?** Between C6 and T2.

2 **What type of lesion would you suspect (most likely first)?** Include: vertebral empyema; sarcocystosis; bilateral fore leg lameness/polyarthritis.

3 What further investigations could be undertaken? Lumbosacral CSF analysis is a sensitive and specific test for an inflammatory lesion causing spinal cord compression, with an increase in lumbar CSF protein concentration from a normal concentration <0.3 g/l (0.03 g/dl) to >1.0 g/l (0.1 g/dl), and frequently >2.0 g/l (0.2 g/dl). There is little increase in the white cell concentration. Radiographic identification of vertebral empyema is difficult even with excellent quality radiographs. Myelography can be performed under general anaesthesia, but is expensive and cannot be justified. The lesion can be confirmed at necropsy by longitudinal section of the vertebral column (**2.12b**, arrow).

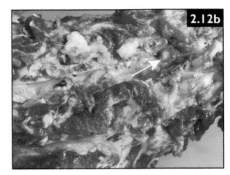

4 What prognosis would you offer? Compressive spinal cord lesions, whether traumatic or infectious in origin, offer a grave prognosis and euthanasia is indicated for animal welfare reasons.

CASE 2.13

1 What action would you take? First consider injection of a NSAID IV to reduce pain, although there is no published evidence at present. (**Note:** Off-label use in many countries.) Extradural xylazine is the better option.

Repulsion of the lamb's head is greatly facilitated after sacrococcygeal extradural lidocaine injection, which blocks the reflex abdominal contractions of the ewe. The more traditional way of repelling a lamb is to enlist the help of an assistant, who suspends the ewe by the hindlegs while the lamb is forced back against the ewe's strong abdominal contractions. This procedure causes considerable distress to the ewe because the weight of the pregnant uterus, rumen and other abdominal viscera are forced against the diaphragm. The risk of trauma to the uterus and vagina are greatly increased if the lamb is forced back into the body of the uterus against such powerful opposition.

The first intercoccygeal space is identified by digital palpation during slight vertical movement of the tail, and a 40 mm (1.6 in) 19 gauge needle directed at 20° to the tail, which is held horizontally. Correct positioning of the needle is determined by the lack of resistance to injection of 0.5–0.6 mg/kg of 2% lidocaine and 0.07 mg/kg xylazine (**Note:** off-label use in many countries) equivalent to 2 ml of 2% lidocaine solution and 0.25 ml of 2% xylazine solution for an 80 kg ewe, respectively.

Correction of this malposture involves repulsion of the head into the vagina, flexing the shoulder and elbow joint of one fore leg, and then carefully

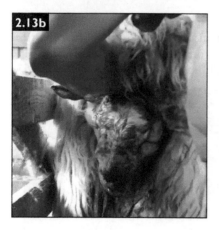

extending the carpus (knee) and fetlock joint in that order, which presents the foot at the pelvic inlet. These manipulations are then repeated for the other fore leg (**2.13b**).

The lamb's head and tongue may remain swollen for a few hours and it is prudent to stomach tube the lamb to ensure that it receives sufficient colostrum (50 ml/kg within the first 2 hours; do it immediately and the task is not forgotten).

CASE 2.14

1 What conditions would you consider? Closantel toxicity; polioencephalomalacia (PEM); basillar empyema.

Closantel toxicity can occur at a low incidence after slight overdosing. The speed of onset and severity of clinical signs appears to be dose dependent. Clinical examination, particularly the lack of pupillary light reflexes, and history narrowed the list of differential diagnoses, with closantel toxicity considered the most likely; pituitary tumours would be unlikely to affect several sheep simultaneously. Sheep affected by PEM have intact pupillary light reflexes. Ovine pregnancy toxaemia would not affect single-bearing and barren ewes.

2 What treatment would you administer? There is no effective treatment for closantel toxicity. Histopathology revealed extensive loss of nerve structure and replacement with fibrosis in the intracanalicular section of the optic nerve. Within the retina there was diffuse loss of the ganglion cell layer and thinning of the photoreceptor layer, especially in the non-tapetal retina.

3 What is this significance of this outbreak? The greater geographical range of *Fasciola hepatica* and the increased incidence of triclabendazole resistance is likely to lead to increased closantel use. Therefore, practitioners should advise clients to limit overdosing by dividing sheep into narrow weight categories at the time of dosing, and be aware of the clinical signs of closantel toxicity.

CASE 2.15

1 What conditions would you consider (most likely first)? Include: carpal hygroma; infected tendon sheath.

2 What further examinations would you take? The carpal swellings are soft, non-painful and restricted to the dorsal aspect of the carpus, thereby consistent with a carpal hygroma. The overlying skin is thickened, with loss of hair. Hygromas can become large (**2.15b**) but do not cause lameness. This condition, although generally bilateral, is common in rams as a consequence of chronic foot lameness (footrot) and long periods spent grazing on their knees. Attempted drainage would be cavalier and unjustified because of the risk of introducing infection. Ultrasonographic examination of any soft tissue swellings using a 5 or 7.5 MHz linear scanner could be undertaken but is not necessary.

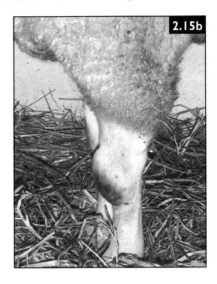

3 What advice would you offer? Carpal hygromas indicate a prolonged period of fore leg lameness and ideally this ram should not have been purchased. Prompt attention to lameness will prevent the development of hygromas.

CASE 2.16

1 What pathogens could be involved? Gangrenous mastitis caused by *Mannheimia* spp. and *Staphylococcus aureus* occurs sporadically during the first 2 months of lactation associated with poor milk supply related to ewe undernutrition and overvigorous sucking by the lambs. Gangrenous mastitis is often preceded by either staphylococcal or orf skin lesions of the ewe's teat. It is most commonly reported in ewes nursing twins or triplets.

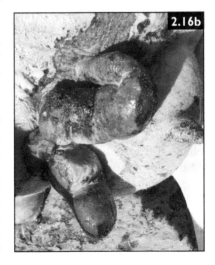

2 What is the prognosis? Despite antibiotic and supportive therapy the prognosis is grave and the gangrenous udder tissue eventually sloughs, leaving a large granulating surface with superficial bacterial infection. Superficial trauma readily causes bleeding. The granulation tissue continues to proliferate (**2.16b**) over the coming months (up to 10–20 cm in diameter) and affected ewes cannot be presented at markets. It is unusual for these lesions to suffer from cutaneous myiasis, but affected sheep are greatly worried by nuisance flies if kept outdoors during the summer and lose a great deal of body condition.

3 What action would you take? These ewes are unsuitable for breeding stock. The infected granulation tissue, and resultant deep inguinal lymph node enlargement, would result in carcass condemnation (and raise genuine welfare concerns). The fleece is very poor because growth has occurred during this period of illness and debility. The ewe should be euthanased for welfare reasons at first presentation.

4 What control measures could be adopted? Control measures include ensuring ewes are well fed. Supply concentrates to ewes and lambs when pasture is poor. Do not expect any ewe to rear triplets. Identify and treat superficial teat lesions with topical antibiotics. Control of orf by skin scarification using live virus vaccine remains largely unproven but is commonly practised.

CASE 2.17

1 What is your diagnosis? The most likely conditions to consider include: visceral caseous lymphadenitis (*Corynebacterium pseudotuberculosis*; CLA); abscess; tuberculosis.

The lamellar appearance of the mediastinal lymph node is typical of visceral CLA. Bacteriology could be undertaken to confirm the diagnosis. Scotland is officially free of bovine tuberculosis.

2 What action would you take? This ram had been purchased 4 years ago and no discharging skin lesions have been noted in the ram group or the flock in general. All other rams in the group are in good body condition. It is likely that the ram had the lesion at the time of purchase and the risk of spread within the group is low. The farmer is advised about the appearance of the cutaneous form CLA (discharging lesion most often involving the parotid lymph node) and to submit any other lean rams for veterinary examination. Serological testing of the ram group could be undertaken, but the farmer was unwilling to cull a fit ram simply on the basis of a seropositive result.

3 What control measures should be adopted in this flock? Strict biosecurity measures with quarantine of all purchased stock, especially rams, is strongly recommended to prevent introduction of many contagious diseases, including CLA, but are not rigorously applied on most UK sheep farms. Visceral CLA is an uncommon cause of emaciation of adult sheep in the UK, a situation that differs from many other countries including the USA and Australia. Commercial interests in promoting CLA control in the UK have deflected resources from other more important diseases such as ovine pulmonary adenocarcinoma and paratuberculosis. CLA is not a major concern for commercial sheep farmers in the UK; strict segregation of affected sheep where it does arise may be all that is required. CLA control in pedigree ram studs, which are housed for long periods and maintained tightly stocked, is more problematic. While this ram would have tested positive for CLA, such infection did not affect its productive life.

CASE 2.18

1 What conditions would you consider (most likely first)? Include: trace element deficiency, particularly cobalt and selenium deficiency; poor grazing; poor parasite control.

2 How would you investigate this problem? Faecal worm egg counts from ten lambs average 100 strongyle epg (no treatment necessary). Serum vitamin B_{12} concentrations from six lambs reveal very low concentrations (mean <160 pg/ml), indicating inadequate cobalt status.

In extreme cases there is pale bone marrow and poor mineralisation of bone (**2.18b**) with spontaneous fractures. Erythrocyte glutathione peroxidase concentrations are within the reference range; selenium assays were not undertaken.

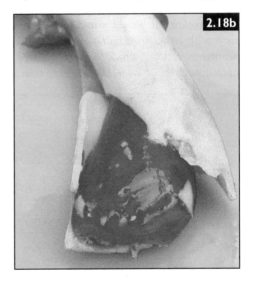
2.18b

3 What treatment would you administer? Treatment involves immediate oral administration with cobalt sulphate. There is often a visible improvement within 2 weeks; monitor liveweight gains over the next 4 weeks and compare with predicted increases. It is possible to leave 10–12 lambs unsupplemented and monitor as a control group provided animal welfare is not compromised. Continue to monitor parasite burdens by analysis of pooled faecal samples every 2 weeks.

4 How would you prevent this problem recurring next year? The cost of supplementing the whole flock with oral cobalt sulphate is cheaper than assaying serum vitamin B_{12} estimations, which can be of doubtful significance anyway. Include advice about cobalt supplementation in the flock health programme for future years.

The low unit cost of cobalt sulphate allows routine inclusion in certain anthelmintic drenches (commercial 'SC' [selenium and cobalt] preparations, or at inclusion rates of 15–30 g per 10 litres of 2.25% benzimadazole or 1.5%

levamisole drench); however, anthelmintic treatment is not indicated at the present time in these lambs on safe grazing.

CASE 2.19

1 What common problems would you consider (most likely first)? The most likely conditions to consider include: coccidiosis; cryptosporidiosis; *Strongyloides papillosus* infection; salmonellosis.

2 How could you confirm your provisional diagnosis? The clinical signs are suggestive of coccidiosis. Oocyst counts can be variable but are usually very high in lambs scouring for more than several days. Identification of the pathogenic species *Eimeria ovinoidalis* or *E. crandallis* is rarely undertaken. Gut smears and histopathology of gut sections are taken from dead lambs. The response to treatment for coccidiosis helps confirm the diagnosis.

3 What treatment would you administer? Treatment options include a single drench with either toltrazuril or diclazuril, or decoquinate added to the lambs' concentrate ration, which can be used as a treatment/preventive measure. Where doubts exist over feed intake, toltrazuril or diclazuril is the treatment

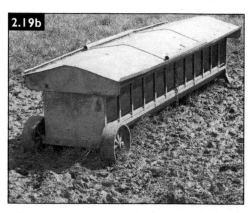

of choice. The feeding areas and water trough area can become very heavily contaminated even when lambs are reared outdoors (**2.19b**), therefore the lambs should be moved to a clean pen/ field immediately.

Medication of the ewe ration with decoquinate will suppress but not totally eliminate oocyst production, therefore this regimen is operated in conjunction with medication of the lamb creep feed.

CASE 2.20

1 What conditions would you consider? The most likely conditions to consider include: contagious ovine digital dermatitis; footrot; white line abscess extending to the coronary band; shelly hoof.

2 What is the likely cause? Contagious ovine digital dermatitis is the most likely cause of lesions originating at the coronary band and causing sloughing of the entire hoof capsule. There is no ready explanation why only one digit of one foot is affected.

3 What action would you take? Isolate all affected lame lambs. Inject all lame lambs with a single injection of tilmicosin or gamithromycin (note off-label use in many countries); oxytetracycline may also be effective. Spray with topical oxytetracycline aerosol. Long-acting amoxycillin has also been shown to be effective but has not been directly compared with a macrolide antibiotic. Convalescence is protracted, especially when the hoof capsule has been shed (**2.20b**; note that both hoof capsules have been shed from the foot on the right-hand side of this image).

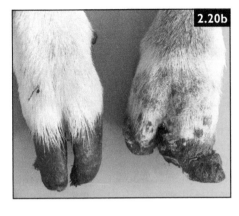

4 How could this condition be prevented? Strict biosecurity should help prevent introduction of the disease. Hoof knives can transmit the causal organism of digital dermatitis between cattle, and this seems likely in sheep as well. Prompt attention (antibiotic injection) to all lame sheep may prevent such advanced painful lesions. Metaphylactic injection could be considered in other sheep in the group.

CASE 2.21

Describe the method you would use to collect CSF from an obtunded sheep. For CSF collection it is necessary to puncture the subarachnoid space in the cerebellomedullary cistern (cisternal sample) or at the lumbosacral site (lumbar sample). In the absence of a focal spinal cord compressive lesion, there is usually no substantial difference between the composition of cisternal and lumbar CSF samples; there are few indications for cisternal collection.

Collection of lumbar CSF is facilitated when the animal is positioned in sternal recumbency with the hips flexed and the hindlegs extended alongside the abdomen. Aversion of the head against the flank may assist in maintaining sternal recumbency during the CSF collection procedure. Sedation of the animal is not usually necessary but can be achieved using 10 µg/kg detomidine injected IV (note off-label use in some countries). Xylazine (0.04–0.07 mg/kg IV) produces very variable sedation and is not recommended.

The site for lumbar CSF collection is the midpoint of the lumbosacral space (**2.21**), which can be identified as the midline depression between the last palpable dorsal lumbar spine (L6) and the first palpable sacral dorsal spine (S2). The site must be clipped, surgically prepared and between 1 and 2 ml of local anaesthetic injected SC. An internal stylet is not required (see Guide below). The needle is

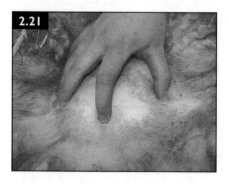

slowly advanced at a right angle to the plane of the vertebral column or with the hub directed 5° caudally. It is essential to appreciate the changes in tissue resistance as the needle point passes sequentially through the subcutaneous tissue, interarcuate ligament then the sudden 'pop' due to the loss of resistance as the needle point finally penetrates the ligamentum flavum into the extradural space. Once the needle point has penetrated the dorsal subarachnoid space, CSF will well up in the needle hub within 2–3 seconds.

One to 2 ml of CSF is sufficient for laboratory analysis and while the sample can be collected by free flow, it is more convenient to employ gentle syringe aspiration over 10–30 seconds. Care must be taken not to dislodge the needle point from the dorsal subarachnoid space when the syringe is attached to the needle hub. Stabilising the position of the needle can be assisted by firmly resting the wrist on the sheep's vertebral column.

Guide to needle length and gauge for lumbar CSF sampling.

Neonatal lambs		1 cm	21–23 gauge
Lambs	<30 kg	2.5 cm	21 gauge
Ewes	40–80 kg	4 cm	19 gauge
Rams	>80 kg	5 cm	19 gauge

CASE 2.22

1 **What conditions would you consider?** The most likely conditions to consider include: chronic copper poisoning; chronic fasciolosis; sulphur toxicity/polioencephalomalacia.

2 **What further tests could be undertaken?** Tests for chronic copper toxicity could include serum liver enzyme assays such as GGT and AST concentrations, which are increased 10–50-fold, indicating severe liver damage. The serum copper concentration may not be elevated above the normal range in toxicity cases.

3 **What actions/treatments would you recommend?** Where available, the treatment plan could include 1.7 mg/kg ammonium tetrathiomolybdate given by slow IV infusion on two occasions 2 days apart (or 3.4 mg/kg injected SC). Three litres of 5% glucose saline can be given IV over 6 hours where cost permits. Oral fluids

could be administered, but the prognosis is guarded and euthanasia is the humane option.

This ram should be euthanased for welfare reasons and the provisional diagnosis confirmed at necropsy, where there is jaundice of the carcass, most noticeable in the omentum. The kidneys are swollen and dark grey (**2.22b**), with dark red urine in the bladder.

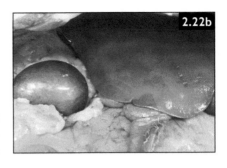

The liver is enlarged and friable. The kidney copper concentration is massively elevated (10–20-fold above normal value of <314 µmol/kg DM). Liver copper concentrations are usually also elevated, but such determinations are not as reliable as kidney copper determination.

4 What control measures could be taken? Sheep must not have access to cattle feed and great care must be taken when considering copper supplementation (e.g. in pregnant ewes to control congenital swayback). No additional source of copper had been administered to this group. Copper antagonists, such as molybdenum, may be required when susceptible breeds are fed high levels of concentrates (especially when rearing studs rams and feeding high levels of supplementary concentrates) despite the content not exceeding 15 mg/kg copper as fed. No extra source of copper was found in this situation and accumulation over time at pasture was considered to be the likely source, but was not proven. Adding a copper antagonist, such as molybdenum, to the ration was recommended. A change of breed should be considered if the problem continues.

CASE 2.23

1 What is the cause of this problem (most likely first)? Several causes in cattle have been suggested such as pharyngeal or reticular irritation, highly acidic rations, vagus indigestion, and high intraruminal pressure. There was no evidence of any of these problems. Rhododendron poisoning is a common cause of acute vomiting in sheep, but there is an obvious source.

2 What action would you take? Without a specific diagnosis, there is no specific treatment.

3 How could you confirm the cause? Necropsy of this case failed to identify any anatomical abnormality.

4 Is this condition heritable? It is not known whether this condition is heritable but it would be prudent not to breed from affected rams. Few farmers keep adequate records to look at the potential heritability of this condition.

CASE 2.24

1 Describe the important postmortem features. The liver is grossly enlarged with multiple haemorrhagic tracts visible under the liver capsule and throughout its substance on cut surface. There is a large amount of organised fibrin on the liver capsule.

2 What is the most likely cause? Severe subacute fasciolosis (*Fasciola hepatica* infection).

3 How could this problem be confirmed in other sheep in the group? Clinical disease is apparent before liver flukes become patent, so a sedimentation test on a faecal sample will not help. Subacute fasciolosis can be diagnosed by the coproantigen ELISA test. Raised serum AST and GLDH concentrations indicate liver damage, but are not pathognomonic for fasciolosis. Increased serum GGT concentrations, which indicate bile duct damage, are also commonly used to aid diagnosis. These three liver enzymes are typically increased by 5–30-fold but, in the case of AST, fall to near normal concentrations within 10–14 days of flukicide treatment. Serum GGT and GLDH remain elevated for at least 1 month after flukicide treatment.

The serum albumin concentration is reduced to 12–20 g/l (1.2–2.0 g/dl) and the serum globulin concentration is massively increased to >65 g/l (6.5 g/dl) and often >75 g/l (7.5 g/dl). There are few bacterial infections that give such a dramatic serum protein profile, and certainly none on a group basis; therefore, serum protein analysis should be included with liver enzymes in the biochemistry profile.

4 What action would you take? Triclabendazole is effective at killing all fluke stages. Drenched sheep should be moved to clean pasture. Re-treatment should be based on risk and may be necessary 3–6 weeks after the first treatment in high risk years where there is no alternative pasture or housing. Thereafter, treatment with closantel should be considered to avoid selecting for triclabendazole resistant strains of liver fluke, but noting that closantel is only effective against developing flukes more than 7–8 weeks post ingestion of metacercariae.

CASE 2.25

1 What conditions would you consider (most likely first)? Dermatophilosis; staphyloccocal dermatitis; psoroptic mange; ringworm.

2 What further tests could be undertaken? Diagnosis of dermatophilosis is based on clinical examination and, if necessary, stained smears from the underside of scabs plucked from the fleece, which reveal coccoid bacteria. Bacteriology is rarely undertaken.

3 What actions/treatments would you recommend? Treatment is rarely indicated, but rams intended for sale are sometimes treated to prevent skin lesions regrowing discoloured wool, which is considered a cosmetic defect at sale. Procaine penicillin

(15 mg/kg IM for 3 consecutive days) effects a cure but it may take several weeks for the scabs to be shed from the growing fleece.

4 What control measures could be taken? A variety of dip solutions have been used in New Zealand and Australia to prevent dermatophilosis following shearing, including 1% potassium aluminium sulphate spray or dip solution. Dermatophilosis is rarely a disease of well-fed sheep; severe disease occurs only in sheep debilitated from another cause, in this case paratuberculosis.

CASE 2.26

1 What conditions would you consider (most likely first)? Include: pleuropneumonia/pleural abscess occupying the right chest; transudate/exudate occupying the right chest; chronic suppurative pneumonia; diaphragmatic hernia; ovine pulmonary adenocarcinoma (OPA); mediastinal abscess caused by caseous lymphadenitis (CLA); visna-maedi.

2 How would you investigate this problem further? Ultrasonographic examination of the chest will allow diagnosis of any respiratory condition, such as pleural abscess/pyothorax or OPA. Note that these respiratory conditions can be largely unilateral. The production of copious clear frothy fluid from nostrils when the ewe's hindquarters are raised (positive wheelbarrow test) is also pathognomic for advanced cases of OPA, but this greatly exacerbates any dyspnoea such that affected sheep should be killed immediately afterwards for welfare reasons. Note that not all OPA cases produces significant fluid.

The ultrasound image of the right chest showed small intestine (**2.26b**) consistent with a diagnosis of diaphragmatic hernia. Sonograms of the left chest revealed normal lung with the heart pushed against the chest wall. A standing lateral radiograph of the right chest showed a fluid line consistent with a diagnosis of diaphragmatic hernia.

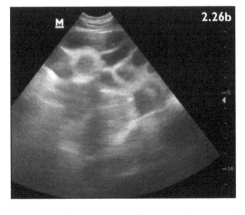

3 What treatment would you administer? The prognosis for diaphragmatic hernia is hopeless and the sheep was killed immediately for welfare reasons.

4 What is the likely cause? The cause of this case of diaphragmatic hernia was not established. There was no history of severe trauma such as a road traffic accident. This was the second case from this flock of 600 breeding sheep in 2 years.

CASE 2.27

1 What conditions would you consider (most likely first)? Elbow arthritis; osteoarthritis of the elbow joint.

Arthropathy of the elbow joint in adult sheep is characterised by extensive enthesophyte formation involving the lateral ligament (*Lig. collaterale ulnae*) following trauma to the mechanism preventing overextension of the elbow joint. Enthesitis is a term used to describe changes occurring at the insertion of a muscle, tendon, ligament or articular capsule where recurring concentration of stress provokes inflammation, with a strong tendency towards fibrosis and calcification. The elbow joint is a typical ginglymus joint, with movements restricted to flexion and extension. The lateral ligament of the elbow is short and strong, and along with tension in the medial collateral ligament and biceps brachii muscle, is largely responsible for limiting the degree of extension of the elbow joint.

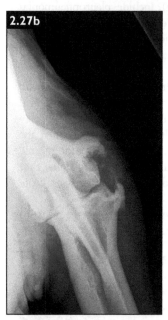

2.27b

2 What further tests could be undertaken? An oblique radiograph of the right elbow (**2.27b**) reveals the characteristic enthesophytic reaction where the two advancing edges are clearly visible.

3 What actions/treatments would you recommend? There is no effective treatment; short-term pain relief (NSAID injection) may be effective but there are no long-term treatment options.

4 What control measures could be taken? Avoid stress/trauma to the elbow joints when performing tasks such as casting, but this is not always easy to achieve. Do not feed young rams excessively to achieve maximum growth rate.

CASE 2.28

1 What conditions would you consider (most likely first)? Partial obstructive urolithiasis; cystitis.

2 What further investigations could be undertaken? Transabdominal ultrasound examination of the right kidney in the right flank can be undertaken to check for hydronephrosis, but may not be necessary because of the relatively short duration of urethral obstruction. Blood urea nitrogen and creatinine concentrations are increased 5–20-fold.

3 What action would you take? The ram should be cast onto its hindquarters and the penis extruded to examine the vermiform appendage (**2.28b**) by straightening the sigmoid flexure. When present, a calculus can be felt within the tip of the vermiform appendage, which is excised with a scalpel blade. After the ram is allowed to stand, a continuous flow of urine is often voided. The ram must be carefully observed for normal urination and appetite over the next few days in case other calculi block the urethra. Spasmolytics (hyoscine) and corticosteroids are often administered but their value remains unproven.

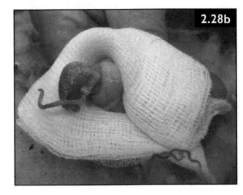

4 What sequelae could result in neglected cases? Early recognition of urethral obstruction is essential because irreversible hydronephrosis develops after approximately 5–7 days due to back pressure within the urinary tract. Re-blockage with further calculi is possible. A tube cystotomy can be undertaken in valuable breeding rams with proximal urethral obstruction. As a salvage procedure, a subischial urethrostomy can be performed under caudal block, but this is not a simple procedure and must be carefully considered because ascending infection of the transected urethra is inevitable.

5 What control measures would you recommend? Control of urolithiasis (struvite crystals) involves feeding a correct ration with a low magnesium content. The salt concentration of the ration can be increased to increase water intake and urine output. Urine acidifiers such as ammonium chloride can also be added to the ration. Good quality roughage should be available *ad libitum*.

CASE 2.29

1 What conditions would you consider (most likely first)? Include: bacterial endocarditis; septic polyarthritis; bluetongue.

2 How could you confirm your diagnosis? Despite vegetative lesion(s) on the heart valve(s), auscultation of both cattle and sheep with vegetative endocarditis often fails to reveal abnormal heart sounds, but the heart rate is usually increased and irregular. Ultrasound examination of the heart with a 5 MHz sector scanner can identify a classical vegetative growth in some cases (**2.29b**, arrow). Arthrocentesis would differentiate joint effusion from sepsis but most joint exudate forms a pannus.

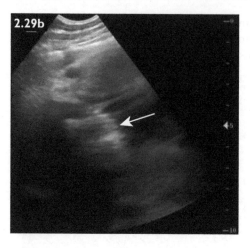

2.29b

3 **What treatment would you administer?** Antibiotic therapy with daily penicillin injections can be attempted, but the response is hopeless because of the advanced nature of the heart valve lesions when presented for veterinary examination. Temporary improvement with reduced joint distension follows a single dexamethasone injection in most cases, but lameness returns within 4–7 days.

4 **What action would you recommend?** The sheep should be euthanased for welfare reasons.

Large vegetative lesions were demonstrated on the mitral valve of this ram. Foci are commonly observed in the kidneys.

5 **What control measures would you recommend?** A primary focus of infection is rarely found at necropsy of adult sheep. Bacterial endocarditis in ewes often occurs 2–3 months after lambing; improved hygiene and prompt treatment of metritis may reduce potential bacteraemia and subsequent endocarditis. In lambs, bacterial endocarditis is occasionally associated with *Erysipelothrix rhusiopathiae* infection.

CASE 2.30

1 **What conditions would you consider (most likely first)?** Include: entropion; infectious keratoconjunctivitis; congenital microphthalmia.

2 **What treatments would you administer?** Treatment involves eversion of the lower eyelid as soon after birth as possible, with regular inspection to ensure it

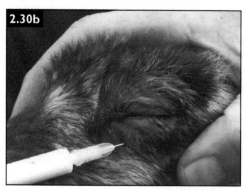

2.30b

remains everted. Topical antibiotic application controls secondary bacterial infection and aids movement of the lower eyelid, thereby reducing the likelihood of inversion.

Subcutaneous antibiotic injection (1 ml of procaine penicillin) can be used to evert the lower eyelid (**2.30b**). Eales clip(s) can be inserted in the skin below the lower eyelid to cause eversion and requires only one operator. Skin suture(s) can be inserted to evert the lower eyelid but this procedure requires two people, one to restrain the lamb and the other to carefully insert the suture.

3 What are the consequences of no action/treatment? Include rupture of the cornea with herniation of the lens and loss of the eye in neglected cases.

4 What preventive measures could be adopted? Entropion has a high hereditary component and rams siring affected progeny should be culled, but this rarely occurs.

CASE 2.31

1 What conditions would you consider? Include: infectious polyarthritis caused by *Erysipelothrix rhusiopathiae*; infectious polyarthritis secondary to tick-borne fever; bacterial endocarditis.

2 What is the likely cause? *Streptococcus dysgalactiae* affects lambs within the first 2 weeks of life, while *E. rhusiopathiae* tends to affect lambs from 2 weeks old.

3 How would you confirm the cause? Samples of synovial membrane from sacrificed untreated cases are preferable to joint aspirates for bacteriological examination. Note that there can be a high seroprevalence to erysipelas in normal healthy sheep.

4 What treatment would you administer? While aggressive penicillin therapy during the early stages of infection effects a good cure rate in many *E. rhusiopathiae* infections, and may render the joints sterile, some infections are not cleared, with the result that progressive and degenerative changes occur within the joint. Indeed, dead bacteria and white blood cells within the joint induce inflammatory changes including proliferation of the synovial membrane and fibrous thickening of the joint capsule. Note that inflammation of the synovium gives the infected joint a pink colour compared with white in the normal joint (inflamed synovium

shown in the left-hand stifle joint in **2.31b**; right-hand side stifle joint is normal). Such joint pathology will not respond to further antibiotic therapy and these lambs should be euthanased for welfare reasons.

5 What control measure(s) would you recommend? Where available, vaccination of the dam with effective passive antibody transfer protects lambs from erysipelas for up to 4–6 months.

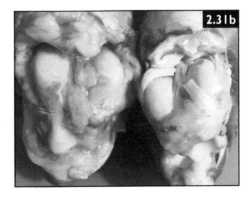

2.31b

CASE 2.32

1 Describe the major radiographic changes. Radiography reveals extensive bone lysis of the femoral head and acetabulum extending to involve the shaft of the ilium. The true extent of bone destruction is best illustrated in 'boiled out' preparations (2.32b, c).

2 What is the likely cause? The septic hip joint probably arose from infection of the proximal femoral growth plate following haematogenous spread. The true incidence of septic physitis is unknown because few lambs are necropsied and it is generally assumed that all chronic severe lameness is caused by joint infection.

3 What treatment would you recommend? The lamb must be euthanased immediately for welfare reasons. This lamb has suffered unnecessarily and the farmer must be made aware of this serious welfare concern.

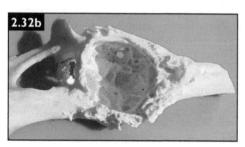

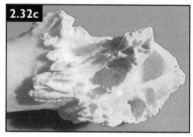

CASE 2.33

1 Describe the sonogram. The broad hyperechoic line present dorsally represents the lung surface (visceral pleura), which is displaced from the chest wall by an extensive hypoechoic area, with a slightly hyperechoic latticework matrix typical of a fibrinous pleurisy extending to 8 cm deep at the ventral margin.

2 What is your diagnosis? The sonographic findings are consistent with a diagnosis of extensive fibrinous pleurisy of the left chest.

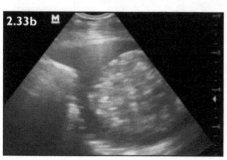

3 What treatment(s) would you administer? There are no reports of diagnosis/successful treatment of such lesions in sheep. The ram was treated with procaine penicillin (15 mg/kg IM daily for 4 weeks) and made a good recovery. After 2 months, the pleural lesion comprised a 5 cm diameter organised fibrin clot (2.33b).

4 What is the origin of this pleurisy? *Streptococcus dysgalactiae* has been isolated from pleurisy lesions in ewes that had numerous large abscesses within the udder parenchyma. The potential source of infection in this ram was not identified.

CASE 2.34

1 Describe the important sonographic findings. The large anechoic area, extending for up to 16 cm, represents fluid distension of the abdomen, with the liver and omentum displaced dorsally. There are numerous large fibrin tags (inflammatory exudate) on the liver capsule extending to the omentum, gallbladder, liver lobe and body wall. The liver is not homogeneous but contains many hyperechoic dots, consistent with inflammatory cell accumulations caused by migrating immature flukes.

2 What tests would you undertake? Abdominocentesis would establish whether the fluid was a transudate or an inflammatory exudate (>30 g/l [3 g/dl]; more likely due to fibrin present).

3 What causes would you consider? The fibrin tags on the liver, and to the adjacent viscera/body wall (**2.34b**), would be consistent with severe subacute fasciolosis and this would indicate late season metacercariae ingestion.

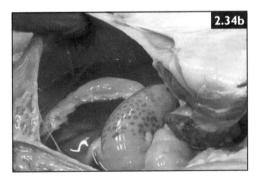

Other conditions to consider include: diffuse peritonitis associated with liver infection (abscessation), although none apparent; ascites associated with transcoelomic spread of small intestine adenocarcinoma, but contains no fibrin tags; uroperitoneum, but has never been reported in a ewe.

4 How would you confirm your diagnosis? Raised serum GGT and GLDH concentrations are consistent with hepatic damage caused by migrating flukes. Changes in albumin and globulin concentrations are not disease specific.

5 What treatment(s) would you administer? The prognosis for this ewe is guarded due to the well-established fibrin adhesions. Antibiotic administration and an injection of dexamethasone could be given in an attempt to treat the peritonitis, and diclabendazole given to treat immature fasciolosis.

6 Are there any control measures to recommend? Treat all sheep in the flock with triclabendazole immediately and 6 weeks later with closantel in case of triclabendazole resistance. Any fluke treatment in May will suffice because all flukes will be mature.

CASE 2.35

1 Briefly list the advantages and disadvantages of flushing.

Advantages:

- Flushing for 4–6 weeks should provide for a 0.5–1.0 unit increase in condition score at mating time.
- Sheep in good body condition will be better able to survive pregnancy if nutrition is poor because of adverse weather, poor management, etc.
- Flushing increases ovulation and implantation rate and eventual pregnancy rate.

Disadvantages:

- Fields must not be grazed for 4–6 weeks to ensure a good (8 cm) grass sward.
- Extra fertiliser may be needed, which is costly.
- Reduced grazing for weaned lambs or purchased store lambs (**2.35b**).
- Flushing increases ovulation and implantation rates in hybrid ewes, resulting in more triplet litters, which suffer much higher perinatal losses.
- Cost and labour involved with rearing orphan lambs.
- Twin- and triplet-bearing ewes are more prone to pregnancy toxaemia, vaginal prolapse and rupture of the prepubic tendon.

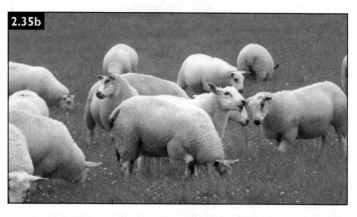

2 List the alternatives that can achieve appropriate body condition scores at mating, and more lambs. Litter size at the normal breeding season can be increased by approximately 15% by the use of melatonin implants. Flushing can ensure appropriate ewe condition score at mating but this can also be achieved by correct management after weaning.

CASE 2.36

1 Interpret the sonogram. The fluid extends for >5 cm from the abdominal wall (2.36b).

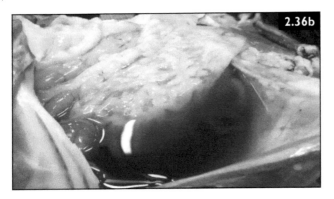

2 What is your diagnosis? This appearance would be consistent with a diagnosis of uroperitoneum.

3 What other structure(s) should be checked sonographically? Uroperitoneum associated with urolithiasis is much more common in lambs than in adult sheep. Bladder rupture is unusual and urine normally leaks across the stretched bladder wall. Detection of a distended bladder (>6–8 cm in a 25–30 kg lamb) would help differentiate uroperitoneum (highly likely) from a transudate (highly unlikely). The absence of fibrin tags rules out an exudate associated with peritonitis. The right kidney should be examined ultrasonographically for evidence of hydronephrosis via the right sublumbar fossa. An increased renal pelvis to cortex ratio indicates hydronephrosis, which develops after more than 5–7 days of urethral obstruction.

4 What further tests could be undertaken? An abdominocentesis sample with a creatinine concentration >2 times the serum concentration indicates uroperitoneum.

5 What action would you recommend? In valuable breeding rams a tube cystotomy could be attempted, but this is not a simple procedure and requires general anaesthesia and long-term case management. A subischial urethrostomy, in an attempt to salvage the carcass value of this lamb, could be undertaken but would not be financially worthwhile and would also present welfare concerns.

CASE 2.37

1 What concerns you about the ram? In-growing horns can cause problems in some sheep breeds and present as a common animal welfare issue in law courts.

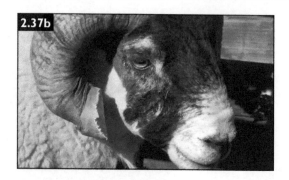

2 **What action would you take?** A conservative length of horn tip has been removed using Gigli wire in this case (**2.37b**) to avoid haemorrhage and possible sensitive areas nearer the horn base. Note that the skin is broken and the horn has been causing a problem for several weeks; this situation is difficult to defend in law courts because of the chronicity of the problem. Occasionally, the horn is broken near its base and becomes misshapen, with the horn tip growing into the cheek or, sometimes, the orbit of the eye.

3 **What advice would you offer the farmer?** Horned sheep must be checked regularly for abnormal horn position/growth and the horn(s) removed, as in **2.37b**, where problems arise.

CASE 2.38

1 **Does routine foot paring reduce lameness, especially footrot?** Foot paring should only be undertaken in lame sheep where the cause of lameness is not obvious and a white line abscess or similar is suspected (**2.38b**). All impacted soil/foreign material

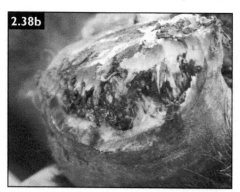

is removed from the interdigital space. Grossly overgrown horn from the abaxial wall and toe of the foot of the lame leg is carefully removed with shears or a sharp hoof knife to check for a white line abscess, toe granuloma, etc. Overparing of the hoof horn of the wall (**2.38a**) must be avoided because this action simply transfers weight to the sole. There is no evidence that routine foot trimming prevents footrot.

2 **Are there any potential disadvantages of routine foot paring?** Underrunning of the horn associated with footrot or contagious ovine digital dermatitis (CODD) is very painful and is best treated with parenteral antibiotics, such as oxytetracycline, or a macrolide drug such as tilmicosin. Field studies show that better results are achieved with tilmicosin, but this drug is restricted to veterinary administration in many countries. Other macrolide antibiotics such as gamithromycin are increasingly used for treating footrot and CODD because no such restriction applies, although there is presently no license for their use in sheep in many countries. It is essential not to damage the sensitive corium, as this will delay regeneration of epithelium and extend healing time. Exposure of the sensitive corium to irritant chemicals, such as formalin in footbaths, may result in excessive granulation tissue and the formation of a toe fibroma. Foot trimming 5–7 days later when the lesions appear less aggressive is not necessary and could delay healing.

3 **What control strategies could be suggested for footrot in this flock?** There are few reported split-flock trials of footrot vaccines in the UK, but there is anecdotal information that vaccination can contribute to footrot control measures in flocks.

Whole flock gamithromycin treatment has produced very encouraging results with footrot elimination and flocks have remained free of disease for up to 2–3 years at the time of publication of this book. The critical factor is that every single sheep must be treated and this appears to require veterinary attendance to ensure no sheep are left untreated.

CASE 2.39

1 **What are these lesions?** Healing fractures at the costochondral junctions.

2 **Comment on the welfare of this lamb with respect to these lesions.** These lesions are likely to have been very painful at the time of injury at delivery and for at least several weeks until full union, which is apparent in **2.39b**.

3 **What is the most likely cause?** Trauma/fractures to the rib cage at the costochondral junctions are a risk when oversized lambs (especially singletons) are delivered in posterior presentation using excessive traction. Fractures of the ribs can severely impair respiratory function and may cause death soon after delivery. It has also been suggested that lambs that sustain rib fractures during assisted delivery are more prone to respiratory infections. Excessive traction can also cause rupture of the liver, resulting in sudden death.

4 **Apart from difficulty with breathing, what other clinical signs may have been present?** Radial nerve paralysis/brachial plexus avulsion may also result from excessive traction of a lamb in posterior presentation.

5 **How could this problem have been avoided?** Perform a caesarean operation when presented with an oversized single lamb in posterior presentation, but clients are rarely prepared to pay for surgery in commercial value sheep. An oversized single lamb in posterior presentation is the most common reason to perform a caesarean operation in pedigree meat breed sheep.

CASE 2.40

1 **Describe the important sonographic findings.** There is marked distension of small intestine and some accumulation of fluid between distended loops of intestine. There are no visible fibrin tags. The sonogram is only an image; observation of the intestines for 30 seconds revealed very poor propulsion of digesta through the intestines.

2 **What conditions would you consider (most likely first)?** Small intestinal torsion around the root of the mesentery; intussusception with distended small intestine proximal to the lesion; ileus caused by grain overload.

3 **What treatment would you administer?** Symptomatic treatment includes 'shock dose' IV fluid therapy. NSAID therapy should also be administered to control pain and likely endotoxaemia. However, these treatments will not correct the primary problem of suspected intestinal torsion and the lamb should be euthanased for welfare reasons, as surgery requires inhalation anaesthesia and a surgeon skilled in abdominal surgery. The torsion was confirmed at necropsy; a similar torsion from a yearling sheep is shown (**2.40b**).

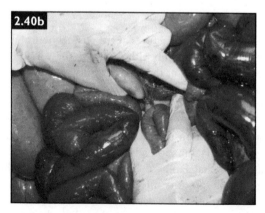

4 **How can this problem be avoided?** Small intestinal torsion around the root of the mesentery occurs sporadically, but the creep feeding may have played a role in the aetiology with limited rumen development. The farmer reported no other cases and was not prepared to compromise lamb growth rates by limiting concentrate feeding.

CASE 2.41

1 What has happened in 2.41a? Death of a foster lamb. Fostering lambs with the aid of the dead lamb's skin generally has good success provided there is good supervision to ensure that the lamb is sucking. Not only has the ewe's lamb died, but also a foster lamb – this situation seriously questions the level of stock supervision on this farm.

2 Is this practice common? In most management systems there is an obvious financial advantage to be gained from ewes nursing twins rather than a single lamb. The perinatal lamb mortality rate is high in many sheep flocks and as a consequence, triplet lambs are often fostered onto those ewes that have lost a lamb, whether stillborn or died from other causes. In addition, lambs are commonly fostered onto ewes that produce a single lamb. No large surveys have been undertaken to determine the number of attempted 'fosterings' in lowground flocks, but are conservatively estimated at greater than 10–15%. Furthermore, this procedure is not as simple as would first appear and the long-term acceptance rate by the ewe is often less than 70%.

3 What advice must be given to farm staff? The ewe and lambs must be carefully supervised to detect early rejection such as not letting the foster lamb suck and pushing the lamb away, and vigorous head butting, which can cause severe chest trauma, and indeed death, of neglected lambs. Ewes with a foster lamb should be clearly marked and allocated to small paddocks for up to 1 week before rejoining the main flock. Adequate supervision is patently lacking in this flock.

4 Are there any alternatives to this practice? Orphan lambs can be very successfully reared on artificial rearing systems using automatic milk dispensers (**2.41b**), which achieve excellent growth rates and a low incidence of digestive disturbances, such as abomasal bloat and/or volvulus, but are expensive.

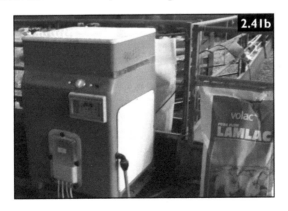

CASE 2.42

1 What conditions would you consider (most likely first)? Include: laryngeal chondritis; laryngeal foreign body; enlarged retropharyngeal lymph nodes compressing the pharynx/larynx; pharyngeal cellulitis/abscess caused by dosing gun injury; pasteurellosis.

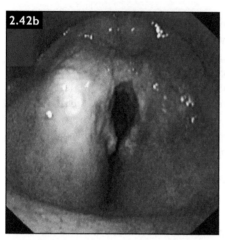

2 How could you confirm your diagnosis? Swelling of the arytenoids, with or without erosion/infection of the underlying cartilage, causing severe narrowing of the larynx can be visualised during endoscopic examination (**2.42b**), but this procedure should not be undertaken in severely dyspnoeic sheep. Sedation is likely to exacerbate the condition.

3 What actions/treatments would you recommend? Treatment includes 10 mg dexamethasone IV immediately to reduce laryngeal oedema. There are few data to indicate which antibiotic is most appropriate; *Trueperella pyogenes* is commonly isolated from lesions. Early recognition and a prolonged primary course of antibiotics are essential; the recovery rate of relapsed cases is low.

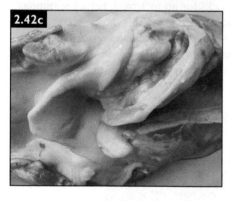

In an emergency situation it may necessary to perform a tracheostomy under local anaesthesia via a ventral midline approach in the mid-cervical region. It may prove difficult fixing the trachea to make the incision between two tracheal rings without aggravating the ram's dyspnoea. Intranasal/transtracheal oxygen administration via a wide bore needle can be supplied if available. Be aware that abscessation of the arytenoid cartilage(s) may be present in many relapsed cases (**2.42c**). No further treatment will successfully resolve this problem and euthanasia is indicated.

4 What controls measures would you recommend? Conformation and turbulent air passage through the oedematous larynx of rams approaching the breeding season leads to erosion of the lining epithelium, with secondary bacterial infection causing swelling and further narrowing of the airway. Reduce level of concentrate feeding when preparing rams for sale. Some breeders believe that there is a strong heritable component, but there are no conclusive pedigree data because most breeders are reluctant to admit to such a problem in their stock.

CASE 2.43

1 How would you achieve effective analgesia for fracture realignment and repair? Effective analgesia can be achieved immediately after lumbosacral extradural injection, using a 21 gauge, 15 mm (5/8 in) hypodermic needle, of 3 mg/kg of 2% lidocaine (note procaine is not licensed for extradural injection) and IV injection of a NSAID such as flunixin before the procedure. There are no injectable general anaesthetic drugs licensed for use in sheep in the UK, but alphaxalone and propofol work very well.

2 How would you repair the fracture? The fracture is easily reduced and immobilised with a fibreglass cast (or similar) applied with slight flexion of the hock joint. The hock angle maintains the cast in place while the 'Softban' or similar padding underneath permits growth over the next 3 weeks before removal. Applying traction to the distal limb without limb paralysis to effect reduction is cruel, largely ineffective and results in overextension of the hock with straightening of the leg and potential for loss of the cast within hours/days (or the cast is applied too tightly). Failure to effectively reduce a metacarpal fracture has resulted in abnormal angulation of the distal limb (valgus) and excessive callus formation (**2.43b**). The bone reaction (exostosis) in this case may extend over time to impact on the fetlock joint.

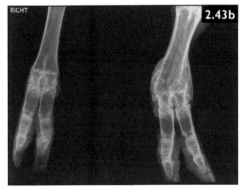

3 What other treatments would you recommend? There is the risk of bacteraemia in neonates, therefore a 10–14 day course of antibiotics is indicated as a precaution against infection of the traumatised (fracture) site.

CASE 2.44

1 What is the likely cause (most likely first)? Footrot, the term commonly used to describe the highly contagious foot disease caused by *D. nodosus,* with extensive under-running of hoof horn; interdigital dermatitis; contagious ovine digital dermatitis.

2 How is the diagnosis confirmed? Diagnosis is based on clinical examination with underrunning of hoof horn of the sole and extending up the wall in severe cases. A polymerase chain reaction-based assay is used to specifically identify and group *D. nodosus* from footrot lesions, although strain typing is rarely undertaken in practice.

3 What treatment would you administer? Foot-bathing is not an appropriate treatment for sheep with footrot, although, when used correctly, it limits the spread of the disease (**2.44b**). The most commonly used treatment for individual sheep with footrot is an injection of long-acting oxytetracycline (20 mg/kg IM) together with removal of all debris from the interdigital space and application of an antibacterial spray. Recent field studies have also demonstrated the efficacy of gamithromycin injection. Treatment of sheep with footrot within 3 days of onset of lameness minimises spread of the disease to other sheep. Pain relief in the form of a NSAID can also be administered where sheep are markedly lame (off-label use in many countries), but there is limited supporting evidence at present. Segregating those sheep with footrot from sound sheep at the earliest opportunity helps to reduce the spread of footrot.

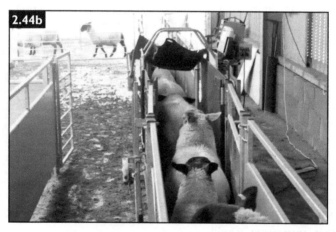

4 What control measures would you include in the flock health plan? Regular foot-bathing is successful in preventing footrot and reducing the spread of footrot and will also treat interdigital dermatitis, but it is not an appropriate treatment for sheep with footrot. There is no evidence that any one type of foot-bath treatment formulation is more effective than another. There is some published information that footrot vaccination can contribute to its control in flocks. There is no scientific evidence that routine foot trimming is beneficial in the treatment or prevention of footrot. Wherever possible, sheep producers should maintain a closed flock to prevent purchasing diseased sheep.

CASE 2.45

1 What is the likely cause? The ewe has suffered from gangrenous mastitis caused by either *Mannheimia* spp. or *Staphylococcus aureus*. The disease peaks around week 6 of lactation when milk demand is highest. It is most commonly reported in ewes nursing twins, but especially in ewes nursing triplets; it is rarely seen in ewes nursing single lambs.

2 What action would you take? This ewe is unsuitable for future breeding because of welfare concerns and the severe damage to mammary tissue. The infected fibrous/granulation tissue, and resultant deep inguinal lymph node enlargement, would result in likely carcass condemnation (and raise genuine welfare concerns at the slaughter plant). The fleece is of poor quality because growth has occurred during this period

of illness and debility. The ewe should have been euthanased for welfare reasons during the peracute phase of disease because it has suffered for months only to be financially worthless. It is not possible to amputate the proliferative fibrous mass(es) because of the profuse blood supply, and their fibrous nature (**2.45b**) means that attempting haemastasis by placing sutures does not generate sufficient pressure to occlude the blood vessels.

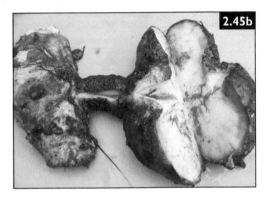

3 What control measures could be adopted? Control measures include ensuring ewes are very well fed during early lactation. Farmers should supply appropriate concentrates to ewes and lambs when pasture growth is poor. Farmers must not expect ewes to rear triplets. Identify and treat superficial teat skin lesions with topical antibiotics.

CASE 2.46

1 Describe the sonogram. There are several compartments to this well-encapsulated structure, which extends up to 30 cm. The extensive anechoic area contains a hyperechoic fibrin matrix.

2 What is this structure (most likely first)? The sonographic findings are consistent with a haematoma, probably sited within the broad ligament. The possibility of an inflammatory exudate could be considered, but the lesion is too extensive considering the lack of clinical signs, the fibrin being too extensive and too organised for peritonitis and no involvement of any abdominal viscera.

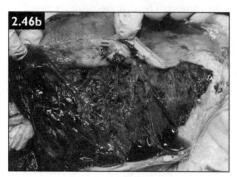

3 What action would you take? The ewe was euthanased for welfare reasons because of the renal adenocarcinoma. The diagnosis of a large haematoma within the broad ligament (or similar) was confirmed at necropsy (2.46b). It is highly unlikely that this volume of organised blood clot would have been resorbed.

CASE 2.47

1 What conditions would you consider (most likely first)? Ovine pulmonary adenocarcinoma (OPA); chronic suppurative pneumonia; pleuropneumonia/pleural abscess; mediastinal abscess caused by caseous lymphadenitis (CLA); visna-meadi.

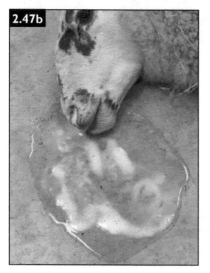

2 How would you confirm the diagnosis? The diagnosis could be confirmed following ultrasonographic examination of the chest. Only about 75% of advanced OPA cases produce copious clear frothy fluid from the nostrils (2.47b; note this sheep is dead) when the ewe's hindquarters are raised (positive wheelbarrow test). However, this 'test' greatly exacerbates any dyspnoea such that all positive sheep should be killed immediately afterwards for welfare reasons.

3 What treatment would you administer? The prognosis for OPA is hopeless and affected sheep must be culled immediately for welfare reasons and to limit further disease spread within the flock.

4 What control measures could be attempted in this flock? Control measures include purchase of flock replacements from known OPA-free sources. During winter housing, when the risk of aerosol transmission is greatly increased, group sheep in age cohorts not on keel marks (anticipated lambing date) to limit spread of OPA. When sheep are grouped by age, infection acquired by older sheep from their pen mates does not present such a problem because these ewes would be voluntarily culled at the end of their productive lives before significant lung pathology had time to develop. Isolate suspected cases immediately and cull as soon as the diagnosis has been established. In endemically infected flocks, it has been recommended that sheep with early OPA lesions can be detected after a period of driving, with any exercise-intolerant or dyspnoeic sheep culled at this early stage. There is presently no commercially available serological test for OPA. Where there is a high prevalence of OPA in one group of sheep, cull that group. In closed flocks, cull the progeny of all clinical OPA cases.

CASE 2.48

1 What is the cause of the lameness? It has been proposed that all lameness in neonates is considered septic until proven otherwise. However, in this case there is a greenstick fracture of the right third metacarpal bone.

2 What other conditions would you consider? Differential diagnoses of moderate lameness would include joint trauma and an early joint infection. Foot abscess and interdigital infections can be readily excluded on clinical examination.

3 How would you correct this problem? Apply a plaster or fibreglass cast extending from the foot to the first joint proximal to the fracture site. Typically, fractures of the third metacarpal bone necessitate immobilisation to the carpus. Plaster casts are removed using an oscillating saw after 3 weeks, by which time the fracture site will be stabilised by callus formation. Recasting is not usually necessary but the two halves of the removed cast can be taped together and left supporting the limb for another 2–3 weeks.

Splints can also be used to stabilise distal limb fractures. Typically, plastic foam-lined splints are applied to the front and rear of the distal limb and taped in position. Such splints are popular with shepherds, as they can be quickly applied in the field without a requirement for hot water and there is no time wasted waiting for the cast to harden. Once removed, these splints can be cleaned and reused.

CASE 2.49

1 What is the cause (most likely first)? Cutaneous myiasis; skin wound and secondary nuisance or head fly activity; severe lice infestation. Clinical inspection eliminates other possible diagnoses.

2 What treatment options would you consider? The lamb can be treated by plunge dipping using a synthetic pyrethroid or organophosphate preparation, but it is

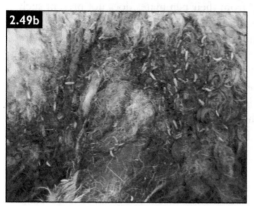

more usual to treat infested sheep with dip wash applied directly to the struck area after first clipping away overlying wool. Antibiotics and a NSAID are indicated in more severely affected individual sheep (**2.49b**), which must be housed to prevent irritation of the skin wound by head flies.

3 What control measures would you recommend to the farmer? Control of parasitic gastroenteritis relies on targeted anthelmintic treatments, which should be part of the veterinary-supervised flock health programme. Where faecal staining of the perineum occurs, this wool must be removed ('dagging' or 'crutching'). Dimpylate (diazinon) and propetamphos are effective against blowfly strike. The synthetic pyrethroids, including high *cis* cypermethrin, have a much higher human safety margin than the organophosphorus compounds and persist in the fleece for up to 8 weeks.

While topical application of high *cis* cypermethrin pour-on preparations provides protection against fly strike, these preparations persist for only 6–8 weeks and require reapplication in most situations. Cyromazine applied before the risk period is effective against blowfly strike for up to 10 weeks after topical application. Dicyclanil provides 16 weeks full body protection against cutaneous myiasis. The extended meat withhold times may help decide which product to use when lambs are close to sale.

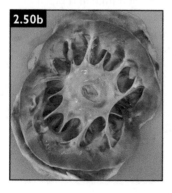

CASE 2.50
1 Describe the sonogram. There is severe hydronephrosis with a fluid-distended renal pelvis and reduced renal cortex (**2.50b**). There is approximately 7–8 cm of fluid separating the kidney from the abdominal wall, which is abnormal. This fluid contains numerous large tags, which are likely to be fibrin strands. There is 1–2 cm of fluid immediately outside the renal capsule (**2.50b**).

2 What has caused this problem? Urethral obstruction results in bladder distension and this back pressure causes bilateral hydroureter and hydronephrosis. The fluid surrounding the right kidney is likely to be urine; haemorrhage and development of a fibrin clot would cause a much larger hyperechoic area than the strands visible in 2.50a.

3 What action would you take? Such renal pathology is irreversible and the ram should be euthanased for welfare reasons.

Hydronephrosis is avoided by prompt identification of the sick ram by the shepherd, with immediate veterinary attention to relieve the urinary tract obstruction. In most cases the urethral obstruction is caused by a calculus within the vermiform appendage, which is simply excised. Obstruction proximal to the sigmoid flexure in a valuable breeding ram is corrected by tube cystotomy. A sub-ischial urethrostomy can be used as a salvage procedure but should be very carefully considered because ascending infection commonly results in cystitis (and pyelonephritis), with clinical signs detected after approximately 6 weeks.

4 How could this problem have been prevented? Correct ration formulation with appropriate mineral supplementation (low magnesium) is the basis for prevention of urolithiasis in intensively reared sheep. Urine acidifiers, such as ammonium chloride, are commonly added to rations. Sodium chloride can be added to rations to promote water intake. Provision of roughage promotes saliva production and water intake. Fresh clean water must always be available.

CASE 2.51

1 What is the lesion? A keloid or keratoma.

2 What is the likely cause? The cause is keratinisation of a skin injury following repeated damage to the skin overlying the poll caused by fighting injury. The role of contagious pustular dermatitis (orf) virus in the aetiology of a keloid has been suggested but not proven.

3 What action would you take? Such lesions grow very slowly and no action is needed. Surgical removal is rarely possible, or advised, due to the broad base and profuse blood supply. Haemostasis would prove difficult; cautery could be attempted but aggravation of the lesion may lead to granulation tissue. Broken skin lesions on the poll attract head flies and a pour-on fly repellent should be applied before, and throughout, the fly season.

CASE 2.52

1 What is the cause of this problem (most likely cause first)? Feeding around head wounds and ear tag injuries (and horn base) by the muscid fly *Hydrotea irritans* causes considerable irritation that frequently results in self-trauma.

Grazing patterns are disturbed and affected sheep often isolate themselves. They may stand with the head held lowered, with frequent head shaking and ear movements. Alternatively, sheep adopt a submissive posture in sternal recumbency with the neck extended and the head held on the ground. Kicking at the head often greatly exacerbates damage caused by head flies around the horn base, and such action may also traumatise the skin of the neck and ears. Head rubbing also causes considerable self-trauma. Bleeding and serum exudation attracts more flies and aggravates the problem. There is rapid loss of condition in severely affected sheep. Myiasis may result in some cases.

2 How can this problem be controlled? Housing is essential for sheep with large skin lesions to allow time for complete healing. Topical emollients and antibiotic preparations are not usually necessary, and skin wounds heal well provided flies are denied access to these areas. Pour-on fly control preparations, such as high *cis* cypermethrin or deltamethrin, must be applied before the anticipated head fly season and especially to horned sheep. Such treatments should be repeated every 3–4 weeks during the fly season or as directed by the data sheet instructions. Following an apparently minor lesion, head flies present a serious welfare issue, which should not be underestimated.

CASE 2.53

1 Comment on the quality of the straw and any associated disease risks to pregnant ewes. *Bacillus licheniformis* is associated with poor quality/mouldy straw stored outdoors and is a recognised pathogen causing late abortion in cattle; there are few reports of such abortion in sheep. However, such poor quality straw will be unsuitable for bedding material for sheep and poor underfoot conditions in the sheep shed may predispose to spread of footrot and an increased incidence of infectious diseases in newborn lambs due to poor hygiene and high environmental bacterial load/challenge.

2 Comment on the silage feeding and any associated disease risks. Punctured silage wraps are a risk factor for listeriosis because ingress of air allows rapid multiplication. It has been postulated that listeria contaminated silage results in numerous latent infections in the intestinal wall, often approaching 100% of the exposed flock, but clinical listeriosis in only a few animals. *Listeria* that are ingested or inhaled tend to cause septicaemia, abortion and latent infection or cause encephalitis via minute wounds in the buccal mucosa, with ascending infection of the trigeminal nerve.

3 How can these disease risks be reduced? Every effort must be taken not to puncture wrapped silage bales during handling and storage, with all punctures sealed immediately. Stores of wrapped silage bales must be fenced against farm stock and vermin. The use of additives at the time of ensiling produces a more acidic pH, which discourages multiplication of *L. monocytogenes*. Outbreaks of listeriosis occur 10–14 days after feeding poor quality silage. Use of that particular silage should be discontinued whenever possible and any spoiled silage (punctured wraps etc.) should be discarded routinely or fed to growing cattle at the farmer's risk. Straw should be stored under cover wherever possible.

CASE 2.54

1 What is the most likely cause of this pathology? Pigmented strain of Johne's disease (paratuberculosis). The grossly thickened and corrugated ileum is typical of Johne's disease; as a simple guide you can read newsprint (font size 14 and above) through stretched overlain normal intestine but not thickened gut affected by Johne's disease. A sample of ileum and mesenteric lymph node should be submitted for histopathology and Ziehl–Neelsen staining where doubt exists over the diagnosis. Pigmented strains of *Mycobacterium paratuberculosis* causing orange discolouration occur in 5–15% of cases.

2 What has this single necropsy revealed? A single necropsy is expensive and gives no indication of disease prevalence.

3 What advice would you offer? Other lean ewes (**2.54b**) should have blood samples analysed for serum protein concentrations because this is the cheapest and most informative initial screening test to determine the significance of the single necropsy result. Sheep with Johne's disease have profound hypoalbuminaemia (serum values <15 g/l [1.5 g/dl]; normal range >30 g/l [3 g/dl]) and normal globulin concentration. These protein concentrations

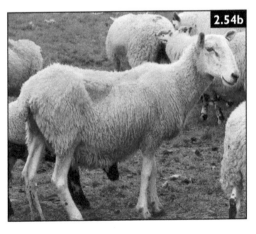

2.54b

may very occasionally be encountered in cases of severe chronic parasitism; protein-losing nephropathies are rare. Typically, in chronic fasciolosis and chronic bacterial infections there is hypoalbuminaemia (<25 g/l [2.5 g/dl]) and a marked increase in serum globulin concentration (>55 g/l [5.5 g/dl]; normal range <45 g/l [4.5 g/dl]). A faecal sample should be checked for fluke eggs (sedimentation) and, where negative, a septic focus should be considered. Be aware that sheep with Johne's disease may have disproportionately high worm egg counts and patent lungworm infection as a consequence of immune system suppression. ELISA tests have a low sensitivity during the early stages of paratuberculosis. A PCR test on a faecal sample could be undertaken but is considerably more expensive than serum protein determinations.

CASE 2.55

1 **What conditions would you consider?** Septicaemia/pasteurellosis predisposed by ovine pulmonary adenocarcinoma (OPA); intestinal torsion or other catastrophic event.

2 **What action would you take?** The prognosis is hopeless if there is evidence of OPA, therefore scan both sides of the chest with a 5 MHz scanner (linear or sector). This examination will take less than 5 minutes, with 100% sensitivity and specificity for OPA lesions >2–3 cm in diameter present at the pleural surface.

3 **What treatment would you administer?** The ewe was euthanased because of extensive OPA lesions identified during ultrasonographic examination, which were subsequently confirmed at necropsy (2.55b). Note that fibrin deposition is present only over lung affected by OPA, presumably because the tumour compromised the

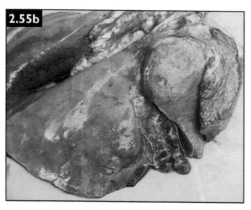

physical lung defences in these areas. There are also widespread petechiae on the lung surface consistent with septicaemia.

Septicaemia secondary to OPA is not uncommon after a stressful event such as housing. Recent veterinary laboratory data show that more than 50% of acute respiratory disease cases in adult sheep are associated with OPA. Always suspect OPA in cases of acute respiratory disease in adult sheep until proven otherwise, even though the tumour may have been growing slowly in the lungs for many months. Failure to clear bacteria from the lower airways in OPA compromised lung may explain the association with septicaemia and sudden illness/death.

CASE 2.56

1 **What is the cause of this problem?** Umbilical infection with *Fusiformis necrophorum* causing hepatic necrobacillosis and associated local peritonitis/adhesions.

2 **Could this problem have been diagnosed?** In some lambs the liver can be palpated extending beyond the costal arch, and digital pressure caudal to the xiphisternum may elicit a painful response. Transabdominal ultrasonography immediately caudal to the costal arch in the ventral midline would identify liver abscesses, but there are no such reports in the literature.

3 **What treatment should have been given?** Prompt recognition and antibiotic treatment of hepatic necrobacillosis may arrest growth of the infective lesions; thereafter, liver regeneration may restore health, although such lambs are unlikely to grow as well as their healthy co-twin. However, this is largely supposition and the extent to which the liver regenerates in hepatic necrobacillosis remains unknown. The causal organism is fully susceptible to penicillin. If there is associated local peritonitis/adhesions to adjacent small intestine (this case), the animal will not respond to antibiotic therapy because the major problem is impaired movement of digesta through the intestines.

4 **Could this problem have been prevented?** The umbilicus (navel) must be fully immersed in strong veterinary iodine BP within the first 15 minutes of life and repeated at least 2–4 hours later. Antibiotic aerosol sprays are much inferior to strong veterinary iodine BP for dressing navels, and are much more expensive. This essential routine procedure can be incorporated into the management routine when the ewe and her lambs are penned soon after birth, and again 2–4 hours later when the shepherd checks that the lambs have sucked colostrum.

CASE 2.57

1 **What are your thoughts on this subject?** There is no reason to castrate a lamb that will reach market weight by 6 months old. After that age, fighting behaviour between male lambs may reduce growth rate and cause individual injury. Castration is now rare in the pig industry and bull beef is standard practice for calves from the dairy industry.

The lamb is more than 1 week old, therefore this means of castration in the UK is illegal, although it is not uncommon to observe this method in lambs older than the legal limit. The lamb shows acute intense pain, frequently lying down with the hindlegs extended, rolling, kicking with its hindlegs and frequent vocalization. There is a large body of evidence that tail docking and castration cause both acute and chronic pain in lambs. An alternative method using a Burdizzo bloodless castrator is unpopular because the method requires two people and the procedure is not 100% effective in many situations because of operator error. Surgical castration again requires two people and risks infection of the open wounds, including tetanus in unvaccinated flocks, and herniation of intestines through the inguinal ring.

Assessment of lamb welfare after castration based on behaviour, serum cortisol and heart rate has sought to evaluate the various methods available. Burdizzo castration followed immediately by local injection into the spermatic cord produced the least pain, but is not considered practical under working conditions on the farm.

Injection of lambs with a NSAID before castration reduces pain but does not completely eliminate it. NSAIDs are being increasingly used to treat a wide range of painful conditions in sheep despite limited data on their clinical efficacy as analgesics. Experimental data are available on the benefits of NSAIDs in treating toxic infections. Although there are no licensed NSAIDs in the UK, they can be administered to sheep under 'the cascade system'.

CASE 2.58

1 What conditions would you consider? Lesion adjacent to, or involving, the optic chiasma such as a pituitary tumour; basilar empyema; cerebral abscess; closantel toxicity. Diagnosis is based on bilateral involvement of cranial nerves II and III. The obtunded mentation could be explained by a large mass causing high intracranial pressure.

2 What treatment would you administer? There is no treatment for a pituitary tumour, although there may be temporary improvement after dexamethasone injection. There is no reported link to long-term exposure to plant poisons such as bracken.

3 What action would you take? The affected sheep was euthanased for welfare reasons and the diagnosis confirmed at necropsy (**2.58b**).

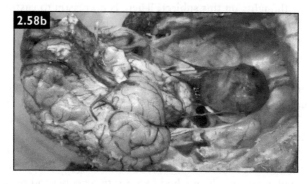

CASE 2.59

1 What conditions would you consider? Infectious keratoconjuctivitis (IKC); periorbital eczema.

2 What treatments would you recommend? The two common causal organisms, *Mycoplasma conjunctivae* and *Chlamydia psittaci*, are susceptible to a wide range of antibiotics including oxytetracycline. Ewes with severe lesions should be injected IM with long-acting oxytetracycline (20 mg/kg). For cost reasons, topical oxytetracycline ophthalmic ointment or powder is applied daily for up to 3 days in mild cases, although there is marked improvement after only one treatment. Ophthalmic powder adheres to the moist conjunctivae, whereas ointment tends to slip off the cornea, especially when the contents of the tube are cold. There is poor immunity and recurrence of IKC is common.

3 What action would you recommend? Ewes in advanced pregnancy with impaired vision in both eyes should be housed, thereby ensuring adequate feeding to prevent ovine pregnancy toxaemia and deaths from misadventure. Ewes should be taken off exposed hill ground when storms are forecast, but this is not always possible. Occasionally, outbreaks of IKC occur associated with concentrate/roughage feeding; in these instances the space allowance should be increased.

CASE 2.60

1 What conditions would you consider (most likely first)? Include: peritonitis causing ileus arising from an umbilical infection; hepatic necrobacillosis; intussusception; abomasal bloat.

2 What treatment would you administer? The lamb is severely dehydrated, therefore fluid therapy is necessary and would best be administered IV; oral fluid therapy, while much cheaper, may exacerbate the abdominal pain. Antibiotics and NSAID therapy should also be administered.

3 What action should be taken? The severity of the clinical signs is such that the prognosis is guarded and the decision was taken to euthanase the lamb for welfare reasons. The provisional diagnosis of peritonitis associated with umbilical infection was shown to be incorrect, with an intussusception revealed at necropsy (**2.60b**, arrow).

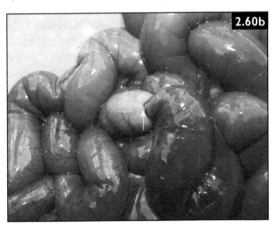

4 How can this problem be avoided? No obvious cause of the intussusception was found, therefore no advice regarding prevention could be given; no further cases were recognised.

CASE 2.61

1 **What is the likely diagnosis?** Include: chronic mastitis – occurs sporadically after weaning but lesions are not usually so extensive; exacerbation of udder infection present during previous lactation.

2 **Are there any consequences of such conditions?** Consequences of udder infection includes bacteraemic spread with secondary lung/pleural abscesses.

3 **What pathogens could be involved?** *Trueperella pyogenes* and *Staphylococcus aureus* are the most common isolates from udder abscesses.

4 **What is the prognosis?** The udder lesions will not resolve despite antibiotic therapy because of the thick-walled abscesses and extensive fibrous tissue reaction. These ewes are unsuitable for breeding stock. Affected ewes can be sent for slaughter but there is the risk of carcass condemnation because of lymphadenopathy, particularly the deep inguinal lymph nodes, and the possibility of abscesses in the parenchymatous organs following bacteraemic spread.

5 **What control measures could have been adopted?** Subcutaneous injection of tilmicosin at weaning has proved successful for the control of post-weaning mastitis in ewes, but such treatment is considered by farmers to be too expensive.

CASE 2.62

1 **What conditions would you consider (most likely first)?** Include: hypocalcaemia; ovine pregnancy toxaemia; acidosis resulting from carbohydrate overfeeding; listeriosis; botulism.

2 **How could you confirm your diagnosis?** In sheep recumbent due to hypocalcaemia, serum calcium concentrations are below 1.2 mmol/l (4.8 mg/dl). Serum 3-OH butyrate concentrations can be elevated, especially if the ewe has been inappetent for more than 12 hours. Appearance of ruminal contents at the sheep's nostrils often leads to a misdiagnosis of pneumonia by farmers.

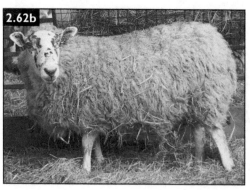

3 **What treatment(s) would you administer?** There is a rapid response to slow IV administration of 30 ml of a 40% calcium borogluconate solution, with eructation and defaecation. This ewe was able to regain her feet (**2.62b**). The response to SC administration of 60–80 ml of 40% calcium borogluconate solution injected over the thoracic wall behind

the shoulder may take up to 4 hours, especially if the solution has not been warmed to body temperature or injected at only one site.

4 What control measures would you recommend? Hypocalcaemia is not uncommon in 3-crop or older ewes during late gestation, but can also occur sporadically during early lactation. 'Outbreaks' of hypocalcaemia can result following errors in formulating home-mix rations with incorrect mineral supplementation and inadequate mixing, stress related events such as dog worrying, severe weather, gathering for vaccination, after ewes are moved on to good pastures before lambing and within 24–48 hours of housing.

CASE 2.63

1 What conditions would you consider? The most likely conditions to consider for the skin lesions include: heavy infestation with the chewing louse *Bovicola ovis*; psoroptic mange (sheep scab); scrapie.

2 How would you establish a specific diagnosis? Large numbers of lice are observed in the fleece, with up to 10–20 lice per fleece parting; very few lice are observed on other sheep in the group. An average count of more than five *B. ovis* per fleece parting is generally considered a heavy infestation. The slow reproductive capacity of *B. ovis* results in a gradual build-up of lice numbers over several months. Lice numbers can be very high on sheep in poor condition; they are the result, rather than a cause, of poor condition.

3 What treatment would you recommend? Lice infestations can be controlled with topical application of high *cis* cypermethrin or deltamethrin. Infested sheep can also be treated by plunge dipping in a synthetic pyrethroid or organophosphate preparation (availability may vary in certain countries). Further investigation revealed that this ewe was suffering from paratuberculosis.

4 What control measures would you recommend? There is no treatment for paratuberculosis and control measures are based on biosecurity/biocontainment and vaccination. Maintenance of a closed flock and effective biosecurity measures will prevent introduction of louse infestation. Annual dipping practices will eliminate this obligatory parasite.

CASE 2.64

Comment on this image (2.64). The term 'mutilation' (deprive of an essential part) is often chosen to refer to tail docking to provoke reaction by farmers because of the acute and chronic pain resulting from this wholly unnecessary procedure. The tails of these lambs have been docked, which is routinely performed in most sheep flocks, to aid in the control of blowfly strike and to present clean sheep at slaughter plants; however, it has clearly proven unsuccessful in this case. It is a legal requirement that sufficient tail remains after docking to completely cover the sheep's anus and vulva (distal to the caudal skin folds). Tail docking has not prevented faecal contamination of the tail and perineum in this situation, and these lambs remain susceptible to the risk of cutaneous myiasis.

Controlling endoparasite-induced diarrhoea by operating safe grazing systems and/or appropriate use of anthelmintics and pour-on insect growth regulators (e.g. dicyclanil), are much more effective measures to control blowfly strike than tail docking, which is a centuries old practice introduced before effective chemical control measures; review is long overdue. Tail docking has long been banned in horses and, more recently, in dogs by enlightened parliaments. Tail docking is banned in piglets unless there are specific issues of tail biting that cannot be controlled by other means. In the longer term, selection of rams for increased resistance to parasitic gastroenteritis may help to reduce faecal contamination of the perineum and tail.

CASE 2.65

1 Describe the important ultrasound findings. Normal aerated lung tissue present dorsally (left of sonogram) reflects sound waves and the lung surface (visceral pleura) appears as a continuous hyperechoic (bright white) line. The uniform hypoechoic (darker) area ventrally represents cellular proliferation/infiltration allowing transmission of sound waves. A broad bright line is readily demonstrable where the sound waves transmitted from the probe head pass through the tumour mass then hit aerated lung. This sharply demarcated hypoechoic area is characteristic of the well-defined tumours of ovine pulmonary adenocarcinoma (OPA).

2 How could you confirm the provisional diagnosis? These sonographic findings are pathognomic for OPA. There is no serological test, such as agar gel immunodiffusion test or ELISA, because infected sheep do not make a detectable antibody response to jaagsiekte sheep retrovirus (JSRV). A PCR test has been used in research on OPA for several years. However, while the test is highly sensitive in laboratory assays, it fails to detect JSRV in most infected sheep other than overt clinical cases. This is because there are few infected cells in the blood during the early stages of disease progression. The sensitivity of a single blood test in field samples identifies only 11% of animals with OPA.

Despite the limitations of the existing blood PCR assay for OPA, testing of a number of animals within a flock should indicate whether the virus is present in the flock.

Copious amounts (50–200 ml) of clear frothy fluid pour from the nostrils of most advanced OPA cases when the hind quarters are raised, but this 'wheel barrow test' is negative in approximately 25% of cases. Large well-defined tumours are revealed at necropsy, occupying the ventral margins of the apical, cardiac and diaphragmatic lung lobes (2.65b).

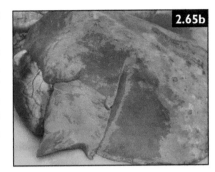

CASE 2.66

1 Comment on the hygiene approach to this common scenario. Farmers must wash their hands and then use arm-length disposable gloves during correction of all dystocias in order to reduce the risk of iatrogenic uterine infection. Obstetrical gel is then liberally applied to the hand of the shepherd's gloved arm; the fingers of the hand are forced together at their tips to form a cone-shape and then gently introduced into the vagina. Careful examination is essential not only for welfare reasons but because the likelihood of infection of the posterior reproductive tract is greatly increased by trauma. Arm-length disposable plastic gloves are cheap and easily carried in pockets,

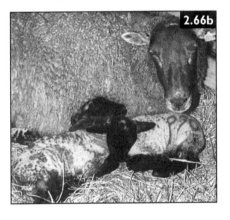

therefore there can be no excuse for non-compliance with such basic hygiene even under extensive flock management systems. Such precautions should also be seen as a minimum standard to limit the risk of potential zoonotic infections such as *Chlamydophila abortus*, *Salmonella* serotypes and Q fever.

Attempted delivery by an unskilled shepherd frequently results in oedema, reddening and bruising of vulval labiae within 1–2 hours. Metritis (2.66b) commonly affects ewes after unhygienic manual interference to correct fetal malpresentation/malposture, causing inappetence and reduced milk production with hungry lambs. All ewes should receive an antibiotic injection after an assisted lambing. Penicillin is the antibiotic most commonly used by sheep farmers and should be administered for a minimum of 3 consecutive days.

Caudal analgesia is strongly recommended for all manipulations undertaken by a veterinary surgeon. This involves extradural injection of 2% per cent lidocaine solution (0.5 mg/kg) at the sacrococcygeal site (caudal block). Blockage of the ewe's reflex abdominal contractions greatly assists corrections/manipulations in dystocia cases and has obvious animal welfare benefits. Reliance on strength by the shepherd to repel the fetus risks serious damage to the ewe.

CASE 2.67

1 What conditions would you consider (most likely first)? Include: bacterial meningoencephalitis; septicaemia; focal symmetrical encephalomalacia; sarcocystosis. Unlike calves, cases of meningoencephalitis are typically encountered in 3–4-week-old lambs.

2 How could you confirm your diagnosis? Collect lumbar CSF under local anaesthesia. Collection using a 21 gauge, 15 mm (5/8 in) hypodermic needle (young lamb) reveals a turbid sample caused by a high white cell concentration, and an frothy appearance visible after sample agitation due to the increased protein content. Laboratory analysis reveals a >100-fold increase in white cell concentration, comprised mainly of neutrophils (neutrophilic pleocytosis), and >five-fold increase in protein concentration (1.5 g/l [150 mg/dl]), consistent with bacterial meningoencephalitis. Culture of lumbar CSF is largely unrewarding and was not undertaken. Inspection of the brain at necropsy rarely yields any gross abnormality because it proves difficult to interpret the significance of congested meningeal vessels.

3 What treatment(s) would you administer? Antibiotic selection could include florfenicol, trimethoprim–sulpha or a fluoroquinolone if the cause was thought to be *Escherichia coli* (product licence regarding use in sheep may vary between countries). Penicillin or amoxicillin would be chosen if a gram-positive cause was considered likely. Dexamethasone (1.0 mg/kg IV) given on the first day by some clinicians is considered controversial.

4 What is the prognosis for this lamb? The normal treatment response rate for bacterial meningoencephalitis in lambs showing seizure activity is very poor. There was no treatment response and the lamb was euthanased for welfare reasons 24 hours later.

CASE 2.68

1 What conditions would you consider (most likely first)? Include: listeriosis; peripheral vestibular lesion with trauma to the right superficial facial nerve; basillar empyema.

2 What laboratory tests could be undertaken to confirm your provisional diagnosis? Gross inspection of lumbar CSF collected under local anaesthesia using a 19 gauge, 50 mm (2 in) hypodermic needle (100 kg ram) reveals no abnormality with listeriosis. Laboratory examination reveals an elevated protein concentration of 1.4 g/l (140 mg/dl) (normal <0.4 g/l [40 mg/dl]), and a slight increase in white cell concentration (pleocytosis) comprised of large mononuclear cells. Serology is not used routinely for diagnosis because many healthy sheep have high *Listeria* titres. In fatal cases, if primary isolation attempts fail, ground brain tissue should be held at 4°C (39°F) for several weeks and recultured weekly.

3 What treatments would you administer? *Listeria monocytogenes* is susceptible to various antibiotics including penicillin, ceftiofur, erythromycin and trimethoprim/sulphonamide. Emphasis should be placed on administering the maximum dose of penicillin cost will permit (up to 300,000 iu/kg) at the first visit rather than the duration of daily penicillin injections thereafter. A single IV injection of soluble corticosteroid (e.g. dexamethasone, 1.1 mg/kg) will reduce the associated severe inflammatory reaction and improve prognosis.

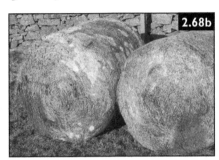

4 What control measures would you recommend? Control involves correct fermentation of grass silage through the use of additives and air-tight storage. When feeding, discard all spoiled silage (**2.68b**) (feed to adult cattle), clean troughs daily and discard refusals.

CASE 2.69

1 What conditions would you consider (most likely first)? Include: ovine pregnancy toxaemia; chronic copper poisoning; polioencephalomalacia; listeriosis; acidosis resulting from excess carbohydrates; impending abortion.

2 How could you confirm your diagnosis? The serum 3-OH butyrate concentration is 4.6 mmol/l (values >3.0 mmol/l are considered to be consistent with pregnancy toxaemia). Plasma glucose and non-esterified fatty acid concentrations are too variable to confirm the presumptive clinical diagnosis.

3 What treatment(s) would you give? Isolate the ewe and offer palatable feedstuffs. Treatments include a concentrated oral electrolyte and dextrose solution or propylene glycol given PO three times daily. Injection with 4 mg dexamethasone promotes appetite and gluconeogenesis (>16 mg after day 135 of pregnancy will induce abortion, which may save the ewe's life). An elective caesarean operation to remove the fetuses is rarely successful because retained fetal membranes and septic metritis invariably result. Recovery is further hindered by a severe fatty liver (**2.69b**).

4 What control measures could be adopted? Control measures include ultrasound scanning, which would identify ewes carrying multiple fetuses. Correct nutrition during gestation is essential, especially for multigravid ewes, which are at most risk from energy deficiency due to fetal demands. Routine monitoring of late gestation

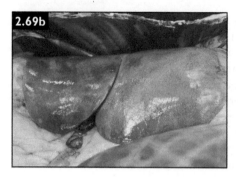

2.69b

nutrition is strongly recommended and the reader is directed to the article by Dr Angus Russel[*], which gives accurate guidelines based upon 3-OH butyrate concentration, fetal number and ewe bodyweight. A veterinary advisory visit undertaken 4–6 weeks before the lambing season is the cornerstone of any flock health programme.

[*] Russel A (1985) Nutrition of the pregnant ewe. *In Practice* 7:23–28.

CASE 2.70

1 **Describe the sonogram.** The broad hyperechoic line representing the lung surface (visceral pleura) has been replaced by a 5 cm diameter anechoic area containing multiple hyperechoic dots bordered distally by a broad hyperechoic capsule.

2 **What is your diagnosis?** The sonographic findings are consistent with a well-encapsulated abscess.

3 **What treatment(s) would you administer?** Published studies have shown that daily treatment with procaine penicillin for up to 42 days is successful in sheep identified with pleural/superficial lung abscesses measuring 2–8 cm in diameter; more extensive lesions and pyothorax cases have a poorer prognosis. The ram was treated with procaine penicillin IM daily for 4 weeks and made a good recovery. It is possible that there were abscesses in other viscera such as the liver and kidneys

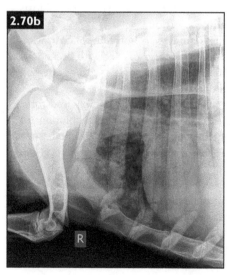

2.70b

as a consequence of bacteraemia, but none were identified. It is not clear why this ram responded to antibiotic therapy when the abscesses appeared to be well-encapsulated; it is possible that other microscopic lesions were not identified.

4 **What other imaging modality could have been used?** Radiography with the left chest against the plate and the leg drawn forward (2.70b) identifies a lesion immediately cranial to the heart but, unlike with ultrasonography, it is not possible to confirm that this structure is an abscess. Smaller lesions cannot readily be identified on the radiograph.

CASE 2.71

1 What conditions would you consider (most likely first)? Include: molar dentition problems (tooth loss, sharp enamel ridges, overgrowth, etc.); listeriosis.

2 How would you investigate this problem? A mouth gag and torch are essential. Be aware that sheep struggle with the mouth gag in place so the shepherd must secure the sheep in the corner of the pen. An oblique lateral view radiograph of the head (plate positioned next to the left side) reveals that all three lower premolars and the first two molars on the left side are missing (**2.71b**). There is considerable bone resorption surrounding the lower third molar tooth on both sides.

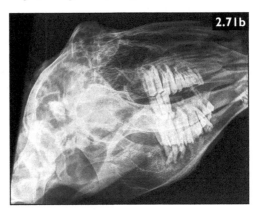

3 What actions/treatments would you recommend? Loss of cheek teeth due to periodontal disease is a common cause of poor body and condition loss in older sheep. Ewes with poor dentition fatten well when fed a high concentrate diet (up to 1.5 kg/head/day) and this is the best commercial option for the farmer. Care must be exercised to avoid acidosis as the ewes are slowly introduced on to a high concentrate ration.

CASE 2.72

1 What common conditions would you consider (most likely first)? Nematodirosis; coccidiosis.

2 What tests could be undertaken to support your provisional diagnosis? Sudden hatching of overwintered infective third-stage larvae (L3) of *Nematodirus battus* after a prolonged period of cold weather can cause sudden-onset profuse diarrhoea, leading to death in young lambs. Faecal samples are usually negative for worm eggs (**2.72b**; large brown *N. battus* egg in centre [arrow]) in acute nematodirosis because the infection is not yet patent. Necropsy reveals

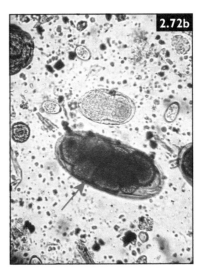

catarrhal enteritis and acute inflammation of the small intestine, with varying numbers of developing larvae and adult worms.

3 What control measures would you recommend? Nematodirosis is a problem where lambs graze pasture used for lambs the previous year. Control by means of safe grazing with alternate years cattle, crops and sheep can rarely be practised on many sheep farms. Prophylactic anthelmintic treatment based on disease risk (weather forecasts) may be necessary to avoid costly disease outbreaks where lambs graze contaminated pastures. Where the timing of prophylactic anthelmintic treatment is in doubt, treat early; such treatment can always be repeated later if considered to be mistimed. Anthelmintic resistance is not a concern with *Nematodirus battus* and Group 1 anthelminitics (benzimadazole anthelmintics), which are otherwise largely ineffective due to resistance in most other nematode species, are commonly administered. Isolated incidents of resistance to benzimadazole anthelmintics have been reported in *N. battus* but this is not a major concern at present.

CASE 2.73

1 What conditions would you consider (most likely first)? Include: contagious pustular dermatitis (CPD, orf, scabby mouth, contagious ecthyma); dermatophilosis; bluetongue; sheep pox (not UK).

2 What treatment would you administer? Intramuscular injection of procaine penicillin for 3–5 consecutive days and topical antibiotic spray can be used to control superficial secondary bacterial infection, but this is not necessary in this situation.

3 What samples would you collect to confirm your diagnosis? CPD virus can be demonstrated by direct electron microscopy of fresh lesions. Bacteriology of the skin lesions to investigate the role of secondary bacteria is of doubtful benefit.

4 What preventive measures could be considered for next year? Orf vaccine must never be used in a clean flock. Vaccination is by scarification of the inner thigh in lambs and the axillary region in ewes. The timing of vaccination is approximately 6 weeks before the anticipated occurrence of disease. Care must be exercised during handling of the live vaccine as it is affected by high temperatures and inactivated by disinfectants. Control thistles, gorse, etc. wherever possible. Orf is a zoonosis, therefore extra care is necessary when handling infected sheep and during vaccination.

CASE 2.74

1 What is the likely cause (most likely first)? Microphthalmia, an autosomal recessive condition recognised in certain breeds, such as the Texel, which can occur at a high prevalence following the introduction of a new ram.

2 What action would you take? Affected lambs should be euthanased for welfare reasons.
3 What advice would you offer? The carrier ram should be identified and culled.

CASE 2.75

1 What conditions would you consider? Include: nephrosis; chronic infection such as suppurative pneumonia; starvation/rejection by dam; coccidiosis.
2 How would you confirm your diagnosis? Laboratory analysis reveals a markedly elevated blood urea nitrogen concentration (54.2 mmol/l [151.8 mg/dl]; normal 2–6 mmol/l [5.6–16.8 mg/dl]) and a low serum albumin concentration (20 g/l [2 g/dl]; normal >30 g/l [3 g/dl]) consistent with a diagnosis of nephrosis. The serum globulin concentration is normal (43 g/l 4.3 g/dl]; normal 35–50 g/l [3.5–5.0 g/dl]), ruling out chronic bacterial infection. Faecal examination for oocysts and strongyle eggs proves negative.

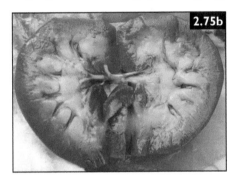
2.75b

3 What is the prognosis for this lamb? The prognosis is hopeless and the lamb should be euthanased for welfare reasons. Necropsy reveals enlarged pale kidneys typical of nephrosis (2.75b). This provisional diagnosis was confirmed on histological examination of stained sections.
4 What control measures would you recommend? There are no specific control measures for nephrosis. For future years the farmer was advised to consider adding decoquinate to the lamb creep to control coccidiosis.

CASE 2.76

1 Describe the important necropsy findings shown. There are widespread petechiae over the myocardium. The lungs appear congested and very oedematous.
2 What is the most likely cause? *Mannheimia haemolytica*, which causes septicaemia in young lambs.
3 How could you confirm your suspicion? Diagnosis is based on bacteriology from various viscera including lung, liver, kidney, spleen, thoracic fluid and heart blood. Histopathology of lung tissue is also advisable.
4 What control measures could be adopted? Vaccination of the dam with a pasteurella vaccine will only provide passively-derived immunity for the first 4 weeks or so of life. Thereafter, vaccination of lambs from 3 weeks old is needed

to provide active immunity. Two vaccinations are required 4–6 weeks apart then annual vaccination 6 weeks pre-lambing. This vaccination protocol may not have prevented disease in this lamb, but is the best available option.

CASE 2.77

1 What is your diagnosis (most likely first)? The most likely conditions to consider include: *Streptococcus dysgalactiae* polyarthritis; polyarthritis caused by another bacterium such as *Escherichia coli*.

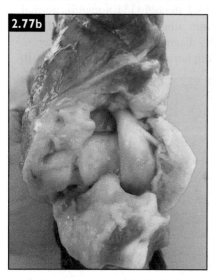

2 How would you confirm your diagnosis? Arthrocentesis often fails to yield sufficient exudate for analysis or bacteriology because chronic joint infection is composed of a pannus (**2.77b**). The lamb will not recover and should be euthanased for welfare reasons. A sample of synovial membrane collected at necropsy yields a higher bacteriology success rate than a joint aspirate. Where possible, samples should be collected from lambs that have not received antibiotic therapy. Radiography would not yield conclusive evidence of joint infection.

3 What treatments would you administer? Recent studies have shown that *S. dysgalactiae* is resistant to oxytetracycline. Procaine penicillin remains the drug of choice for all streptococcal infections in farm animals. A minimum of 5–7 consecutive days of IM procaine penicillin should be administered because this drug is time-dependent. Long-acting penicillin preparations are not appropriate and should not be used as a convenient alternative. As with cases of atlanto-occipital joint infection caused by the same bacterium, there is a rapid and dramatic response to dexamethasone administered on the first day of antibiotic therapy. This response is much better than a NSAID. (**Note:** *S. dysgalactiae* causes >90% of joint infections in lambs, therefore the corticosteroid injection is given at the same time as an effective antibiotic.)

4 What preventive measures could be adopted? The shepherd had immersed the lambs' navels in strong veterinary iodine on three occasions within the first 6 hours of life. Hygiene measures in the lambing shed and ensuring passive antibody transfer often fail to reduce ongoing problems of *S. dysgalactiae* polyarthritis. Changing the lambing accommodation is rarely possible other than turning housed ewe out to pasture, but this increases the risks from hypothermia and causes problems catching ewes with dystocia problems. In an emergency situation of high disease prevalence, prophylactic penicillin injection of lambs around 24 hours old is often effective but unsustainable.

CASE 2.78

1 How will you deal with this case? Vaginal prolapse is a common condition of late gestation but it is concerning that this sheep is recumbent and unresponsive on approach. The major complications associated with vaginal prolapse could include: rupture of a middle uterine artery and extensive haemorrhage; hypocalcaemia; fetal death/autolysis/resultant toxaemia.

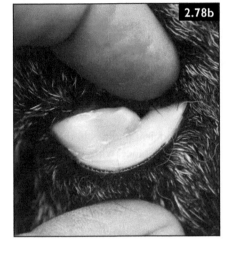

Examination of the conjunctivae reveals very pale mucous membranes (**2.78b**) indicating severe anaemia/haemorrhage.

2 What is the future management of this sheep? The ewe should be euthanased immediately for welfare reasons. Greater patience should be exercised when sheep with prolapses are gathered from the field with dogs, as it is assumed that the uterine artery ruptures when the sheep is running away from the dogs/farmer's quad bike.

CASE 2.79

1 What conditions would you consider? The most likely conditions to consider would include: polioencephalomalacia (PEM; syn. cerebrocortical necrosis, CCN); focal symmetrical encephalomalacia; meningitis/brain abscess; sarcocystosis; listerial meningitis.

2 What treatment would you administer? Treatment for PEM includes injection of thiamine (10 mg/kg IV twice daily on the first occasion, then IM twice daily for 2 more days). There is evidence from field studies that IV injection of dexamethasone (1 mg/kg), or a similar short-acting corticosteroid, aids recovery by reducing brain swelling.

3 What is the prognosis for this case? The prognosis is good when sheep are presented early in the clinical course; this sheep made a rapid recovery.

4 How can the diagnosis be confirmed? Diagnosis is confirmed by the rapid response to timely thiamine treatment. Diagnostic biochemical parameters for

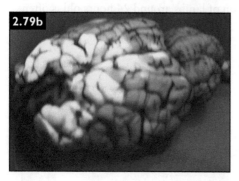

PEM include thiaminase activities in blood; rumen fluid or faeces are rarely used in farm animal practice. At necropsy affected areas of the cerebral cortex may exhibit a bright white autofluoresence when cut sections are viewed under ultraviolet light (Wood's lamp; 365 nm) (**2.79b**). This property has been attributed to the accumulation of lipofuchsin in macrophages, but not all PEM cases fluoresce. Definitive diagnosis relies

on the histological findings in the cortical lesions of vacuolation and cavitation of the ground substance, with astrocytic swelling, neuronal shrinkage and necrosis.

5 What control measures would you recommend? Disease occurs sporadically and there are no specific control measures. Prompt recognition and veterinary treatment are essential for a full recovery.

CASE 2.80

1 What conditions would you consider (most likely first)? Small intestinal torsion around the root of the mesentery; bloat (choke is rare in sheep); ileus caused by grain overload; except for uterine perforation/infection, peritonitis is uncommon in sheep.

2 What further investigations would you undertake? Transabdominal ultrasound examination takes only 2 minutes. Typically, with abdominal catastrophes, there is much reduced gut motility with marked distension of intestinal loops and perhaps an increased amount of fluid/exudate within the peritoneal cavity.

3 What treatment would you administer? A very high heart rate and toxic mucous

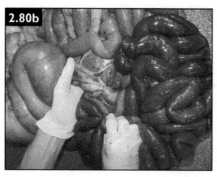

membranes afford a grave prognosis. Symptomatic treatment could include 'shock dose' IV fluid therapy. NSAID therapy should also be administered to control pain and likely endotoxaemia. However, these treatments will not correct the primary problem of suspected intestinal torsion and the ewe should be euthanased for welfare reasons. The torsion was confirmed at necropsy (**2.80b**).

4 How can this problem be avoided? Small intestinal torsion around the root of the mesentery is uncommon in adult sheep, but recent exposure to lush pasture and concentrate feeding may have played a role. The farmer reported having never encountered any similar cases over the past 5 years and was unwilling to change his flock management, which was aimed at achieving high lamb growth rates ahead of breeding sales.

CASE 2.81

1 What is the cause of this problem? Ulcerative posthitis; wool or other material adherent to the glans; trauma; obstructive urolithiasis.

The vermiform appendage could not be identified because of the dried blood and foreign material adherent to the glans. Surprisingly, the ram was able to urinate normally. Attempts to gently soak the penis in warm water and remove dried blood from the glans resulted only in profuse haemorrhage, with the foreign material remaining firmly adherent. It was not possible to decide whether the superficial bacterial infection on the prolapsed penis was the cause of the paraphimosis or a consequence. While the preputial ring was oedematous, there was no evidence of ulcerative posthitis (sheath rot). This condition is caused by *Corynebacterium renale*, which contains the enzyme urease capable of breaking down urea in the urine to release ammonia, which is caustic to the epithelium of the prepuce.

2 What action would you take? It was not possible to replace the penis within the sheath. Strapping the penis in a sling close to the ventral abdominal wall to restrict the dependent oedema was thought to likely cause more trauma when the ram lay down.

3 What treatment would you administer? Daily IM penicillin therapy was started on the assumption that *Corynebacterium renale* was a likely secondary bacterial invader. A single injection of dexamethasone was administered on day 1 to reduce oedema. The prolapsed tissues were bathed in very dilute povidone–iodine solution followed by topical corticosteroid and antibiotic cream applied four times daily.

4 What is the prognosis? The prolapsed tissue remained largely unchanged after 5 days treatment, so the treatment was continued. By day 8 the ram was able to withdraw most of his penis into the sheath, and completely by day 10. There was no obvious reason for the sudden improvement, as the treatment had not changed.

CASE 2.82

1 What is the reasoning behind this management decision? Poor or reduced grazing is thought by farmers to speed up the 'drying off' process and reduce the incidence of mastitis, but there is little evidence that this management practice works.

2 **What are the alternative management strategies?** There are no licensed long-acting intramammary antibiotic preparations for sheep in many countries, although preparations for cattle are used 'off-label' at weaning to eliminate/reduce chronic infections and prevent establishment of new infections in the udder during the dry period. Care must be exercised with intramammary infusion in sheep because iatrogenic infections are common when the procedure is undertaken in wet or unhygienic conditions. Appropriate teat disinfection before antibiotic infusion is essential. The intramammary syringe nozzle is held against the teat orifice; it must not be forced into the streak canal.

Encouraging results have been reported for the treatment of mild cases of mastitis that have been acquired during that lactation using tilmicosin at weaning, but the low prevalence and high cost of whole group therapy mean that only pedigree flocks use this protocol. Treatment based on individual ewe monthly milk somatic

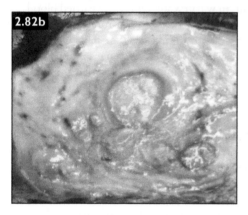

cell counts could be undertaken in milking ewes, as practised in dairy cattle.

Treatment of chronic mastitis that has progressed to abscessation within the gland is not usually undertaken because of the hopeless prognosis and associated loss of normal mammary tissue and lactogenesis. Ewes with chronic mastitis and abscesses (**2.82b**) should be culled following identification at weaning or at the pre-breeding check.

CASE 2.83

1 **What advice would you give?** Testing for triple resistance (Groups 1–3) could be undertaken using a faecal egg count reduction test (FECRT), but your client considers this too much work and expense. Furthermore, the lambs were purchased from multiple sources. The FECRT uses approximately 10 sheep randomly allocated to control and treatment groups (one for each class of anthelmintic to be tested). A faecal worm egg count is then undertaken for all sheep and repeated 10 days later for 2-LV group sheep and 14 days later for control sheep, 1-BZ and 3-ML groups. Anthelmintic resistance is suspected where the mean faecal worm egg count is less than 95% of the percentage reduction in the control group.

Quarantine arrangements are considered essential to reduce the risk of introducing anthelmintic-resistant worms of species such as *Haemonchus contortus* and *Teladorsagia circumcincta*. Current best practice involves sequential full-dose treatments with either 4-AD monepantel (Zolvix®) or 5-SI derquantel and abamectin (Startec®), and moxidectin. All introduced sheep should be grazed separately from the main flock for at least 1 month. As no resistance has been reported to date to Groups 4 and 5 in the UK, including moxidectin for store lambs seems excessive and could be omitted.

Whether 10% of the strongest lambs should be left untreated to carry some anthelmintic-susceptible worms over onto the new pasture to reduce selection for anthelmintic-resistant worms is debatable, because all lambs will be slaughtered within 3–4 months, and the field will be used for silage next season.

Lambs may not need to be treated again with an anthelmintic for up to 8–10 weeks; however, this will depend on the amount of infection carried over, the stocking rate and weather conditions (large numbers of lambs left untreated, high stocking rates and wet weather increase challenge). Monitoring of pooled faecal worm egg counts every 7–10 days after 4–6 weeks with fresh faeces collected from around 10 lambs after gathering into a corner of the field can help to decide whether anthelmintic treatment is necessary. Flukicide treatment would be based on where the lambs were sourced and whether a high risk year was predicted following a wet summer. Treatment against very early stage immature flukes would necessitate the use of triclabendazole. It would be advisable to regularly weigh lambs to ensure target growth rates are being met.

CASE 2.84

1 What are these lesions? Paramphistome infections reside in the ventral walls of the rumen and are now considered common in sheep in the UK. *Calicophoron daubneyi* affects cattle and sheep and was probably introduced into the UK with cattle imported from Europe. *C. daubneyi* has a similar two-host life cycle to *Fasciola heptica* but uses a different intermediate snail host.

2 Are these lesions important? Adult flukes are not thought to cause clinical signs, although large numbers of migrating immature rumen flukes may cause transient diarrhoea. Mature rumen flukes are readily identified at necropsy (**2.84**). Eggs of *C. daubneyi* can be detected by the same sedimentation technique as *F. heptica*.

3 What action would you recommend? Treatment is not considered necessary because rumen flukes are thought to cause little clinical disease.

CASE 2.85

1 What conditions can cause sudden death in growing lambs (most likely first)? *Mannheimia haemolytica* infection, which causes septicaemia in young lambs; *Bibersteinia trehalosi* infection, which causes septicaemia in 4–9-month-old lambs (systemic pasteurellosis); lamb dysentery and pulpy kidney in lambs that have not received sufficient passive antibody.

2 How could you confirm your suspicion? Diagnosis is based on postmortem findings and bacteriology from lung, liver, kidney, spleen, thoracic fluid and heart blood. In peracute cases there are widespread petechiae over the myocardium, spleen, liver and kidney, with enlarged lymph nodes and congested and oedematous lungs. Less acute cases often show a considerable fibrinous pleurisy at necropsy. It may prove difficult to differentiate autolytic change from true lung pathology; diseased lung sinks, while normal aerated lung floats (**2.85b**). There is excess fluid in the body cavities and pericardium, often containing fibrin clots, in sheep that have died from clostridial disease such as pulpy kidney.

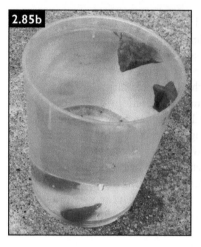

3 What control measures could be adopted? Vaccination of the dam with a pasteurella vaccine will only provide passively derived immunity for the first 4 weeks or so of life. Thereafter, vaccination of lambs from 3 weeks old is needed to provide active immunity. Two vaccinations are required 4–6 weeks apart and at least 2 weeks before any stressful event such as weaning or sale. Vaccinated lambs often obtain a premium at breeding sales.

CASE 2.86

1 What are these ribbon-like segments? Tapeworm segments of the genus *Monezia* are readily recognised in faeces of young lambs as white ribbon-like structures up to 10 mm wide.

2 What action is necessary? Treatment is not considered necessary because tapeworms are non-pathogenic. Only members of the benzimadazole group (1-BZ) are effective against adult tapeworms.

3 What control measures would you recommend? No control measures are necessary for tapeworms of the genus *Monezia*.

CASE 2.87

1 What advice would you give? Anthelmintic treatment of all breeding females pre-tupping is rarely necessary. The ewes look to be in very good body condition and there is no faecal staining of the perineum visible to suggest a history of parasitic gastroenteritis. Dosing all ewes pre-tupping may select for anthelmintic resistant strains, especially if ewes are moved immediately to safe grazing for flushing. Faecal egg counts will indicate whether ewe anthelmintic treatment is necessary. In general terms, anthelmintic treatment should be targeted at leaner ewes, sheep pregnant for the first time or those sheep with faecal staining of the perineum. Indeed, it may be a sound selection policy to sell lean ewes and not breed from them, as these sheep are likely to have smaller litters in the next breeding season. Note the difference in body condition of the two ewes shown in **2.87b**. The ewe on the right is in much poorer body condition and has faecal staining of the perineum. The farmer elected to keep this sheep, which lost further body condition, subsequently shown to be caused by Johne's disease.

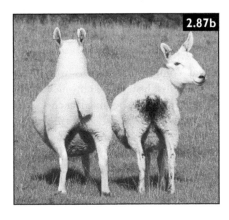

It is not unusual for sheep with paratuberculosis to have high worm eggs counts and diarrhoea due to immune system suppression.

Rams are often neglected at this time and a faecal worm egg count will decide whether pre-tupping anthelmintic treatment is necessary in this group.

Flukicide treatment may be necessary with risk based on weather data throughout the summer and autumn, as described more than 50 years ago by Ollerenshaw (the Ollerenshaw Index). While there are a lot of flukicide/anthelmintic combination products on the market, these are rarely needed and a flukicide product only should be used.

CASE 2.88

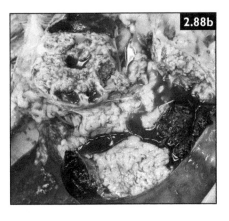

1 Describe the sonogram. The irregular structure is 10 cm in diameter and appears well-encapsulated. There are irregular pockets of fluid at the periphery and beneath the capsule.

2 What is this structure (most likely first)? The sonographic findings are not consistent with any normal viscus. The structure could be: neoplasia involving the kidney; neoplasia involving the uterus; neoplasia involving the bladder.

3 **What action would you take?** While it would be possible to obtain an ultrasound-guided fine needle aspirate of the structure, the prognosis is hopeless and the ewe should be euthanased for welfare reason. Serum BUN, creatinine and proteins would give an accurate assessment of renal function, but are not necessary. A renal carcinoma was confirmed at necropsy (**2.88b**).

CASE 2.89

1 **What common conditions would you consider (most likely first)?** Parasitic gastroenteritis; lush grass; chronic fasciolosis.

2 **What tests could be undertaken to support your provisional diagnosis?** Clinical examination reveals no abnormality and there is no anaemia suggestive of haemonchosis. Faecal samples are taken from six rams, revealing an average worm egg count of 1,800 epg (range 800–2,400) using the McMaster technique; there are a few coccidian oocysts visible on the slide. Sedimentation is negative for liver fluke eggs.

3 **What control measures would you recommend?** The farmer is aware of the risk of anthelmintic resistance and treats his ewes only once a year with an anthelmintic before lambing time to reduce the periparturient rise. His lambs are treated with an anthelminitc only when they fail to reach target growth rates (targeted selective treatment) and then weaned onto safe grazing to avoid the peak of the mid-summer rise of infective larvae on contaminated pasture. The farmer assumed that rams, like ewes, would be largely immune to parasite challenge except under periods of prolonged stress. Unfortunately, rams remain susceptible to parasitic gastroenteritis throughout their lives and regular faecal egg count monitoring is important, with treatment as necessary to maintain body condition. As the rams are rarely drenched at present, triple resistance would seem unlikely, but it would be prudent to undertake a faecal worm egg count reduction test. As this pasture is likely to be highly contaminated with infective larvae for the remainder of the summer and into autumn, movement to safe pasture where available would be advisable. Where possible, the pasture should be grazed by cattle for the remainder of the year.

CASE 2.90

1 **Are there any risks to these young lambs?** Yes, sarcocystosis and coenurosis.

Sarcocystis species are obligate two-host parasites. The two potentially pathogenic microcyst species in sheep (*S. arieticanis* and *S. tenella*) have either a sheep–dog or a sheep–fox cycle. *Coenurus cerebralis* is the larval stage of the tapeworm *Taenia multiceps*, which infests the small intestine of carnivores.

2 **What clinical signs would be expected?**
All ages of sheep may be affected,
but neurological signs of spinal cord
disease are more commonly observed in
6–12-month-old lambs. The prevalence of
neurological disease caused by *Sarcocystis*
spp. in the UK is probably underdiagnosed
because the clinical signs are easily
mistaken for vertebral empyema. Affected
sheep remain bright and alert with a
normal appetite. Hindleg paresis has been
described with affected sheep adopting a
dog-sitting posture (**2.90b**). Some sheep

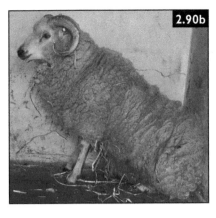

recover with supportive care. Seizure activity followed quickly by death has been
reported attributed to massive challenge.

Acute coenurosis has been reported in 6–8-week-old lambs where clinical
signs ranged from pyrexia, listlessness and head aversion to convulsions and
death within 4–5 days. Chronic coenurosis presents as a slowly progressive focal
lesion of the brain, typically involving one cerebral hemisphere in 80% of cases,
the cerebellum in approximately 10% and affecting multiple locations in 8%.
Compulsive circling behaviour is commonly observed in sheep with coenurosis.
The presence of a cyst in one cerebral hemisphere causes blindness/loss of the
menace response in the contralateral eye.

3 **What signs may be noted in these lambs at slaughter?** Macroscopic *Sarcocystis*
spp. lesions are commonly observed at slaughter plants in the oesophagus,
diaphragm and heart muscle. *Cysticercus tenuicollis* cysts, the intermediate stage
of *Taenia hydatigena*, may be observed adherent to the omentum and indicate poor
parasite control (tapeworms) in dogs accessing the sheep's grazing.

4 **What simple hygiene measures would you recommend?** The dogs should be
kennelled in a separate building away from other animals. Control is based on
preventing completion of the sheep–dog life cycle, including prevention of faecal
contamination of pasture and bedding material by dogs, especially litters of
puppies, correct disposal of sheep carcasses (a legal requirement in some countries)
and not feeding uncooked sheep meat or offal to dogs. The hay should be provided
in racks off the ground and replenished daily. Dogs should be regularly treated
with an anthelmintic effective against tapeworms.

CASE 2.91

1 **What is the lesion (most likely first)?** A well-encapsulated 4 cm diameter
lesion with a heterogeneous 'snowstorm' appearance with a distinct capsule

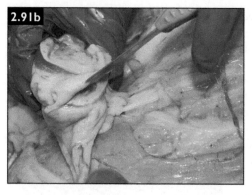

can be seen. This sonographic appearance is consistent with an abscess. A tumour within the omentum would likely appear more heterogeneous. It is unlikely that there would be four tumour masses of similar size.

2 What is the significance of these lesions? Adhesions between the abscess capsule and small intestine will likely slow the rate of propulsion of digesta through the gut and be responsible for the weight loss; however, the abscesses are largely enveloped by omentum.

3 What action would you recommend? The ewe was euthanased for welfare reasons. Necropsy confirmed the lesions to be abscesses with associated chronic fibrous peritonitis (**2.91b**).

CASE 2.92

1 What conditions would you consider (most likely first)? *Bibersteinia trehalosi* infection, which causes septicaemia in 4–9-month-old lambs (systemic pasteurellosis); pulpy kidney in lambs that have not received sufficient passive antibody.

2 What treatment would you administer? Unlike cattle, most pasteurellae causing respiratory disease in sheep are sensitive to oxytetracycline, which should be given IV. A NSAID or dexamethasone should also be given IV to counter the toxaemia; there are no comparative field studies. Confirmation of the diagnosis is based on postmortem findings and bacteriology from lung, liver, kidney, spleen, thoracic

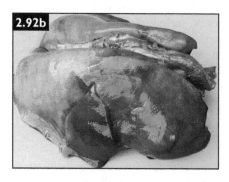

fluid and heart blood. In peracute cases there are widespread petechiae over the myocardium, spleen, liver and kidney, with enlarged lymph nodes and congested and oedematous lungs (**2.92b**). It may prove difficult to differentiate autolytic change from true lung pathology; a simple test is that diseased lung sinks while normal aerated lung floats. Histopathology of lung tissue should be undertaken wherever cost allows. There is excess fluid in the body cavities and pericardium, often containing fibrin clots, in sheep that have died from clostridial disease such as pulpy kidney.

3 What control measures could be adopted? Vaccination of the dam with a pasteurella vaccine will only provide passively derived immunity for the first 4 weeks or so of life. Thereafter, vaccination of lambs from 3 weeks old is needed to provide active immunity. Two vaccinations are required 4–6 weeks apart and must be completed ahead of the major risk of weaning, often accompanied by change of diet and sometimes sale through a market and long journey times. Metaphylactic injection with either oxytetracycline or tilmicosin could be considered after several more cases, but mortality rarely exceeds 2%, which means there is no financial benefit to the farmer. Lush pasture is considered a risk factor for pasteurellosis and clostridial disease in unvaccinated lambs, but is essential to achieve good lamb growth rates.

CASE 2.93

1 What is the cause of this problem? Umbilical/urachal infection with associated omental and bladder adhesions. Umbilical infection usually tracks to the liver (hepatic necrobacillosis) but can occasionally involve the urachus (**2.93b**)

2 Where would you extend your necropsy examination? Urachal infection can ascend via the bladder to the kidney but this is unusual in lambs. Propulsion of digesta can be significantly impaired if strong adhesions form to the intestines, but in this case the adhesions involve only the omentum (**2.93a**). Rupture of the infected urachal remnant causing uroperitoneum has occasionally been reported in calves but not been recorded in sheep.

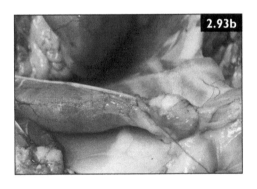

2.93b

3 Could this problem have been prevented? Urachal infection can be prevented by fully immersing the umbilical remnant in strong veterinary iodine BP within the first 15 minutes of life and repeating at least 2–4 hours later. Antibiotic aerosol sprays are much inferior to strong veterinary iodine BP for dressing navels, and are much more expensive. This essential procedure can be incorporated into the management routine when the ewe and her lambs are penned soon after birth, and again 2–4 hours later when the shepherd checks that the lambs have sucked colostrum.

CASE 2.94

1 What conditions would you consider (most likely first)? Include: brachial plexus avulsion (possibly caused by the keel harness); radial nerve paralysis following trauma in the mid/distal humeral region; trauma of the shoulder/elbow joints; severe foot lesion (foot abscess, septic pedal arthritis); exacerbation of an elbow arthritis lesion.

2 What treatment(s) would you administer? Clinical examination failed to reveal any evidence of a fracture and there are no joint swellings. The injury occurred 1 week ago, therefore a corticosteroid injection to reduce any associated soft tissue swelling would be unlikely to have much beneficial effect. The ram was isolated indoors to aid recovery and help restore body condition.

3 What is the prognosis for this ram? The ram showed no signs of improvement after 3 months and was culled for welfare reasons. It can prove difficult to differentiate between radial nerve paralysis and brachial plexus avulsion, the latter having a much poorer prognosis.

CASE 2.95

1 What has happened to this sheep? Ear loss following severe oedema and skin necrosis associated with photosensitisation; septicaemia and ischaemic necrosis.

In sheep, photosensitisation occurs either as a primary condition or secondary to hepatotoxic damage resulting in retention of the photosensitising agent phylloerythrin. Primary photosensitisation follows ingestion of photodynamic agents, for example hypericin from St. John's Wort (*Hypericum perforatum*). In Norway, ingestion of bog asphodel (*Narthecium ossifragum*) is reported to cause photosensitisation in large numbers of lambs. In New Zealand, facial eczema is caused by ingestion of the toxin sporidesmin, which is produced by the saprophytic fungus *Pithomyces chartarum*, which proliferates in vegetation during the autumn months. Sporidesmin is absorbed and accumulates in the liver and bile, where

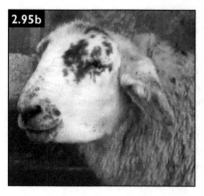

2.95b

metabolic changes result in the release of free radicals, with consequent damage to the biliary tree and reduced excretion of phylloerythrin.

2 Could anything have been done to prevent this situation? Typical cases of primary photosensitisation occur sporadically in white-faced breeds. Initially, affected animals are dull and attempt to seek shade. The ears in particular are affected and become swollen, oedematous and droopy (**2.95b**). The response to protection from sunlight and corticosteroid therapy to reduce oedema at this stage is generally good, although some cases do slough the ears. The prevalence of primary photosensitisation in a particular group of sheep rarely exceeds 2% and the source/cause is often not determined.

3 Should this sheep be kept for future breeding? This case was considered to be one of primary photosensitisation and the current excellent body condition of the sheep would indicate that any significant liver pathology (secondary photosensitisation) would be unlikely. There is no reason to cull this sheep.

CASE 2.96

1 Comment on the radiographs. The dorsoplantar view of the right stifle joint shows extensive loss of the articular surfaces. The lateral view shows complete loss of articular surfaces and extensive osteophytosis.

2 Comment on the animal welfare implications of these findings. This sheep would have been severely lame for at least 6–9 months and presents as a serious welfare concern.

3 What are the expected necropsy findings? At necropsy, the right stifle joint shows extensive erosion of articular cartilage with exposure of subchondral bone; the normal left stifle joint is shown for comparison (**2.96c**). There is synovial membrane hypertrophy, giving the incised affected joint a red colour compared with the white colour of the normal joint.

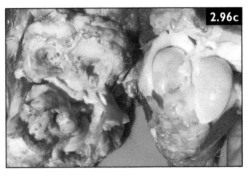

4 What advice should be given to the farmer? Every lame sheep that does not return to normal within 5–7 days of treatment should be examined by a veterinary surgeon; there is no excuse whatsoever that this ewe has suffered such severe lameness for such an extended period.

CASE 2.97

1 What advice would you offer regarding flock biosecurity? All introduced sheep, especially rams from pedigree breeders, should be assumed to be potential sources of resistant strains of helminth parasites and be treated with an effective anthelmintic or combination of products on arrival on the farm. Quarantine arrangements are essential to reduce the risk of introducing anthelmintic-resistant strains of *Haemonchus contortus* and *Teladorsagia circumcincta*. These rams should then be yarded for 48 hours to ensure that any viable nematode parasite eggs have been voided before they are turned onto pasture. After quarantine treatment, the rams should be turned out onto pasture that has been grazed by sheep this season so that any parasites left after treatment make up a very small percentage of an otherwise (assumed) susceptible population 'in refugia'.

The current recommendation is to use a combination of anthelmintic drugs with different mechanisms of action. Current best practice involves sequential full-dose treatments with either 4-AD monepantel (Zolvix®) or 5-SI derquantel and abamectin (Startec®), and moxidectin.

Quarantine treatment with a flukicide is based on risk analysis and the choice will depend on the likely stage of migrating/adult flukes. Tricalbendazole is the only product effective against early migrating stages of liver fluke. However, it would be prudent to use closantel 6–8 weeks after the use of triclabendazole because of the suspected widespread occurrence of resistance to this flukicide.

All introduced sheep should be grazed separately on contaminated pasture from the main flock for at least 1 month. This quarantine period allows inspection for a range of other common diseases and infections that can be introduced onto the farm but are not visible at sale, such as sheep scab, lice and footrot. Most pedigree sheep flocks are monitored for visna-maedi virus and caseous lymphadenitis, although these diseases are not of major significance for commercial sheep farmers. In flocks where only rams are purchased, veterinary ultrasound scanning of purchased rams to detect early lung lesions of ovine pulmonary adenocarcinoma, with immediate culling before significant virus shedding, is a major step in tackling this disease.

CASE 2.98

1 What is the likely cause (most likely first)? Interdigital dermatitis (scald). Interdigital dermatitis is an acute necrotising infection of the interdigital skin caused by *Dichelobacter nodosus* and predisposed by wet conditions and trauma to the interdigital skin. It is most commonly seen affecting intensively managed and densely stocked lambs, causing considerable lameness. Footrot is the term commonly used to describe the highly contagious foot disease with extensive underrunning of hoof horn also caused by *D. nodosus*.

2 What treatment would you administer? If possible, the flock should be moved to dry pasture where spontaneous recovery may occur, but this is not an option in most situations. In the UK, the method of choice is to turn over every lamb and treat all affected feet with topical oxytetracycline aerosol, but this is very labour intensive. Surprisingly, despite the severe lameness there is return to full soundness within 1–2 days of a single treatment.

The use of 5% formalin footbaths produces acceptable results but young lambs do not go through a footbath easily. Farmers sometimes add straw to the formalin solution to encourage sheep to enter the footbath (**2.98b**), but this practice will largely negate the bacteriocidal action of the formalin. Footbaths should be cleaned out and replenished before use. The caustic nature of formalin on eroded skin means that lameness is often worse for several days after formalin foot bathing before improving. Zinc sulphate, as a 10% solution with sodium

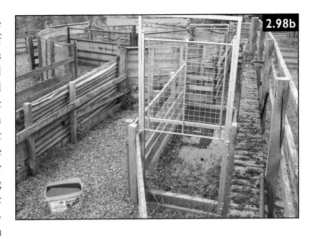

2.98b

lauryl sulphate added as a wetting agent, has largely replaced formalin footbaths.

3 What control measures would you include in the flock health plan? Some farmers report that where there are fewer ewes with footrot, epidemics of interdigital dermatitis in lambs occur less frequently. Regular foot bathing is successful in preventing footrot and reducing the spread of footrot and will also treat interdigital dermatitis. There is no evidence that any one type of footbath formulation is more effective than another. The lack of adequate foot bathing facilities within ready access to grazing means that footbaths are used much less often than is optimal for foot health.

CASE 2.99

1 Do you agree with the decision to undertake a caesarean operation? The cervix and vagina appear thickened and oedematous such that successful digital dilation of the cervix after replacing the cervicovaginal prolapse under low extradural block would be high unlikely. Any delay is likely to compromise viability of the lambs (if they are still alive). Cost is a factor in many situations; is the cost of surgery likely to be greater than the financial value of the ewe and her lamb(s)? Published studies show that successful surgical outcome is >98% when the lambs are alive. The prognosis is very poor if there is a foetid discharge, and euthanasia is perhaps the best option as peritonitis is common due to leakage of uterine content into the peritoneal cavity during surgery. Furthermore, toxins can leak across compromised uterine wall, causing peritonitis.

2 What anaesthetic protocol would you adopt? Excellent analgesia of the flank for caesarean operation can be achieved after lumbosacral extradural injection of 3–4 mg/kg of 2% lidocaine solution and is indicated during first-stage labour associated with a vaginal prolapse. The prolapsed tissues can be readily replaced even

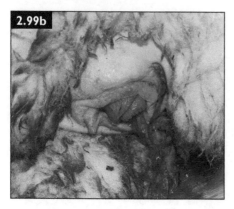

2.99b

when the ewe is in lateral recumbency (2.99b) and there is complete analgesia of the flank for surgery. The only disadvantage is paralysis of the ewe's hindlegs for 2–3 hours, therefore care of the newly delivered lambs is paramount including ensuring passive antibody transfer. It is not essential to place a Buhner suture afterwards but it may be prudent to do so; this was not undertaken in this case and prolapse did not recur.

CASE 2.100

1 **What conditions would you consider?** The most likely conditions to consider include: septic pedal arthritis; white line abscess extending to the coronary band; interdigital infection/cellulitis.

2 **How would you confirm your diagnosis?** The combination of widening of the interdigital space and swelling above the coronary band on the abaxial aspect of the hoof wall is consistent with septic pedal arthritis. Diagnosis could be confirmed by radiography in chronic cases but this is cost-prohibitive in most practical situations. Arthrocentesis is rarely undertaken because there is only a small amount of pannus within the joint; rarely is there a large amount of fluid pus within the joint.

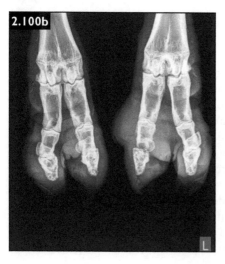

2.100b

3 **How long has this ram been lame?** There is no obvious erosion of articular surfaces or osteophytosis on radiography (2.100b), but the soft tissue reaction (2.100a) would indicate that the infection has been present for 2–3 weeks at least.

4 **What treatment would you recommend?** Flunixin meglumine is injected IV before surgery. Lidocaine 2% solution (5–7 ml) is injected into the superficial vein running on the craniolateral aspect of the third metatarsal bone (recurrent metatarsal vein) after application of a strong rubber band tourniquet below the

hock (IVRA). Analgesia is achieved within 2 minutes. The interdigital skin is incised as close to the infected tissue as possible and the incision extended for the full length of the interdigital space to a depth of 1.5 cm. A length of embryotomy wire is introduced into the incision and the medial digit removed at the level of mid P2. In chronic cases where there is extensive osteophytosis extending onto distal P1, excision through mid P1 is recommended. A melolin dressing is applied to the wound and a pressure bandage applied. Analgesics and antibiotics are administered for 4 days. The dressing is changed after 4 days.

Joint lavage through an indwelling catheter has been recommended as an alternative treatment and has the advantage of maintaining both digits, but this takes more time, is more expensive and takes longer for resolution of lameness.

CASE 2.101

1 Comment on the radiograph. There is obvious soft tissue swelling of the elbow region. The articular spaces of the shoulder and elbow joints are perhaps wider than normal, but comparison should be made with the contralateral normal joints. There is no convincing evidence of joint infection in this radiograph.

2 What action would you take? Clinical examination suggests joint involvement of the right shoulder and elbow joints despite lack of radiographic changes. The lamb has not responded to antibiotic therapy, although this may have been started too late. Euthanasia followed by necropsy reveals a pannus in both joints, with early articular cartilage erosion of the humerus (**2.101b**). Radiography is of very limited use in confirming a provisional diagnosis of early septic arthritis in young lambs; clinical examination is much more informative, bearing in mind that joint effusion is limited and the major inflammatory component is a pannus. Crepitus will not be appreciated, if at all, until there is significant articular cartilage erosion and osteophytosis, which may take 4–6 months. Lambs with polyarthritis that remain lame after appropriate antibiotic therapy should be euthanased for welfare reasons because they will not recover. Where *Streptococcus dysgalactiae* is the major joint pathogen, the most appropriate antibiotic therapy is procaine penicillin (15 mg/kg IM for 7–10 consecutive days) remembering that penicillin is a time-dependent antibiotic – duration of therapy not dose rate is the critical factor. A single injection of long-acting penicillin is

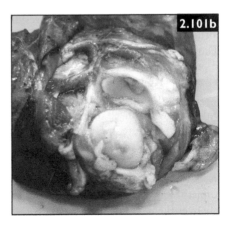

not an appropriate treatment. There is no advantage in administering a penicillin and streptomycin combination; indeed such preparations contain only two-thirds of the concentration of penicillin compared with a penicillin-only preparation. A single corticosteroid injection on the first day of antibiotic therapy reduces joint exudation, inflammation of the synovium and lameness.

CASE 2.102

1 What conditions would you consider? Sheep scab mite infestation (*Psoroptes ovis*); louse infestation; keds; severe dermatophilosis.

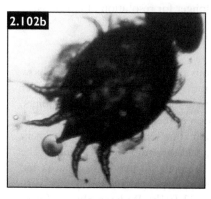

2 How would you confirm the diagnosis? Skin scrapings taken from the periphery of the lesion demonstrate large numbers of mites under ×100 magnification (**2.102b**). Lice and keds can be visualized on careful examination of the skin, but are not seen in these sheep.

3 What treatment would you administer? One injection of doramectin is effective against sheep scab mite infestation, but two injections of ivermectin 1 week apart are needed for scab treatment. Two injections of moxidectin 1%, 10 days apart, are needed for scab treatment. Subcutaneous injection of moxidectin 2% at the base of the ear provides 60 days protection against sheep scab.

Ivermectin provides no significant residual protection against reinfestation from a contaminated environment, therefore it is essential that sheep are not returned to the same pastures/buildings for at least 17 days post treatment. Although doramectin and moxidectin do have residual action against reinfestation, it would be prudent to apply this rule to all systemic endectocide treatments.

Dimpylate (diazinon), flumethrin and propetamphos-containing dips treat and prevent sheep scab, while high *cis* cypermethrin-containing dips are effective for treatment only if used a second time 14 days later. Treatment for sheep scab necessitates that sheep are immersed in the dip wash for 60 seconds with the head submerged twice. Sheep dipped in high *cis* cypermethrin-containing dips must not be returned to infested pastures after dipping because of the limited residual action against scab mites.

Occasionally, severely affected sheep may develop seizures during handling, caused by an anaphylactic reaction. These sheep should be treated with IV dexamethasone. Affected sheep recover in 15–30 minutes but further seizures are likely over the next few days if handled.

CASE 2.103

1 What are the possible causes of this problem? Reduced lamb birthweight can occur when placental development has been limited by competition in the uterus for caruncles, resulting in a reduced number of placentomes per fetus. This situation is not uncommonly encountered in multiple litters where the birth of twins with disproportionate weights (e.g. 5.5 kg versus 3.5 kg) probably indicates that three embryos implanted and underwent early fetal development, but one fetus failed to develop further and was resorbed. The limited number of caruncles available to the remaining fetus in the ipsilateral horn results in poor growth and a reduced birthweight compared with the co-twin, which developed without competition in the contralateral horn. While the placentomes can increase in size and blood flow, these compensatory mechanisms often fail to overcome their reduced number. Severe subacute fasciolosis has been associated with fetal resorption, a much reduced scanning percentage and low lamb birthweights. Inadequate energy supply during late gestation results in similar low birthweight within litters and a low ewe BCS (<2/5).

2 What action can be taken? There is no reported management to correct this problem. A review of flock nutrition during mid-gestation where litter size disparity is approximately >5–10% has failed to reveal any major problems in this author's experience.

CASE 2.104

1 Describe the important features in the sonogram. The distal lobe is a well-encapsulated mass with an anechoic appearance containing multiple hyperechoic dots consistent with an abscess. Note the 1.5 cm distance from the probe head to the abscess capsule, representing thickened skin and subcutaneous oedema (see **2.104b**).

2 What conditions would you consider (most likely first)? Sperm granuloma; epididymitis; orchitis. Sperm granulomas (**2.104b**) are a coincidental finding in rams several years after vasectomy. This ram was vasectomised 3 years previously and was left in the group to test you out!

3 What action would you take? No action is necessary; the ram is in excellent condition and the scrotal contents are not painful.

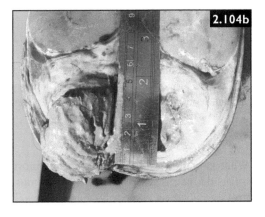

The presence of a sperm granuloma does not appear to affect the function of a teaser ram despite testicular atrophy. Attempted collection of a semen sample by electroejaculation would be contraindicated.

CASE 2.105

1 What is the significant finding? There has been total resorption of perirenal fat, with the kidney now clearly visible. This contrasts markedly with a well-fed lamb where the kidney is embedded in fat (**2.105b**). The cause of fat mobilisation is starvation, whether due to poor dam milk supply or mismothering.

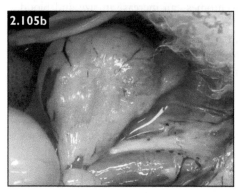

2 What other supporting evidence would you check for in the cadaver? In well-fed lambs there will be large milk clots in the abomasum. If the lamb has been artificially fed immediately before death, the milk may not have had time to clot and will be liquid.

3 What other supporting evidence would you check for on the farm? Hungry lambs are readily identified by their gaunt appearance. Colostrum, then milk, in the lamb's abomasum immediately caudal to the costal arch can readily be detected by gentle transabdominal palpation. Transabdominal ultrasonographic examination of the abomasum of neonatal lambs provides a reliable method to determine whether lambs have sucked.

Venous blood samples collected into lithium heparin vacutainers can be spun down in a microhaematocrit centrifuge and total plasma protein concentration determined using a hand-held refractometer. The plasma protein concentration of lambs that have not sucked sufficient colostrum is <45 g/l (4.5 g/dl) compared with >60 g/l (6 g/dl) for lambs that have sucked adequate colostrum within the first 12 hours. Such tests are accurate, inexpensive and very informative.

Ewe nutrition during late gestation can be judged from BCSs. Lamb birthweight will also give an accurate assessment of late gestation ewe nutrition, with values >1 kg below normal indicative of dietary energy deficiency.

CASE 2.106

1 What conditions would you consider (most likely first)? Include: contagious pustular dermatitis virus and *Dermatophilus congolensis* causing 'strawberry footrot'; granulation tissue following a deep skin cut; sheep pox (not UK).

2 What treatments would you administer? Procaine penicillin (15 mg/kg IM for 7–14 consecutive days) and topical antibiotic spray should be used to control the superficial secondary bacterial infection, but response to treatment is poor and may take several months. Remove both lambs from this pasture and isolate from the group to prevent spread. Housing is preferable; be aware of possible cutaneous myiasis in animals left at pasture. Healing takes many months and lesions may not completely resolve; marked enlargement of the drainage (popliteal) lymph node would raise concerns at the slaughter plant and could result in hindquarter/carcass condemnation.

3 What samples would you collect? Contagious pustular dermatitis virus can be demonstrated by direct electron microscopy of fresh lesions. Bacteriology of the skin lesions is of doubtful benefit as *D. congolensis* is a common skin commensal.

4 What preventive measures could be considered for next year? Disease is introduced into a flock by carrier sheep with no obvious skin lesions. Infection can remain viable in dry scab material for many months and is the likely reason for persistence of infection from year to year on the same premises. The benefit of vaccination is debatable and is undertaken by scarification of the inner thigh in lambs and the axillary region in ewes. The timing of vaccination is approximately 6 weeks before the anticipated occurrence of disease, which could not have been predicted in these purchased lambs of unknown health status. Care must be exercised during handling the live vaccine as it is affected by high temperatures and inactivated by disinfectants. Limit skin trauma by controlling thistles, gorse, etc. in pastures wherever possible.

CASE 2.107

1 How will you deal with this case? The vaginal prolapse is cleaned and replaced under low extradural block in the standing ewe. The first intercoccygeal space is identified by digital palpation during slight vertical movement of the tail, and a 1 inch 19 gauge needle directed at 20° to the tail, which is held horizontally. Correct position of the needle is determined by the lack of resistance to injection of 0.5–0.6 mg/kg of a 2% lidocaine solution and 0.07 mg/kg xylazine (equivalent to 2 ml of 2% lidocaine and 0.25 ml of 2% xylazine for an 80 kg ewe, respectively.

The vaginal prolapse almost always contains urinary bladder, which is emptied by gently elevating the prolapse relative to the vulva. This relieves the kink in the urethra and urine freely drains from the distended bladder. The much reduced size of the prolapse is then replaced by gentle pressure. Topical sugar is claimed to reduce the size of the prolapse and aid replacement.

A perivulval Buhner suture of 5 mm umbilical tape is inserted and tied with an opening of two fingers width to allow urination. The ewe is treated with procaine penicillin for 3–5 consecutive days. The suture should be untied after a few days

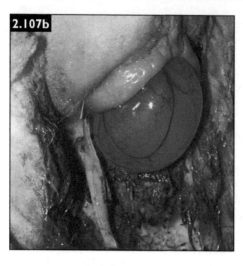

and not delayed until there are signs of first stage labour (**2.107b**).

2 What is the future management of this sheep? Risk factors for vaginal prolapse include excessive body condition, housing, lack of exercise, multigravid, high-fibre diets and lameness; however, these risk factors apply to the majority of sheep that are not affected by this condition. Affected ewes must not be kept for future breeding, as recurrence is common.

CASE 2.108

1 Describe the important sonographic findings. The liver is not homogeneous but contains many hyperechoic dots with distant shadowing consistent with inflammatory cell accumulations caused by migrating immature flukes. The ultrasound findings are consistent with subacute fasciolosis.

2 What tests would you undertake? Raised GGT and GLDH concentrations (5–30-fold) are consistent with hepatic damage caused by migrating flukes (**2.108b**). Changes in albumin and globulin concentrations are not disease-specific. The coproantigen ELISA test detects digestive enzymes produced by migrating (late immature) and adult flukes, which are released into the bile and detected in faeces, thereby confirming active infection. Fluke infection can be detected after

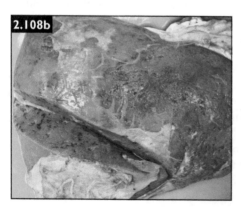

3–4 weeks but more reliably after 6–9 weeks, 2–3 weeks before eggs can be detected in faeces

3 What treatment(s) would you administer? Treat all sheep in the flock with triclabendazole immediately and 6 weeks later with closantel in case of triclabendazole resistance. Use a different fluke treatment in spring, which need only be effective against adult flukes, thereby further reducing the risk of selecting for flukicide resistance.

4 What could be a major consequence of this problem? Fetal death/resorption causing high barren rates and much lower litter size is reported after severe subacute liver fluke infection. Indeed, where disease has not been seen before, very poor scanning results may be the first indication that there is a serious liver fluke problem on the farm. This problem may be limited to only one group of sheep depending on its autumn/winter grazing.

CASE 2.109

1 What is your diagnosis (most likely first)? The most likely conditions to consider include: delayed swayback; vertebral empyema C1 to C6; *Streptococcus dysgalactiae* infection of the atlanto-occipital joint causing cord compression, although much older than usual cases; injection site infection tracking to the cervical spinal canal; muscular dystrophy (white muscle disease).

In the delayed form of swayback (enzootic ataxia) the lambs are normal at birth but show progressive weakness of the hindlegs from 2–4 months of age. Signs are often first noted during gathering or movement when affected lambs lag behind the remainder of the flock. The hindlegs are weak with reduced muscle tone and reflexes, and show muscle atrophy. Lumbar CSF protein concentration is normal, ruling out significant cord compression from an inflammatory focus.

2 What treatments would you administer? There is limited evidence that copper supplementation of lambs with enzootic ataxia slows the progress of the condition; treatment was unsuccessful in this case.

3 How could you confirm your diagnosis? Delayed swayback was confirmed by histopathological examination of the spinal cord after euthanasia for welfare reasons.

4 What preventive measures could be adopted? Prevention of swayback by copper supplementation of ewes during mid-pregnancy must very carefully consider the prevalence of confirmed or suspected swayback cases in the flock, breed of sheep, supplementary feeding during gestation, whether the sheep will be housed during late gestation, and the geological area including soil analysis.

CASE 2.110

1 Comment on the major radiographic findings. There is marked soft tissue swelling of the interdigital space extending over the abaxial aspect of the lateral claw. There is considerably widening of the articular space of the distal interphalangeal joint, with effective disarticulation and erosion of articular surfaces. There is also osteophytosis of distal P1, and more so involving P2.

2 What condition would you consider? Septic pedal arthritis with disarticulation of the distal interphalangeal joint.

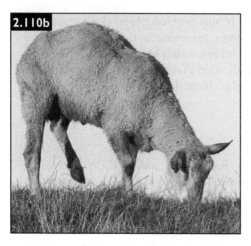

3 How long has this ram been lame? This degree of bone destruction/reaction would likely have taken 2 months at a conservative estimate, during which time the ram would have been severely lame (**2.110b**).

4 What treatment would you recommend? Digit amputation through distal P1 (see **Case 2.100** for a detailed description of the procedure).

CASE 2.111

1 What conditions would you consider (most likely first)? Vertebral empyema affecting the spinal cord in the region from T2 to L3; sarcocystosis; trauma; nutritional myopathy (selenium/vitamin E deficiency/white muscle disease); delayed swayback.

2 How would you confirm your diagnosis? A lumbar CSF sample collected under local anaesthesia reveals a protein concentration of 1.7 g/l, with a slight increase in white cell concentration comprised almost exclusively of neutrophils. A diagnosis of a compressive lesion of the spinal cord is based on >4-fold increase in lumbar CSF protein concentration (normal range <0.3 g/l). Culture of lumbar CSF is unrewarding because the swelling and infection are extradural.

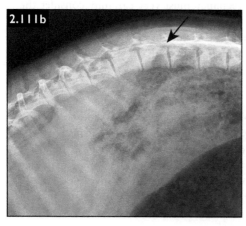

A normal protein concentration but increased white cell count with predominance of eosinophils would suggest sarcocystosis.

Plain radiographs often fail to reveal bone lysis caused by the empyema except in severe (chronic) lesions. Myelography will clearly identify the site of the lesion (**2.111b**, arrow) but is costly and requires general anaesthesia and therefore is rarely undertaken. In this case, where the lamb weighed 22 kg, 4 ml of CSF was slowly removed from the lumbar site and an equivalent amount of contrast medium injected over 1 minute. The lamb's hindquarters were raised for 5 minutes before the lateral radiograph was taken.

3 What action would you take? The extent of bone destruction is so severe when clinical signs present that antibiotic treatment is unsuccessful and the lamb should be euthanased for welfare reasons. In this case the farmer insisted on a definitive diagnosis; the lamb was euthanased while still anaesthetised.

CASE 2.112

1 What are the important features? The significant lesions involve the left temporomandibular joint, where there is severe erosion and remodelling of subchondral bone and osteophytosis affecting the articular condyle of the mandible (**2.112a**) and the zygomatic process of the temporal bone (**2.112b**).

2 What clinical signs would this sheep have presented with? Sheep spend up to 10 hours per day ruminating, thus placing considerable wear and tear on the temporomandibular joint. Osteoarthritis is a degenerative disease of joints characterised by the destruction of articular cartilage and osteophyte formation causing pain. Affected sheep might be expected to show quidding and resultant chronic weight loss, leading to emaciation.

3 What advice would you offer? A slaughterhouse survey of cull sheep from this flock would be required to assess the incidence of this disease and its significance in weight loss leading to involuntary culling. This pathology has not been reported to date in other breeds of sheep, although difficulties accessing the temporomandibular joint at necropsy limits the necropsy data available for analysis.

CASE 2.113

1 What might this structure be (most likely first)? Toe fibroma; keratoma; squamous cell carcinoma; footrot. A toe fibroma is comprised solely of exuberant granulation tissue.

2 What factors contribute to this condition? Toe fibromas usually arise from overzealous hoof trimming exposing an area of corium at the toe (**2.113b**) coupled with misuse/overuse of formalin footbaths exacerbating granulation tissue formation. In some cases, footrot can play an important role in exposing and damaging the corium.

3 What would you do to correct this problem? A toe fibroma is comprised solely of exuberant granulation tissue without a nerve supply, therefore it can be excised level with the sole using a No. 22 scalpel blade without the need for local anaesthesia. Melolin, or similar topical dressing, must be applied directly onto the exposed corium, followed by abundant cotton and a pressure bandage.

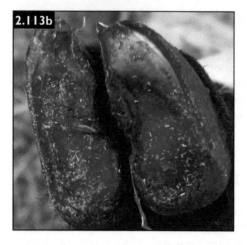

2.113b

A second pressure bandage may be needed after 3–4 days in some cases. The role of cautery (hot disbudding iron) and/or copper sulphate to prevent regrowth of the fibroma is controversial because further damage to the corium delays epithelialisation.

4 What advice would you offer about future control? Foot trimming is not recommended in the treatment of footrot. When undertaken, for example to pare out a white line abscess, paring the hoof horn must not expose the sensitive corium. Topical antibiotic spray with parenteral oxytetracycline or tilmicosin is the preferred treatment for footrot; foot bathing in formalin solutions is restricted to the prevention of footrot. If a small area of the corium is exposed, the lesion should be sprayed topically with oxytetracycline aerosol and not put through a footbath. If a large area of the corium is exposed, a pressure bandage should be applied for 4–5 days and the foot rechecked.

CASE 2.114

1 What is your differential diagnosis? Fetal death/autolysis; undetected dystocia/dead lambs; uterine torsion/dead lambs; intestinal torsion; peritonitis.

Potential abortifacient agents that could contribute to this clinical presentation include: salmonellae including *S. montevideo* and *S. typhimurium*; *Chlamydophila abortus* (enzootic abortion of ewes; EAE). Other common causes of abortion (*Campylobacter fetus intestinalis, Listeria monocytogenes, Pasteurella* spp.) cause abortion often without signs of illness in the ewe.

2 What further tests could be carried out? Transabdominal ultrasound examination of the uterus can be undertaken to check the integrity of the uterus and whether the lambs are alive (fetal heartbeat). Ultrasound examination of the abdomen will also identify fluid-filled loops of intestine in cases of torsion.

3 What treatment/action would you consider? The ewe could be treated symptomatically with IV oxytetracycline and an NSAID. However, the prognosis is hopeless, therefore the ewe should be euthanased for welfare reasons. Fetal death and autolysis are confirmed at necropsy (**2.114b**).

4 What investigations would you undertake? The farmer was advised to isolate aborting ewes immediately and for up to at least 6 weeks depending on laboratory findings. The farmer was also advised regarding the zoonotic risk of some of the common causes of abortion and to adopt strict personal hygiene when handling sick sheep.

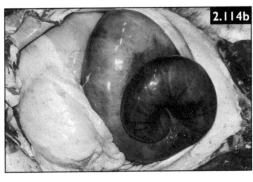

The fetuses and placentae, or fetal stomach contents and samples of placentae, should be sent to the nearest diagnostic laboratory. A blood sample collected for EAE and *Toxoplasma* serology could be collected before euthanasia of the ewe. *S. typhimurium* was isolated in pure culture from the fetal stomach contents in this case.

CASE 2.115

1 What conditions would you consider (most likely first)? Trichostrongylosis, particularly *Trichostrongylus vitrinus*; other causes of parasitic gastroenteritis; liver fluke; yersiniosis; salmonellosis.

2 How would you investigate this problem? Faecal egg counts (McMaster technique) are routinely used to aid diagnosis of nematode infestations. As a general rule, a trichostrongyle egg count of 400 epg is considered moderate, while 700–1,000 epg is considered high and worthy of anthelmintic treatment. However, the faecal egg count may not always accurately reflect potential parasite damage because disease can be caused by developing larvae. Liver fluke infections do not usually cause diarrhoea.

3 What action would you take? There are five different anthelmintic groups that could be used to treat trichostrongylosis:

- 1-BZ: benzimidazoles, probenzimidazoles (white wormers).
- 2-LM: imidazothiazoles, tetrahydropyrimidines (yellow wormers). Levamisole and tetramisole are imidazothiazoles. Morantel and pyrantel are tetrahydropyrimidines.
- 3-AV: avermectins, milbemycins (clear wormers). Preparations that contain avermectins include doramectin and ivermectin; moxidectin is an example of a milbemycin.
- 4-AD: monepantel (orange wormers).
- 5-SI: derquantel and abamectin (dual active) (purple wormers).

Resistance to benzimidazoles has been recognised as being widespread in the UK and resistance to all members of groups 1–3 ('triple or multiple resistance') has been identified since 2001. It would be prudent to do a pooled faecal worm egg count 7–10 days after treatment to check anthelmintic efficacy. Group 4 and 5 anthelmintics are generally held in reserve should resistance problems arise to the other three groups.

CASE 2.116

1 How will you deal with this case? Administer a low extradural block by identifying the first intercoccygeal space by digital palpation during slight vertical movement of the tail. A 25–40 mm 19 gauge needle is directed at 20° to the tail, which is held horizontally. The correct position of the needle is determined by the lack of resistance to injection of 1.5 ml of 2% lidocaine (0.5–0.6 mg/kg) and 0.2 ml xylazine (Rompun 2%®, 0.07 mg/kg) for a 60 kg ewe. The uterine prolapse is replaced 5–10 minutes after combined sacrococcygeal extradural injection. It is important not to penetrate the vaginal mucosa when inserting the Buhner suture of 5 mm umbilical tape.

The ewe is injected with dexamethasone to reduce perivulval oedema. Procaine penicillin (15 mg/kg IM for 5 consecutive days) is given to counter bacterial infection. NSAIDs, such as ketoprofen or flunixin meglumine, could also have been given for their analgesic properties, but extradural lidocaine gives immediate analgesia and the xylazine component provides analgesia for up to 36 hours. The Buhner suture is removed after 2–3 days. The lamb should be monitored closely because it may require supplementary milk over the next few days.

Unlike vaginal prolapse cases, prolapse of the uterus in subsequent pregnancies is uncommon and culling is not necessary.

CASE 2.117

1 List the potential advantages of management systems using a vasectomised ram. Vasectomised rams are widely used to induce ovulation and synchronise oestrus in ewes before the introduction of fertile rams, thereby compacting the lambing period, optimising seasonal labour and reducing the consequences of disease build-up as the lambing season progresses. It is common practice to introduce the vasectomised ram for 1 week starting 2 weeks before the breeding season. This management practice will generally induce ovulation in ram-responsive ewes within 2–3 days, with normal behavioural oestrus around 17 days later (i.e. around 6 days after the introduction of fertile rams).

2 What analgesia/anaesthesia would you employ? A NSAID is given IV before surgery. Spinal analgesia is induced using an extradural lidocaine injection (3 mg/kg) at the lumbosacral site.

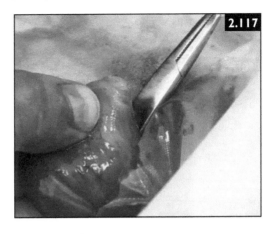

3 How is the vas deferens identified during surgery? The spermatic cord is exteriorised following blunt dissection and the vas deferens localised medially within the spermatic cord between the thumb and index finger. The vaginal tunic is nicked with the scalpel blade point (2.117) and a 6 cm length of vas deferens is ligated twice and the 4–5 cm section between the ligatures removed.

4 How is successful vasectomy confirmed? The two lengths of vasa deferentes are submitted for histological confirmation in correctly labelled containers of formal saline. Alternatively, material contained within the excised material is expressed onto a microscope slide to check for spermatozoa.

5 What is the minimal interval between vasectomy and introduction of the teaser ram to a group of ewes? There are no published guidelines; 2 weeks would seem a safe interval, as significant sperm survival within the remaining sections of vasa deferentes is limited.

CASE 2.118

1 What conditions would you consider (most likely first)? Vertebral empyema affecting the spinal cord in the region from T2 to L3; delayed swayback; sarcocystosis; trauma/fracture.

2 What is the origin of this problem? The infection has originated from bacteraemia, with initial localisation in an articular facet and spread to the vertebral body causing osteomyelitis/empyema with subsequent compression of the spinal cord.

3 What is the significance of no ticks on the lamb? On many hill farms, vertebral body abscessation and polyarthritis are not uncommon sequelae to tick-borne fever and tick bite pyaemia, but this farm is not in a tick area and there are no ticks on this lamb. Septic foci are not usually found to be the potential source of the bacteraemia, except for minor superficial wounds associated with castration, tail docking and ear tags.

4 What treatments would you now administer? Treatment of vertebral empyema with antibiotics is never successful because of the extensive bone destruction

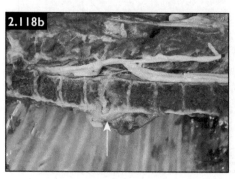

present when clinical signs appear (**2.118b**, arrow). The lamb must be euthanased for welfare reasons once a definitive diagnosis has been established by demonstrating a >4-fold increase in lumbar CSF protein concentration (normal range <0.3 g/l). Culture of lumbar CSF is unrewarding because the swelling and infection are extradural. Except in severe (chronic) cases, plain radiographs fail to reveal the bone lysis caused by the empyema. Myelography will clearly identify the site of the lesion but is costly and requires general anaesthesia and therefore is rarely undertaken.

5 How can this condition be prevented? There are no specific control measures as the condition occurs sporadically (for example 1 case per 500 lambs), unless caused by tick-borne fever and tick bite pyaemia.

CASE 2.119

1 What conditions would you consider (most likely first)? Include: peripheral vestibular lesion; trauma involving the middle ear/facial nerve; listeriosis; acute gid (*Coenurus cerebralis*).

2 What is the likely cause? The vestibular system helps the animal maintain orientation in its environment and the position of the eyes, trunk and limbs with respect to movements and positioning of the head. Unilateral peripheral vestibular lesions commonly arise from ascending bacterial infection of the eustachian tube. There may be evidence of otitis externa and a purulent aural discharge in some cases, but rupture of the tympanic membrane is not a common route of infection. *Pasteurella* spp, *Streptococcus* spp. and *Trueperella pyogenes* have been isolated from infected lesions.

3 What treatment would you administer? A good treatment response is achieved with 5 consecutive days treatment with procaine penicillin, although other antibiotics, including oxytetracycline and trimethoprim–sulphonamide combination, can be used.

4 What is the prognosis for this case? The prognosis is very good in acute cases. The prognosis is poor in neglected cases where infection has extended into bone (empyema).

CASE 2.120

1 What conditions would you consider? The most likely conditions to consider include: endotoxaemia (watery mouth disease); septicaemia; *Escherichia coli* enteritis (enterotoxigenic strains); starvation/mismothering/exposure (SME complex).

The diagnosis of endotoxaemia is based on clinical findings; clinical chemistry typically reveals low plasma glucose concentration and leucopenia, but elevated lactate and BUN concentrations.

2 What treatments would you recommend? Despite abomasal distension, oral rehydration solution administration (50 ml/kg four times daily) by stomach tube is essential. Many lambs showing clinical signs are also bacteraemic, therefore a broad-spectrum antibiotic such as amoxicillin should be injected IM. Flunixin meglumine should be given IV, where possible, to counter the endotoxaemia.

3 What control measures would you instigate? Studies have shown that failure of passive antibody transfer is not a major contributor to this disease. Control measures include improving hygiene standards in the lambing shed. Paraformaldehyde powder should be applied daily to the straw bedding. Individual pens should have a concrete base and must be cleaned out completely, disinfected and allowed to dry between ewes.

The role of probiotics in the prevention of endotoxaemia is unproven, but colonisation of the neonatal gut by lactobacilli and *Streptococcus faecium*, which competitively block *E. coli* strains, seems a good idea. In the early clinical stages of watery mouth disease, soapy water enemas and mild laxatives/purgatives are often effective.

The single most effective means of preventing endotoxaemia is administration of an oral antibiotic preparation (an aminoglycoside such as spectinomycin) within 15 minutes of birth; however, such prophylactic use of antibiotics is unsustainable and likely to come under increasing scrutiny. Indeed, recent field investigations have reported multidrug resistance (including spectinomycin but not neomycin) in enterotoxigenic K99 *E. coli*.

CASE 2.121

Comment on the welfare of this group of fattening lambs at the end of winter (2.121a). Assessment of the welfare of farm animals is largely based on the Farm Animal Welfare Council's Five Freedoms.

Freedom from hunger and thirst by ready access to fresh water and a diet to maintain full health and vigour. These lambs have been grazing kale, which is now limited to very fibrous stalks. The ration is limited to *ad-libitum* cereals in hoppers with no roughage, and while this diet promotes rapid growth, it would not be considered a 'natural' ruminant diet (otherwise why does a sheep have such a large rumen). Unless the diet is managed correctly, *ad-libitum* cereals have the potential to cause ruminal acidosis.

Freedom from discomfort by providing an appropriate environment including shelter and a comfortable resting area. The lambs are very muddy because of the wet areas around the hoppers, which are strategically sited in the lowest part of the field, and the lack a suitable dry lying area. There is shelter provided from the wood seen on right-hand side of the image, but not on the other three sides of this field.

The lambs should be offered roughage such as hay or silage sited in a raised and well-drained area of the field. There should be access to a dry run-off area, preferably a grass field. However, there has been very limited preference testing in lambs and where lambs are offered a choice, it is not unusual for them to choose to lie on bare earth rather than a grass field (**2.121b**).

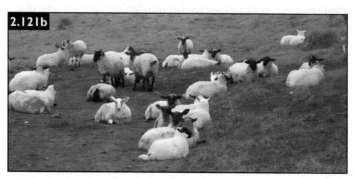

2.121b

CASE 2.122

1 What conditions would you consider (most likely first)? Include (depression extending to stupor): severe cobalt deficiency; sulphur toxicity; coenurosis; early polioencephalomalacia; cerebral abscess.

2 How would you investigate this problem? Serum vitamin B_{12} analysis. Response to vitamin B_{12} injection and oral cobalt supplementation. As a general guide, a growth response is expected when the mean plasma vitamin B_{12} concentration falls below 500 pg/ml, and is likely to be significant below 250 pg/ml.

3 What treatment will you administer? Treatment is more quickly effected by a combination of IM injection of vitamin B_{12} and drenching with up to 1 mg/kg bodyweight of cobalt sulphate than with oral supplementation alone. Thereafter, monthly drenching with cobalt sulphate should ensure normal weight gain.

4 How would you prevent this problem recurring next year? Oral cobalt supplementation is very cheap and certain anthelmintic preparations belonging to Group 1-BZ and Group 2-LM may already contain a cobalt supplement ('SC' preparations). Monthly dosing from around 3 months old should supply sufficient cobalt to growing lambs in most situations.

CASE 2.123

1 What is the cause of this condition? Woolslip occurs sporadically in sheep and most commonly starts 2–4 weeks after recovery from ovine pregnancy toxaemia, infectious causes of abortion/metritis or other serious disease. Surprisingly, the sheep are typically in very good body condition when the fleece is being shed and despite previous serious illness.

2 What action would you take? There is no treatment and the new fleece is normal in appearance, although there will be no requirement for shearing that year. Adopt preventive strategies (e.g. vaccinate for infectious causes of abortion where possible) and correct nutrition to prevent pregnancy toxaemia etc.

Multiple choice questions

Turn to page 318 for the answers.

1 The dental formula in sheep is:
A 2(incisors 4/4, premolars 3/3, molars 3/3)
B 2(incisors 0/4, premolars 3/3, molars 3/3)
C 2(incisors 0/4, premolars 4/4, molars 3/3)
D 2(incisors 0/4, premolars 3/3, molars 4/4)
E 2(incisors 0/4, premolars 3/3, molars 2/2)

2 Which one of the following assays is the most specific test for confirmation of chronic liver toxicity in sheep?
A Kidney copper concentration
B Liver copper concentration
C Serum copper concentration
D Plasma copper concentration
E Serum AST concentration

3 Sudden onset tetraparesis in a 5-day-old lamb is most likely caused by which one of the following conditions?
A Muscular dystrophy
B Infection of the atlanto-occipital joint
C Cervical spinal abscess
D Cerebellar hypoplasia
E White muscle disease

4 A 10-day-old collapsed 40 kg (88 lb) calf with a history of profuse diarrhoea requires how much bicarbonate to successfully correct the acidaemia?
A 20 mEq
B 50 mEq
C 100 mEq
D 200 mEq
E 400 mEq

5 The conception rate in a flock of healthy sheep should be in the region of:
A 50%
B 60%
C 70%
D 80%
E 90%

6 The target barren rate in a flock of healthy sheep after a 5-week service period should be:
A <2%
B >4%
C <6%
D <10%
E <20%

7 Caudal analgesia in sheep is achieved after sacrococcygeal extradural injection of:
A 0.1 mg/kg of 2% lidocaine solution
B 0.2 mg/kg of 2% lidocaine solution
C 0.5 mg/kg of 2% lidocaine solution

D 5 mg/kg of 2% lidocaine solution

E 10 mg/kg of 2% lidocaine solution

8 Which of the listed potential causes of abortion in sheep presents the greatest zoonotic risk?

A *Chlamydophila abortus*

B *Salmonella montevideo*

C *Campylobacter fetus intestinalis*

D *Listeria monocytogenes*

E *Pasteurella* spp.

9 The scrotal circumference of a purchased yearling ram should be greater than:

A 32 cm

B 36 cm

C 38 cm

D 40 cm

E 44 cm

10 The best analgesic approach to ram vasectomy under field operating conditions is:

A General anaesthesia

B Spinal analgesia using extradural lidocaine injection at the lumbosacral site

C Local infiltration of the spermatic cord

D Xylazine sedation and local infiltration of the spermatic cord

E Local infiltration of the spermatic cord and subcutaneous NSAID injection

11 A sperm granuloma is most commonly seen in rams:

A Associated with orchitis

B Associated with epididymitis

C Several years after vasectomy

D Associated with obstructive urolithiasis

E Following testicular atrophy

12 A lamb should ingest how much colostrum within the first 2–6 hours of life:

A 10 ml/kg

B 20 ml/kg

C 30 ml/kg

D 40 ml/kg

E 50 ml/kg

13 Which of the following strategies is the best treatment for a comatose 12-hour-old lamb?

A Placing the lamb in a warming box

B Intraperitoneal injection of 25 ml of 20% glucose solution followed by placing the lamb in a warming box

C Stomach tubing with colostrum followed by placing the lamb in a warming box

D Stomach tubing with colostrum

E Intravenous antibiotic injection

14 Plasma samples for measurement of protein concentrations used to evaluate passive antibody transfer should be collected from:

A Newborn lambs

B Lambs 1–4 hours old

C Lambs 5–8 hours old

D Lambs >24 hours old

E Two-week-old lambs

15 Outbreaks of polyarthritis in 1-week-old lambs is most commonly caused by which one of the following bacteria?

A *Streptococcus agalactiae*

B *Streptococcus dysgalactiae*

C *Trueperella pyogenes*
D *Escherichia coli*
E *Fusobacterium necrophrum*

16 At necropsy in sheep that have
    died from grain overload, the
    rumen pH is typically:
A <6.5
B <5.5
C <3.5
D >7.5
E >8.5

17 Marked free fluid accumulation
    (transudate) within the
    abdominal cavity in an individual
    adult sheep is most likely
    caused by:
A Liver abscesses
B Right-sided heart failure
C Paratuberculosis
D Intestinal adenocarcinoma
E Protein-losing nephropathy

18 A serum albumin concentration
    of 12 g/l (1.2 g/dl) and globulin
    concentration of 45 g/l (4.5 g/
    dl) would be most consistent
    with which of the following
    conditions?
A Chronic mastitis
B Pleural abscesses
C Paratuberculosis
D Liver abscessation
E Chronic parasitic gastroenteritis

19 A faecal sample from an emaciated
    adult ewe without diarrhoea or
    anaemia reveals a worm egg count
    of 4,000 epg, including 500 epg
    Nematodirus battus, and a patent

Dictyocaulus filaria infestation.
Which of the following conditions
may be associated with such
findings?
A Chronic mastitis
B Pleural abscesses
C Cobalt deficiency
D Liver abscessation
E Paratuberculosis

20 In cases of vegetative endocarditis,
    a heart murmur is most often
    auscultated:
A Over the tricuspid valve
B Over the mitral valve
C Over the aortic valve
D Over the pulmonary valve
E There is no audible heart murmur
    in most cases of vegetative
    endocarditis

21 Septicaemia in 4–9-month-old
    lambs is most often caused by
    which one of the following
    bacteria?
A *Bibersteinia trehalosi*
B *Pasteurella multocida*
C *Mannheimia haemolytica*
D *Clostridium perfringens* type D
E *Histophilus somni*

22 Transmission of jaagsiekte sheep
    retrovirus occurs predominantly
    via which of the following
    routes?
A Colostrum
B Milk
C Direct contact
D By inhalation of infected
    respiratory secretions
E By contaminated needles

23 Early clinical cases of ovine pulmonary adenocarcinoma can be reliably identified by:

A ELISA serology
B Radiography
C 'Wheelbarrow test'
D Transthoracic ultrasonography
E Auscultation of the lungs

24 Which area of the brain is primarily concerned with fine coordination of voluntary movement?

A Cerebrum
B Vestibular system
C Brainstem
D Cerebellum
E Mid-brain

25 Which area of the brain is primarily concerned with mental state, behaviour and vision?

A Cerebrum
B Vestibular system
C Brainstem
D Cerebellum
E Mid-brain

26 Brainstem dysfunction is characterised by:

A Multiple cranial nerve deficits
B Head tilt and loss of balance
C Ataxia and dysmetria
D Blindness and altered behaviour
E Tetraparesis

27 Which needle length and gauge should be selected for lumbar CSF sampling in a 70 kg (155 lb) ewe?

A 25 mm 21 gauge
B 25 mm 19 gauge
C 40 mm 21 gauge
D 40 mm 19 gauge
E 60 mm 16 gauge

28 Which cell type is found in CSF following destruction of cerebral tissue?

A Macrophages
B Neutrophils
C Eosinophils
D Lymphocytes
E Red blood cells

29 A polymorphonuclear intrathecal inflammatory response is most likely to be found in which of the following conditions?

A Listeriosis
B Sarcocystosis
C Coenurosis
D Brain abscess
E Bacterial meningoencephalitis

30 Swayback is associated with low status of which trace element in the dam and/or growing lamb?

A Selenium
B Cobalt
C Copper
D Iodine
E Calcium

31 Which disease of weaned lambs is characterised by blindness, initial depression and aimless wandering, dorsiflexion of the neck, progressing rapidly to hyperexcitability, seizures and opisthotonus, but with a good response to thiamine.

A Polioencephalomalacia
B Focal symmetrical encephalomalacia

C   Listeriosis
D   Bacterial meningoencephalitis
E   Lead poisoning

32 At necropsy, which disease
    causes emission of a bright white
    autofluorescence when cut sections
    of the brain are viewed under
    ultraviolet light?
A   Lead poisoning
B   Focal symmetrical encephalomalacia
C   Listeriosis
D   Bacterial meningoencephalitis
E   Polioencephalomalacia

33 A large number of weaned lambs
    fed high levels of concentrates
    show depression and bilateral
    lack of menace response but not
    hyperaesthesia, nystagmus,
    dorsiflexion of the neck or
    opisthotonus. Which of the
    following is the most likely cause?
A   Sulphur toxicity
B   Lead poisoning
C   Chronic copper poisoning
D   Selenium toxicity
E   Urea poisoning

34 Bacterial meningoencephalitis most
    commonly affects lambs aged:
A   2–3 days
B   4–7 days
C   1–2 weeks
D   2–4 weeks
E   2–4 months

35 *Coenurus cerebralis* is the larval
    stage of which tapeworm?
A   *Taenia multiceps*
B   *Taenia hydatigena*

C   *Echinococcus granulosus*
D   *Monezia expansa*
E   *Cysticercus tenuicollis*

36 *Sarcocystis* species are obligate
    two-host parasites; the two
    potentially pathogenic microcyst
    species in sheep (*S. arieticanis* and
    S. tenella) have:
A   A sheep–dog cycle
B   A sheep–badger cycle
C   A sheep–cat cycle
D   A sheep–deer cycle
E   A sheep–sheep cycle

37 Listeriosis is primarily a winter–
    spring disease most commonly, but
    not exclusively, associated with:
A   Silage feeding; less alkaline pH of
    spoiled silage (pH <8.0) increases
    risk
B   Silage feeding; less acidic pH of
    spoiled silage (pH >5.0) increases
    risk
C   Feeding mouldy hay
D   Access to poultry manure
E   Feeding high-grain rations

38 Listeric encephalitis causes
    a localised infection of the
    brainstem that occurs when:
A   *L. monocytogenes* ascends the
    facial nerve
B   *L. monocytogenes* ascends the
    optic nerve
C   *L. monocytogenes* ascends the
    trigeminal nerve
D   Haematogenous spread of
    L. monocytogenes from the gut
E   *L. monocytogenes* ascends the
    eustachian tube

311

39 Pregnancy toxaemia can most reliably be confirmed by:
A Serum 3-OH butyrate concentration >5.0 mmol/l (52.5 mg/dl)
B Serum glucose concentration <2.0 mmol/l (36 mg/dl)
C Serum non-esterified fatty acid (NEFA) concentration >1.0 mmol/l (28 mg/dl)
D BUN concentration >10 mmol/l (28 mg/dl)
E Serum fructosamine concentration >1.0 mmol/l (>0.18 mg/dl)

40 A pituitary tumour would most likely present with which of the following collection of neurological signs?
A Multiple bilateral cranial nerve deficits, especially V and VII
B Bilateral cranial nerve II and III deficits
C Head tilt
D Ataxia
E Hypermetria

41 A spinal lesion causing reduced forelimb reflexes (lower motor neuron signs) and increased hindlimb reflexes (upper motor neuron signs) would be present at:
A C1–C5
B C6–T2
C T3–L2
D L4–S2
E S1–S3

42 Footrot in sheep is caused by:
A *Dichelobacter nodosus*
B A spirochaete
C *Fusobacterium necrophorum*

D *Bacteroides nodosus*
E *Trueperella pyogenes*

43 Whole flock injection with which antibiotic has successfully eradicated footrot from sheep flocks?
A Oxytetracycline
B Tilmicosin
C Amoxycillin
D Penicillin
E Gamithromycin

44 In sheep, infection usually gains entry to the distal interphalangeal (pedal) joint:
A Haematogenously
B From a punctured sole
C Extension from an interdigital lesion
D Associated with footrot
E Direct extension of a contagious ovine digital dermatitis lesion

45 An infected distal interphalangeal (pedal) joint is best treated by:
A A prolonged course of antibiotics
B Digit amputation under intravenous regional anaesthesia
C Digit amputation under a ring block
D Lavage and ankylosis
E Culling the sheep

46 Infectious arthritis with high morbidity and moderate to severe lameness typically affecting growing lambs aged 6 weeks to 4 months is most likely caused by which of the following organisms?
A *Erysipelothrix rhusiopathiae*
B *Streptococcus dysgalactiae*

C *Staphylococcus aureus*
D *Streptococcus agalactiae*
E *Fusobacterium necrophorum*

47 For diagnostic purposes in suspected cases of infectious polyarthritis, the best samples to collect are:
A Arthrocentesis samples from acute cases prior to antibiotic treatment
B Arthrocentesis samples from treated cases that have failed to recover with antibiotic therapy
C Synovial membrane at necropsy from two or three severely lame lambs that have failed to recover with antibiotic therapy
D Synovial membrane at necropsy from two or three severely lame lambs that have not received any antibiotic therapy
E Samples of pannus from two or three severely lame lambs that have failed to recover

48 The best antibiotic therapy for erysipelas polyarthritis is:
A Ceftiofur for 3 consecutive days
B Three consecutive days of marbofloxacin
C A single long-acting injection of oxytetracycline
D Penicillin (44,000 iu/kg once daily) for at least 5 consecutive days
E Amoxycillin/clavulanic acid for at least 5 consecutive days

49 In obstructive urolithiasis in adult rams, high urinary back pressure within the bladder most commonly causes:
A Bladder rupture

B Hydroureters and bilateral hydronephrosis
C Kidney rupture
D Uroperitoneum
E Rupture of the penis

50 Ulcerative posthitis (sheath rot) is caused by which of the following bacteria?
A *Trueperella pyogenes*
B *Corynebacterium pseudotuberculosis*
C *Corynebacterium renale*
D *Escherichia coli*
E *Fusobacterium necrophorum*

51 Caseous lymphadentitis is characterised by abscessation of which lymph node?
A Parotid
B Mesenteric
C Mediastinal
D Deep inguinal
E Popliteal

52 Which of the following products provides the longest protection against flystrike?
A High *cis* cypermethrin pour-on preparations
B Cyromazine pour-on preparation
C Dicyclanil pour-on preparation
D Ivermectin injection
E Diazinon dips

53 Which of the bacteria listed below is the most common cause of gangrenous mastitis in sheep?
A *Bibersteinia trehalosi*
B *Pasteurella multocida*

C *Mannheimia haemolytica*
D *Escherichia coli*
E *Streptococcus uberis*

54 The birth of weakly lambs with markedly swollen thyroid glands (goitre) suggests a deficiency of which trace element during gestation?

A Cobalt
B Copper
C Selenium
D Manganese
E Iodine

55 Which of the bacteria listed below is the most common cause of gangrenous mastitis in cows?

A *Staphylococcus aureus*
B *Pasteurella multocida*
C *Mannheimia haemolytica*
D *Escherichia coli*
E *Streptococcus uberis*

56 The conception rate in a healthy beef herd should be in the region of:

A 50%
B 60%
C 70%
D 80%
E 90%

57 Caudal analgesia in a cow is achieved after sacrococcygeal extradural injection of:

A 1 ml of 2% lidocaine solution
B 2 ml of 2% liocaine solution
C 3 ml of 2% liocaine solution
D 4 ml of 2% lidocaine solution
E 5 ml of 2% lidocaine solution

58 A 45 kg (100 lb) calf should ingest how much colostrum within the first 2–6 hours of life?

A 0.5 litres
B 1 litre
C 2 litres
D 3 litres
E 5 litres

59 Marked free fluid accumulation (transudate) within the abdominal cavity in an individual adult cow is most likely caused by:

A Liver abscesses
B Right-sided heart failure
C Paratuberculosis
D Intestinal adenocarcinoma
E Protein-losing nephropathy

60 A serum albumin concentration of 22 g/l (2.2 g/dl) and globulin concentration of 65 g/l (6.5 g/dl) would be most consistent with which one of the following conditions?

A Coliform mastitis
B Vagus indigestion
C Paratuberculosis
D Chronic suppurative pneumonia
E Chronic parasitic gastroenteritis

61 Which needle length and gauge should be selected for lumbar CSF sampling in a 40 kg (88 lb) calf with suspected bacterial meningoencephalitis?

A 25 mm 23 gauge
B 25 mm 20 gauge
C 40 mm 21 gauge
D 40 mm 19 gauge
E 60 mm 16 gauge

62 Middle ear infection in 2–6-month-old calves is most often caused by which one of the following bacteria?
A *Bibersteinia trehalosi*
B *Pasteurella multocida*
C *Mannheimia haemolytica*
D *Mycoplasma bovis*
E *Histophilus somni*

63 Bacterial meningoencephalitis most commonly affects calves aged:
A 1–2 days
B 3–7 days
C 1–2 weeks
D 2–4 weeks
E 2–4 months

64 In dairy cows, infection usually gains entry to the distal interphalangeal (pedal) joint:
A Haematogenously
B From a sole ulcer
C From an interdigital lesion
D From a sole abscess
E By direct extension of a digital dermatitis lesion

65 Congenital dwarfism (congenital joint laxity and dwarfism) is associated with low status of which trace element in the dam during gestation?
A Selenium
B Cobalt
C Copper
D Iodine
E Manganese

66 Calf diphtheria is caused by which of the following bacteria?
A *Trueperella pyogenes*
B *Corynebacterium pseudotuberculosis*
C *Staphylococcus aureus*
D *Escherichia coli*
E *Fusobacterium necrophorum*

67 The best antibiotic therapy for chronic suppurative pneumonia in adult dairy cows is:
A Ceftiofur for 3 consecutive days
B Three consecutive days of marbofloxacin
C A single long-acting injection of gamithromycin
D Penicillin once daily for at least 30 consecutive days
E Amoxycillin/clavulanic acid for at least 5 consecutive days

68 Basillar empyema would most likely present with which of the following collection of neurological signs?
A Multiple bilateral cranial deficits, especially II, III, V and VII
B Bilateral cranial nerve X and XII deficits
C Head tilt and Horner's syndrome
D Ataxia and hindlimb weakness
E Hypermetria, wide-base stance and preservation of strength

69 In cattle, the liver can readily be visualised ultrasongraphically from:
A One-third the way down the 9th to 12th intercostal spaces on the right side

B   One-third the way down the 9th to 12th intercostal spaces on the left side

C   One-third the way down the 6th to 8th intercostal spaces on the right side

D   One-third the way down the 6th to 8th intercostal spaces on the left side

E   The ventral midline immediately caudal to the xiphisternum

70 Peritoneal sampling from a cow with traumatic reticulitis will typically reveal a sample with:

A   Normal protein and white cell concentrations

B   A low protein concentration but increased white cell count comprised almost exclusively of neutrophils.

C   A high protein concentration but low white cell count

D   A high protein concentration and increased white cell count comprised almost exclusively of lymphocytes

E   A high protein concentration and increased white cell count comprised almost exclusively of neutrophlils

71 Manual transrectal examination of a dairy cow identifies a blind-ended 20 cm diameter viscus extending into the pelvis. The most likely cause is:

A   Caecal distension

B   Abomasal volvulus

C   Torsion of the small intestine

D   Right-sided distension of the abomasums

E   Vagus indigestion

72 Enterotoxigenic *E. coli* typically affects calves at what age?

A   1–3 days old

B   4–7 days old

C   7–14 days old

D   14–21 days old

E   >21 days old

73 Rotavirus diarrhoea typically affects calves at what age?

A   1–3 days old

B   4–7 days old

C   7–14 days old

D   14–21 days old

E   >21 days old

74 Diarrhoea caused by *Salmonella* serotypes typically affects calves at what age?

A   1–3 days old

B   4–7 days old

C   7–14 days old

D   14–21 days old

E   >21 days old

75 Coccidiosis affecting calves at pasture is most commonly caused by which one of the following *Eimeria* species?

A   *E. zuernii*

B   *E. bovis*

C   *E. alabamensis*

D   *E. crandallis*

E   *E. ovinoidalis*

76 At what stage during gestation does bovine viral diarrhoea virus infection of the fetus cause congenital abnormalities?

A Between 30 and 60 days
B Between 60 and 90 days
C Between 90 and 150 days
D Between 150 and 200 days
E Between 200 and 250 days

77 Malignant catarrhal fever in cattle necessitates contact with which species?

A Badgers
B Sheep
C Ticks
D Pigs
E Midges

Answers to multiple choice questions

1	B	21	A	41	B	61	B
2	A	22	D	42	A	62	D
3	B	23	D	43	E	63	B
4	D	24	D	44	C	64	B
5	E	25	A	45	B	65	E
6	A	26	A	46	A	66	E
7	C	27	D	47	D	67	D
8	A	28	A	48	C	68	A
9	B	29	E	49	B	69	A
10	B	30	C	50	C	70	E
11	C	31	A	51	A	71	A
12	E	32	A	52	C	72	A
13	B	33	A	53	C	73	C
14	D	34	D	54	E	74	E
15	B	35	A	55	A	75	C
16	B	36	A	56	C	76	C
17	D	37	A	57	E	77	B
18	C	38	C	58	D		
19	E	39	A	59	B		
20	E	40	B	60	D		

Reading list

General texts that the reader may find useful:

Aitken I (2007) (ed.) *Diseases of Sheep*, 4th edn. Blackwell Publishing, Oxford.

Andrews AH, Blowey RW, Boyd H, Eddy RG (2004) (eds.) *Bovine Medicine: Diseases and Husbandry of Cattle*, 2nd edn. Blackwell Publishing, Oxford.

Ball PJH, Peters AR (2004) *Reproduction in Cattle*, 3rd edn. Blackwell Publishing, Oxford.

Divers T, Peek S (2007) (eds.) *Rebhun's Diseases of Dairy Cattle*, 2nd edn. Elsevier, Amsterdam.

Maxie MG (2007) (ed.) *Jubb, Kennedy and Palmer's Pathology of Domestic Animals (Volumes 1–3)*, 5th edn. Saunders, Philadelphia.

Radostits OM (2001) *Herd Health: Food Animal Production Medicine*, 3rd edn. Saunders, Philadelphia.

Radostits OM, Gay C, Hinchcliff KC, Constable PD (2007) *Veterinary Medicine: A Textbook of the Diseases of Cattle, Horses, Sheep, Pigs, and Goats*, 10th edn. Saunders, Philadelphia.

Scott PR (2015) *Sheep Medicine*, 2nd edn. CRC Press, London.

Scott PR, Penny CD, Macrae A (2011) *Cattle Medicine*. CRC Press, London.

Smith BP (2008) (ed.) *Large Animal Internal Medicine*, 4th edn. Mosby, New York.

Index: Cattle

Note: References are to case numbers, not page numbers.

Index: Sheep

Note: References are to case numbers, not page numbers.

Also available in the Self-Assessment Color Review series:

T - #0366 - 101024 - C344 - 210/148/19 - PB - 9781498747370 - Gloss Lamination